MW01121696

ANALYZING

DISCOURSE IN

COMMUNICATIVELY

IMPAIRED ADULTS

**THE REHABILITATION INSTITUTE OF CHICAGO
PUBLICATION SERIES**

Don A. Olson, PhD, Series Coordinator

Functional Rehabilitation of Sports and Musculoskeletal
Injuries

Spinal Cord Injury: A Guide to Functional
Outcomes in Physical Therapy Management

Lower Extremity Amputation: A Guide to Functional
Outcomes in Physical Therapy Management, Second Edition

Stroke/Head Injury: A Guide to Functional
Outcomes in Physical Therapy Management

Clinical Evaluation of Right Hemisphere Dysfunction,
Second Edition

Spinal Cord Injury: A Guide to Functional
Outcomes in Occupational Therapy

Spinal Cord Injury: A Guide to Rehabilitation Nursing

Head Injury: A Guide to Functional Outcomes in
Occupational Therapy Management

Speech/Language Treatment of the Aphasias: Treatment Materials
for Auditory Comprehension and Reading Comprehension

Speech/Language Treatment of the Aphasias: Treatment Materials
for Oral Expression and Written Expression

Rehabilitation Nursing Procedures Manual

Psychological Management of Traumatic Brain Injuries
in Children and Adolescents

Medical Management of Long-Term Disability

Psychological Aspects of Geriatric Rehabilitation

Clinical Management of Dysphagia in Adults and Children,
Second Edition

Cognition and Perception in the Stroke Patient: A Guide to
Functional Outcomes in Occupational Therapy

Spinal Cord Injury: Medical Management and Rehabilitation

Clinical Management of Communication Problems in Adults
with Traumatic Brain Injury

Rehabilitation of Persons with Rheumatoid Arthritis

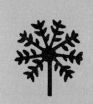

Rehabilitation
Institute of
Chicago
PROCEDURE
MANUAL

ANALYZING

DISCOURSE IN

COMMUNICATIVELY

IMPAIRED ADULTS

Leora Reiff Cherney, PhD, CCC-SLP,
BC-NCD
Clinical Educator/Researcher
Center for Clinical Excellence,
Rehabilitation Institute of Chicago
Associate Professor
Physical Medicine and Rehabilitation
Northwestern University Medical School
Chicago, Illinois

Barbara B. Shadden, PhD, CCC-SLP,
BC-NCD
Professor
Program in Communication Disorders
University of Arkansas
Fayetteville, Arkansas

Carl A. Coelho, PhD, CCC-SLP,
BC-NCD
Department of Communication Sciences
University of Connecticut
Storrs, Connecticut

AN ASPEN PUBLICATION®
Aspen Publishers, Inc.
Gaithersburg, Maryland
1998

The authors have made every effort to ensure the accuracy of the information herein. However, appropriate information sources should be consulted, especially for new or unfamiliar procedures. It is the responsibility of every practitioner to evaluate the appropriateness of a particular opinion in the context of actual clinical situations and with due considerations to new developments. Authors, editors, and the publisher cannot be held responsible for any typographical or other errors found in this book.

Library of Congress Cataloging-in-Publication Data

Cherney, Leora Reiff.
Analyzing discourse in communicatively impaired adults / Leora
Reiff Cherney, Barbara B. Shadden, Carl A. Coelho.
p.   cm.
Includes bibliographical references and index.
ISBN 0-8342-0632-3
1. Language disorders. 2. Discourse analysis. I. Coelho,
Carl A. II. Shadden, Barbara B. (Barbara Bennett) III. Title.
RC423.C53   1998
616.85´506—dc21
98-18602
CIP

Aspen Publishers, Inc., grants permission for photocopying for limited personal or internal use. This consent does not extend to other kinds of copying, such as copying for general distribution, for advertising or promotional purposes, for creating new collective works, or for resale. For information, address Aspen Publishers, Inc., Permissions Department, 200 Orchard Ridge Drive, Suite 200, Gaithersburg, Maryland 20878.

Orders: (800) 638-8437
Customer Service: (800) 234-1660

About Aspen Publishers • For more than 35 years, Aspen has been a leading professional publisher in a variety of disciplines. Aspen's vast information resources are available in both print and electronic formats. We are committed to providing the highest quality information available in the most appropriate format for our customers. Visit Aspen's Internet site for more information resources, directories, articles, and a searchable version of Aspen's full catalog, including the most recent publications: **http://www.aspenpublishers.com**
Aspen Publishers, Inc. • The hallmark of quality in publishing
Member of the worldwide Wolters Kluwer group.

Editorial Services: Nora Fitzpatrick
Library of Congress Catalog Card Number: 98-18602
ISBN: 0-8342-0632-3

Printed in the United States of America

1 2 3 4 5

Table of Contents

Contributors

Leora Reiff Cherney, PhD, CCC-SLP, BC-NCD
Clinical Educator/Researcher
Center for Clinical Excellence,
Rehabilitation Institute of Chicago
Associate Professor
Physical Medicine and Rehabilitation
Northwestern University Medical School
Chicago, Illinois

Carl A. Coelho, PhD, CCC-SLP, BC-NCD
Department of Communication Sciences
University of Connecticut
Storrs, Connecticut

Betty Z. Liles, PhD
Department of Communication Sciences
University of Connecticut
Storrs, Connecticut

Barbara B. Shadden, PhD, CCC-SLP, BC-NCD
Professor
Program in Communication Disorders
University of Arkansas
Fayetteville, Arkansas

Preface

It is with great excitement that I write this Preface to *Analyzing Discourse in Communicatively Impaired Adults*. This book is the culmination of many years of collaboration between Barbara Shadden, Carl Coelho and myself. We initially met together in the early 1990s, when we began to develop a two-day continuing education course on discourse production impairments in the neurologically impaired adult. At that time, we each were using various discourse analysis procedures in our own independent research. However, most practicing speech-language pathologists were unaware of these analysis techniques and the important clinical information they could potentially yield. The course, sponsored by the Rehabilitation Institute of Chicago, was taught first in 1992, and then several times thereafter. Much of the content of *Analyzing Discourse in Communicatively Impaired Adults* is an expansion of the material presented in these early courses.

We are convinced that, for many of our communicatively impaired patients, the analysis of discourse production can provide an important level of understanding about their communication problems that cannot be obtained from our typical observations and standard assessment tools. However, discourse assessment is a complex area with multiple options for analyses available. Although we each have our own preferences about the tasks and analyses we like to use, we have tried to adopt an eclectic approach so that a variety of procedures are included in this book. Our intent is to provide the practicing clinician with an arsenal of clinically relevant techniques. For any given patient, the clinician then will select those tasks and analyses that are most appropriate.

In Chapter 1, discourse is defined within the framework of pragmatics and a brief introduction to the types of discourse, methods of elicitation, and analysis is provided. Chapter 2 expands on methods of elicitation, and discusses the variables to be considered when obtaining a discourse sample. Guidelines for the transcription and initial preparation of the discourse sample are provided. Particular emphasis is given to the rules for segmenting the discourse sample into T-units prior to further analysis.

Chapters 3 through 7 discuss the specific procedures that are available for the analysis of discourse production. Chapter 3 focuses on the surface-level analyses including the analysis of syntactic accuracy and semantic structure and diversity. Methods for quantifying verbal fragmentation or disruption are discussed, as well as their relationship to word retrieval difficulties. Chapter 4 outlines the procedures for the microstructural analysis of cohesion. These procedures have been refined over many years of research experience with cohesion analyses. We are indeed fortunate to be able to draw on the expertise of Betty Liles and include these procedures. Chapter 5 summarizes the variety of techniques used to analyze informational content. Chapter 6 focuses on procedures that are specific to one type of discourse—the narrative—and presents guidelines for analyzing the structure of the story. Similarly Chapter 7 highlights one type of discourse, conversation, and discusses the procedures that are relevant for analyzing this most commonly occurring type of discourse.

Finally, Chapter 8 is an attempt to help the clinician keep up with the ever-growing number of research studies in the area of discourse and the communicatively impaired adult. The chapter is primarily an annotated bibliography of relevant research that has been conducted with four populations: aphasia, right-hemisphere damage, traumatic brain injury, and dementia. This bibliography is intended to be a quick guide to the key articles and their major findings. The reader is urged to consult the original article if more detailed information is desired. Since the number of published articles is increasing rapidly, the bibliography will, no doubt, have omissions soon after going to press. Therefore, several blank pages have been provided so that the reader can add any new relevant literature as he or she reads it.

It is important to note that the scope of *Analyzing Discourse in Communicatively Impaired Adults* is limited to the evaluation of discourse production. We never intended for this book to be a guide for the treatment of discourse deficits. However, when formulating a treatment plan, treatment goals that focus on each of the identified discourse deficits can be developed.

There are two issues related to discourse analysis that, as researchers, we have continually struggled with and which require mention here. First, the analysis of discourse is relatively new and as such, there is a lack of data regarding normal performance on many of the tasks and measures discussed throughout this book. Second, inter-rater reliability is often difficult to accomplish without extensive training and practice. Despite these issues, we contend that discourse analysis remains a viable and useful tool for clinical practice. At the outset, the decision about whether discourse is impaired or not can be made by comparing each patient's performance to that of a family member or a peer. Then, throughout treatment, each patient serves as his or her own control subject with respect to assessing progress. We are confident that, with time, objective normative data will be forthcoming.

The issue of reliability can be addressed in clinical practice by each clinician ensuring that they are at least consistent with themselves in their scoring. Clinicians then can be sure that any changes in performance are a function of progress and not of errors in scoring. We hope that this book will assist clinicians in achieving intra-rater reliability by addressing many of the common questions that are raised and by providing opportunities for practice. Furthermore, we hope that this book will serve as a hands-on guide to help with the selection of appropriate tasks and the application and interpretation of the relevant discourse production analyses.

The best way to learn the methodologies is to actually do them. Each chapter has provided samples of completed analyses to review. In addition, the Appendixes at the end of the book give the reader a large number of examples elicited from a variety of patients using several different tasks. We hope that you will enjoy practicing your newly learned skills on these samples.

Leora Reiff Cherney, PhD, CCC-SLP, BC-NCD

CHAPTER 1

Pragmatics and Discourse: An Introduction

Leora Reiff Cherney

In recent years, there has been a proliferation in the number of research studies published in the area of discourse and in the number of books devoted to discourse in clinical populations. Titles such as *Discourse Ability and Brain Damage* (Joanette & Brownell, 1990), *Narrative Discourse in Neurologically Impaired and Normal Aging Adults* (Brownell & Joanette, 1993), and *Discourse Analysis and Applications: Studies in Adult Clinical Populations* (Bloom, Obler, DeSanti, & Ehrlich, 1994) have piqued the interest of clinicians working in the area of communication sciences and disorders. Yet clinicians are still attempting to understand more precisely what discourse is and why it is important to consider discourse skills in the management of communicatively impaired individuals. Furthermore, there is little consensus on how to evaluate and analyze discourse, and even less agreement about how to treat problems in discourse. The purpose of this chapter is to define discourse within the broad framework of language and pragmatics and to provide a rationale for the importance of including discourse analysis procedures in our management of adults with neurologically based communication problems.

PRAGMATICS AND DISCOURSE

Language has been conceptualized as having three primary dimensions: the form that it takes, its content or meaning, and its use in various communicative contexts (Bloom & Lahey,

1978). Clinicians have long been concerned with the form and content of language. According to Bloom and Lahey (1978), the form or structure of language involves the subsystems of *phonology* (the rule system for the way in which the sounds of a language are combined), *morphology* (the rules for the way in which the words of a language are formed), and *syntax* (the rules for combining words into meaningful sequences such as sentences). The content of language, or *semantics*, refers to the linguistic representation of an individual's knowledge of objects, events, and relationships (Bloom & Lahey, 1978).

It was not until the 1980s, however, that clinicians began to focus on the third dimension of language, *pragmatics*, or how language is used in context. As a result of the increased interest, a variety of different pragmatic frameworks were proposed, tests were developed to evaluate different aspects of pragmatics, and pragmatically based treatment procedures were devised for different clinical populations.

Pragmatics has been defined as the set of rules that governs the use of language in context (Bates, 1976) or the study of the relationships between language and the contexts in which language is used (Davis, 1986). It is the pragmatic dimension of language, then, that determines "why a speaker says something, when the speaker says it, to whom the speaker says it, and how it is said" (Newhoff & Apel, 1990, p. 222). Therefore, pragmatics is concerned with the social appropriateness of language. According to

Davis (1986), three aspects of the communicative situation determine the social appropriateness of language: the extralinguistic, paralinguistic, and linguistic contexts.

Extralinguistic Context

The *extralinguistic context* refers to aspects of the environment that are separate from the actual utterance itself. The extralinguistic context may be external, related to the physical and temporal setting, or internal and related to the participants in the communicative exchange. External determiners include the physical surroundings, the time of day, and the number and location of the participants. For example, communicative interactions that occur in a church will differ from interactions that occur in a bar, particularly with regard to content, choice of words, and interactive style. Conversations around the breakfast table, when everyone is rushing to leave the house, may differ from those around the dinner table, when the family has more time to talk about what was accomplished during the day.

Internal determiners relate to the participants themselves. Participants who identify with each other as a group, either professionally or culturally, may have presupposed knowledge of each other as well as conceptual knowledge of the topic at hand. For example, if a group of physicians are conversing about a medical issue, they will assume that each participant has a basic level of knowledge of the topic. When a physician is conversing with an individual who is not in a medically related field, the same level of knowledge cannot be assumed; therefore, more explanations, using simpler terminology, must be provided. Similarly, our values and beliefs influence how we interact with individuals from the same or different cultural backgrounds.

The roles of each of the individual participants also influence the interchange. This is particularly related to perceived social status, which is determined by factors such as authority, age, and power. For example, an employer-employee exchange will require certain formalities, as will a teacher-student interchange, a parent-child in-

terchange, or a physician-patient interchange. When the individuals are perceived as equal, such as two friends or a husband and wife, the exchange may be less formal.

Another internal factor relates to the movements and body language of the participants. This includes gestures, facial expressions, and proxemics, or the distance between speakers. Movements may be determined in part by the emotional status of the participants. The movements of individuals who are angry and hostile may hinder an interaction, whereas those of individuals who are cooperative or friendly may facilitate the interaction.

Paralinguistic Context

The *paralinguistic context* has been defined as the "trappings" surrounding the verbal production. It includes the prosodic and suprasegmental characteristics of the verbal production and as such is an integral part of the verbal output. The paralinguistic context is used for a variety of purposes. Prosodic inflections such as increased volume or pitch may reflect the emotional state of the speaker. A rising or falling pitch at the end of a sentence may facilitate syntactic analysis by identifying the utterance as a question or a statement. Use of stress, indicated by pauses or changes in inflection, may signal semantic interpretations (e.g., *récord* versus *recórd*) or identify new information.

Linguistic Context

The *linguistic context* refers to the verbal behavior itself or the discourse. *Discourse* has been defined as continuous stretches of language or a series of connected sentences or related linguistic units that convey a message. The length of the discourse is determined by the communicative function. Although typically discourse is longer than a word, it has been argued that when a word alone expresses a message, it may be considered discourse (Ulatowska, Allard, & Chapman, 1990). This is particularly relevant for the aphasic population, in which the unit of analysis may be as short as a word.

Discourse involves both comprehension and production. Specific rules apply to each participant as the speaker and as the listener. For effective and efficient communication, both must have a knowledge of discourse form and of the rules for participating in discourse.

Discourse also may be oral or written. However, oral and written discourse may differ because of the constraints of each modality. For example, in oral face-to-face discourse, a speaker can use pauses, intonation, gaze, posture, and gesture to indicate meaning; in a telephone conversation, the speaker can rely only on pauses and intonation; and in written discourse, none of these signals are available but writers have at their disposal the use of such linguistic devices as punctuation, paragraph indicators, and headings. The focus of this book is on oral production of discourse, although many of the analyses can be applied to written discourse.

MULTILEVEL ANALYSIS OF DISCOURSE

There are a variety of genres or types of discourse based on differences in the function they serve. Exhibit 1–1 lists the major discourse types. Each genre requires different cognitive and linguistic skills. Since cognition and language may be differentially impaired in different neurological populations, the analysis of discourse performance can provide the clinician with valuable information about the level of breakdown and help define the focus of treatment. A comprehensive evaluation entails a multilevel analysis that (a) assesses patient performance *across* discourse tasks that require different cognitive and linguistic skills and (b) assesses different aspects of discourse performance *within* the same task. Therefore, the clinician must be familiar with the types of discourse that may be elicited and their relative cognitive and linguistic demands, as well as with the variety of discourse analysis procedures that are available.

Types of Discourse

Descriptive discourse involves the listing of static concepts, attributes, and relations without an obligatory temporal sequence. Examples of descriptive discourse include describing an object or describing a picture. In contrast, narrative discourse is ordered in a chronological or temporal sequence. It is usually recounted in the first or third person (*I/we* or *he/she/they*) and may be defined as a representation in language of either real or imagined actions or events that unfold in time. Examples include telling a story from a series of pictures or from a complex action picture (e.g., a Norman Rockwell picture); retelling a story that was heard, read, or seen on television; or retelling a personal experience.

A primary function of narrative discourse is to entertain (Ulatowska et al., 1990). In contrast, the primary function of procedural discourse is to inform or instruct. In procedural discourse, the focus is not on what was done and who did it but rather on how a procedure is done. It includes instructions or directions that are specified in a particular order, either conceptually or chronologically. Therefore, the demands for explicitness and clarity may be greater in procedural discourse than in any other type of discourse.

Whereas procedural discourse requires a more basic level of cognitive skills (such as organizational skills), persuasive and expository discourse require higher-level reasoning skills. Persuasive discourse involves expressing an opinion on a topic and providing reasons, examples, or facts to support that opinion. Expository discourse requires talking about a topic and includes comparison and contrast, cause and effect, and generalization. For example, explaining why you believe that there should be a law that all motorcycle riders should wear helmets is persuasive discourse. Talking about the advantages and disadvantages of motorcycle helmets, comparing and contrasting the effects of a state versus a federal helmet law, and comparing the value of helmets in preventing serious injuries in bicycle accidents versus motorcycle accidents would involve expository discourse.

Exhibit 1–1 Types of Discourse

DESCRIPTIVE
  Lists static concepts, attributes, and relations
NARRATIVE
  Conveys actions and events that unfold in time
PROCEDURAL
  Provides instructions or directions specified in a particular order

PERSUASIVE
  Gives reasons or facts to support an opinion
EXPOSITORY
  Provides factual and interpretative information about a topic
CONVERSATIONAL
  Communicates thoughts, ideas, and feelings to others in an interactive and cooperative way

Perhaps the most common context of discourse is conversational discourse. Grice (1975) has defined *conversation* as a cooperative endeavor requiring adherence to four basic maxims or rules. The *maxim of quantity* states that the speaker must be as informative as required, giving neither too much nor too little information. The *maxim of quality* refers to the veracity of the information: the speaker should not say what is believed to be false or give information that is lacking evidence. According to the *maxim of relation*, the speaker must provide information that is relevant to the aims of the ongoing conversation. Finally, the *maxim of manner* refers to the clarity of the information and the need to avoid ambiguity. Furthermore, Wilson and Sperber (1981) described conversation as having an equal distribution of "speaker rights." Each participant in the conversation has equal rights to initiate, interrupt, respond to, or change topics.

Since there are so many different types of discourse with differing cognitive and linguistic demands, it is important that the clinician understand the many variables affecting discourse production. These variables may be related to the task, such as the stimulus modality; to the genre, such as the degree of specificity; or to the individual, such as personal relevance. Consideration of these variables, which are discussed further in Chapter 2, will help guide the selection of appropriate discourse tasks.

Discourse Analysis Procedures

We have, at this point, defined discourse as the verbal aspect of pragmatics. Therefore, any tool that evaluates pragmatics, should, by definition, also assess discourse skills. However, such an assumption is not as simple as it seems. First, despite some general agreement on a definition of pragmatics, there is some inconsistency about what pragmatics encompasses. In a recent survey (Goldsmith & Mackisack, 1992), 127 speech-language pathologists cited 59 different pragmatic communication behaviors as most crucial to include in an assessment of adults with neurogenic communication disorders. The inconsistency among clinicians stems, in part, from differences that have been cited in the literature. For example, Penn's Profile of Communicative Appropriateness (1988) includes 40 pragmatic skills under the general headings of nonverbal communication, sociolinguistic sensitivity, fluency, cohesion, control of semantic context, and responsiveness to the interlocuter. Prutting and Kirchner (1987) classified 30 pragmatic behaviors into the three general categories of verbal aspects, paralinguistic aspects, and nonverbal aspects. Roth and Spekman (1984) divided pragmatic abilities into communicative intentions, presuppositions, and social organization of discourse. In contrast, Halper, Cherney, Burns, and Mogil (1996) focused on the categories of nonverbal communication, verbal communication, and completeness of narrative discourse in their Pragmatic Rating Scale, which was developed for individuals with right-hemisphere damage.

Most tools for assessing pragmatic behaviors have relied on rating scales. Although studies of reliability have been undertaken during the development of these scales, it is more difficult to ensure the ongoing reliability of the rating scales when used in clinical settings by clinicians with different levels of experience. In addition, when a major purpose is to measure progress over time, the use of rating scales may be less desirable. *Observer drift* refers to the tendency for observers to alter the way that they apply observational procedures over time. *Observer expectancy and feedback* refers to the bias that may be present when there are expectations of change. Because of these issues, more objective measures of discourse should be readily available for the practicing clinician.

The procedures that have been used to analyze discourse more objectively in the neurologically impaired population can be categorized according to their level of analysis. *Microstructural analyses* focus at the local level of the word or sentence. They are concerned with the small elements in a text and the relations between these small elements. The identification and coding of cohesion devices is an example of a microstructural analysis. *Macrostructural analyses* focus at the level of the entire text. These analyses are more global in that they look at the gist, theme, or main ideas of the discourse. Informational content analysis occurs at the level of the macrostructure. *Superstructural analysis* overlies the text and includes the analysis of story grammar.

Brain-damaged individuals may show differential impairments at each level. For example, one patient may be able to maintain the superstructure but may be impaired at the local level of discourse (cohesion). In contrast, another patient may be able to identify and provide the main ideas or gist of a story but may not be able to organize it into the sequential steps or superstructure. Therefore, it is important for the clinician to use a variety of different analyses to identify the specific discourse impairments of the patient. Each of these types of analyses is discussed in detail in the following chapters.

Discourse and Functional Communication

The proliferation of research on discourse analysis has occurred concomitantly with changes in health care that emphasize the need for determining *functional* communication goals for communicatively impaired patients and measuring *functional outcomes* in clinical practices. Therefore, the emphasis on pragmatics and discourse is timely because discourse *IS* functional communication. Functional communication has been defined as the dynamic, complex, and purposeful use of language in a specific environment (Hartley, 1995). The environment determines the nature of the communication; if the environment changes, the communication changes accordingly. Functional communication goals for a specific client can be determined only with respect to that client's own social and physical setting and therefore can be defined only with respect to the individual (Hartley, 1995). Discourse analysis provides the clinician with an objective means of measuring communicative performance, regardless of the individuality of the functional communication goal. Because measures of discourse performance can be employed in the individual's specific environment, they are an important means of assessing baseline performance, guiding the setting of functional communication goals, and measuring changes over time (during and after treatment) to determine if the communication goals are met.

In summary, discourse analysis procedures provide the clinician with a set of evaluation tools that (a) describe the impairment in objective and measurable terms, (b) help identify the underlying cognitive or linguistic processes that contribute to the discourse impairment, (c) assist in treatment planning, and (d) are sensitive to changes over time. In addition, once a clinician is familiar with a discourse analysis procedure, quick and easy ways of adapting the procedure to analyze discourse for clinical purposes are available. Therefore, discourse analysis can be time- and cost-effective.

It is important to consider the discourse of all patients with neurological communication impairments. However, the systematic application of discourse analysis procedures may not be warranted for all patients, particularly if the communication problem is severe and output is limited. Therefore, for each patient, clinicians must make decisions about when and what kind of discourse should be sampled and how the discourse should be analyzed. Exhibit 1–2 lists some of the questions that should be asked for every patient to help guide the decision-making process. The following chapters (Chapters 2–7) provide practical guidelines to help follow through with these clinical decisions. Chapter 8 provides an annotated bibliography and quick reference source, summarizing our current knowledge about discourse in adults with neurological disorders.

Exhibit 1–2 Questions To Guide Your Decisions

The following questions can help the clinician determine whether discourse should be elicited, analyzed, or treated.

1. Does the patient have any verbal output, either spontaneously or when elicited?

   NO—Reassess periodically; treatment goals may focus on facilitating increased verbal output.
   YES—Elicit and record the verbal output. Note that the eliciting and recording of discourse is not necessarily a commitment to analyze the discourse at this time. Samples may be recorded and then kept for later analysis if needed.

2. What type of discourse should be elicited? What kinds of stimuli should be used to elicit that type of discourse?

   Consider eliciting and recording a variety of different types of discourse. At the very least, a narrative and conversational discourse should be elicited. Specific tasks may be determined by clinician preference, whereby clinicians develop a set of discourse tasks that they routinely like to give. Patient variables must be considered: for example, if the patient is visually impaired, it is better not to use visual stimuli to elicit the discourse.

3. Should the discourse samples be analyzed? If so, when? What analyses would be appropriate?

   Consider whether the results of the analyses will provide necessary information. For example, analyzing the discourse of the high-level patient who performs well on formal testing may help identify areas of deficit and provide a baseline measure against which to measure progress.

4. Given the results of the analyses, should the identified discourse deficits be treated? If so, what goals should be developed? What treatment tasks would be appropriate?

   Develop treatment goals with the patient, and select functional communicative tasks that are relevant to the patient's environment.

REFERENCES

Bates, E. (1976). *Language in context.* New York: Academic Press.

Bloom, L., & Lahey, M. (1978). *Language developments and language disorders.* New York: John Wiley.

Bloom, R.L., Obler, L.K., DeSanti, S., & Ehrlich, J.S. (Eds.). (1994). *Discourse analysis and applications: Studies in adult clinical populations.* Hillsdale, NJ: Lawrence Erlbaum.

Brownell, H.H., & Joanette, Y. (1993). *Narrative discourse in neurologically impaired and normal aging adults.* San Diego, CA: Singular Publishing Group.

Davis, G.A. (1986). Pragmatics and treatment. In R. Chapey (Ed.), *Language intervention strategies in adult aphasia* (2nd ed.). Baltimore: Williams & Wilkins.

Goldsmith, T., & Mackisack, E.L. (1992, November). *Current practice in pragmatics assessment: National survey results.* Paper presented at the annual meeting of the American Speech-Language-Hearing Association, San Antonio, TX.

Grice, H.P. (1975). Logic and conversation. In P. Cole & J.L. Morgan (Eds.), *Syntax and semantics: Vol. 3. Speech acts* (pp. 41–58). New York: Academic Press.

Halper, A.S., Cherney, L.R., Burns, M.S., & Mogil, S.I. (1996). *RIC evaluation of communication problems in right hemisphere dysfunction—revised (RICE-R).* Gaithersburg, MD: Aspen Publishers, Inc.

Hartley, L.L. (1995). *Cognitive-communicative abilities following brain injury: A functional approach.* San Diego, CA: Singular Publishing Group.

Joanette, Y., & Brownell, H.H. (1990). *Discourse ability and brain damage: Theoretical and empirical perspectives.* New York: Springer-Verlag.

Newhoff, M., & Apel, K. (1990). Impairments in pragmatics. In L. LaPointe (Ed.), *Aphasia and related neurogenic language disorders* (pp. 221–233). New York: Thieme Medical.

Penn, C. (1988). The profiling of syntax and pragmatics in aphasia. *Clinical Linguistics and Phonetics, 2,* 179–208.

Prutting, C.A., & Kirchner, D.M. (1987). A clinical appraisal of the pragmatic aspects of language. *Journal of Speech and Hearing Disorders, 52,* 105–119.

Roth, F.P., & Spekman, N.J. (1984). Assessing the pragmatic abilities of children: Part I. Organizational framework and assessment parameters. *Journal of Speech and Hearing Disorders, 49,* 2–11.

Ulatowska, H.K., Allard, L., & Chapman, S.B. (1990). Narrative and procedural discourse in aphasia. In Y. Joanette & H.H. Brownell (Eds.), *Discourse ability and brain damage: Theoretical and empirical perspectives* (pp. 180–198). New York: Springer-Verlag.

Wilson, D., & Sperber, D. (1981). *On Grice's theory of conversation and discourse: Structure and interpretation.* New York: St. Martin's.

CHAPTER 2

Obtaining the Discourse Sample

Barbara B. Shadden

As Chapter 1 has illustrated, discourse tasks and behaviors are extraordinarily diverse. As a result, obtaining a discourse sample is not a simple process. With clients for whom discourse has been identified informally as a critical domain for assessment and intervention, the clinician must make a variety of important decisions before beginning the elicitation of the sample. These decisions pertain primarily to the selection of tasks that will sample a diverse range of behaviors and will further tap into areas of known or suspected deficit for the individual client. These deficit domains may be directly linguistic, or they may reflect underlying disruptions in related cognitive processes.

TASK VARIABLES

A variety of task-related variables can be used to distinguish among discourse tasks and to make decisions about tasks to be selected for assessment and intervention. These variables, along with the characteristics of a sampling of three discourse tasks, are shown in Table 2–1. The Rooster Story is a brief story-retelling task in which the client first hears a story and then must recount it (Ulatowska, Freedman-Stern, Doyle, Macaluso-Haynes, & North, 1983; Ulatowska, North, & Macaluso-Haynes, 1981). In the Cat Story, the client tells a story from four cartoon pictures showing a girl whose cat has become trapped in a tree. Her father attempts to save the cat, but the cat jumps to safety, and the

father ends up hanging off one limb and must be rescued by a fireman (Ulatowska, Freedman-Stern, et al., 1983). The Grocery Store procedural task asks the client to explain how to use an American supermarket to someone unfamiliar with this country (Ulatowska, Doyle, Freedman-Stern, & Macaluso-Haynes, 1983). The descriptions of each task's attributes are based in part upon work by Shadden, Burnette, Eikenberry, and DiBrezzo (1991) and Ulatowska and Chapman (1989) and in part upon simple analyses of task demands. Each variable warrants further brief commentary.

Stimulus Variables

The stimulus upon which the task is based can play a critical role in discourse performance (see Correia, Brookshire, & Nicholas, 1988; Potechin, Nicholas, & Brookshire, 1987). In this instance, *stimulus* refers to whether there is any visual or auditory stimulus, the specificity of the linguistic model, its complexity, and the presence or absence of shared reference. For example, a story that is told on the basis of a series of visible sequenced pictures will present different stimulus and memory challenges than a story that must be retold on the basis of auditory input from the examiner's initial telling. Further, story retelling after auditory input provides a very specific linguistic model but will present varying challenges to the language system depending on the linguistic complexity of this model. A re-

Table 2–1 Variables Affecting Performance across Three Discourse Tasks

Task Variable	Rooster Story (Narrative Retelling)	Cat Story (Narrative Generation)	Grocery Store (Procedure)
Stimulus			
Modality	Auditory	Visual	None
Linguistic specificity and complexity	High—due to model	Limited—no model, but pictures may require search for words. Syntactic complexity low to moderate	Low in terms of no model and options. Syntactic complexity moderate
Stimulus complexity	High	Low	None
Shared reference	High (in memory)	Always present	None, except through personal experience
Cognitive Complexity			
Memory demands	Major memory constraints	No memory constraints	Low memory constraints
Sequencing and organizational demands	Requires recognition and use of storytelling principles, high levels of cohesion, little inference	Requires recognition and elective use of storytelling principles, moderate inference and cohesion	Requires memory and organization of procedural steps with multiple options; potential cohesion demands high
Level of Task Constraint	High	Moderate	Low
Instructions	Constraining only due to request to replicate model	Constraining only due to request to tell story	Suggests formulation of message with no presuppositions about listener
Personal Relevance	Low	Variable	Variable
Syntactic Complexity	Moderate (due to model)	Low-to-Moderate	Moderate-to-High
Anticipated Disruption	May be high due to attempt to replicate model	May be low due to ease of following visual model (except where specific word-finding problems exist)	Variable due to memory and organizational demands and strategy in attempting task
Option for Exercise of Personal Style	None	Limited, but task can be personalized	Considerable

quest for production of procedural discourse may provide the client with more flexibility in word selection or organization, as may conversation (e.g., Easterbrook, Brown, & Perera, 1982). However, this very flexibility and open-endedness may create problems for some brain-damaged clients. In general, there is some evidence that syntactic complexity varies from task to task on the basis not only of stimulus attributes but also of the fundamental information to be communicated. For example, action-oriented tasks (in terms of either storytelling or procedural sequences) may elicit more adverbial subordinate clauses than do more straightforward descriptive tasks, which may elicit more adjectival subordinate clauses (Shadden et al., 1991).

Pictures also vary in complexity. A composite picture like a Norman Rockwell illustration may present many specific items and/or events in contrast to a simple line drawing of a single event or series of such events. A good example of this contrast can be found in the single Nicholas and Brookshire (1993) drawing of the basic elements of the Cat Story versus the four-part sequential cartoon drawing used by Ulatowska et al. (1981). In the case of the single stimulus, the creation of a story is dependent upon the speaker's imagination and understanding of the sequential elements of story grammar. Those same elements are laid out for the speaker in the sequenced drawings.

Finally, shared reference can have a major impact on the client's discourse behaviors, although the nature of this impact can be variable (Bottenberg & Lemme, 1990; Brenneise-Sarshad, Brookshire, & Nicholas, 1991). For example, if a client viewed a filmstrip without the clinician present and then was asked to tell the clinician the story, one would expect very different assumptions about what the clinician knew and thus different word selections and cohesive strategies than if the clinician was present during the viewing. In contrast, if the examiner told the client a story that then had to be retold, the client either might feel some pressure to be precise in the language (depending on instructions) or

might assume that the examiner knew many key elements of the story and might abridge or eliminate them.

Cognitive Complexity

Discourse tasks also vary considerably in terms of the cognitive challenges posed by each task (Ulatowska & Chapman, 1989). These challenges specifically involve memory demands and/or constraints, as well as the sequencing and organizational requirements of a particular discourse form. Memory constraints may result from the nature and specificity of the model provided, the time interval between model and discourse production, or the degree to which the client must access personal memories of an event or a task to perform effectively on the discourse task.

Sequencing and organizational constraints apply in varying degrees to all discourse forms and involve the macro- and superstructural levels of performance in particular. For example, a procedural discourse task requires the individual to search personal memory stores in order to recall not only all relevant and necessary steps to complete a procedure but also the correct sequence of such steps to effect the desired end product. Narrative storytelling tasks impose an entirely different set of organizational demands, although there is a time sequence requirement. As described in Chapter 1 and later in this book, stories have an episode structure that is considered essential to the effective generation or retelling of a true story. The speaker must have the mental schema for this structure and be able to assign story elements accurately to each component in order to communicate effectively.

Conversation appears, on the surface, to be the least organized and therefore least cognitively constrained of discourse tasks. However, clear "rules" apply to the initiation, maintenance, and termination of topics, to the management of conversational breakdown and repair, and to basic turn-taking behaviors (see Gerber & Gurland, 1989; Roth & Spekman, 1984a, 1984b). In reality, probably the least cognitively challenging discourse task is simple picture description, in which the client may opt to itemize picture elements without integrating them in any other fashion. For this reason, caution must be exercised in using picture description as the primary basis for assessing discourse behaviors. However, even this task requires organizational strategies that can be revealed in task performance.

Together, memory, sequencing, and organizational demands impose varying levels of constraint upon task performance. Coupled with stimulus attributes and challenges, overall task constraint can be said to vary considerably across discourse samples. Individual clients may be differentially affected by variables constraining performance. Some may benefit, while others may find task constraint highly taxing to impaired cognitive or linguistic abilities.

Anticipated Disruption

Aspects of the stimulus (particularly linguistic specificity and shared reference) and cognitive complexity also play a role in the degree of verbal disruption or fragmentation expected in a specific task. The term *verbal disruption* is used to refer to the degree to which the client exhibits repetitions, revisions, excessive pausing, and other breaks in the smooth flow of information (see Chapter 3). Although degree of verbal disruption is not always as predictable as other task variables, certain patterns can be anticipated. For example, if a client with any form of specific linguistic deficit is engaged in story retelling based upon an auditory stimulus, moderate verbal fragmentation may be anticipated, since the attempt to replicate the model may tax the language system. That same client may experience less disruption in a procedural discourse task where the vocabulary and syntactic constraints are low. Another client with specific cognitive deficits related to organization of information may show particular difficulties in generating a story based on a single composite picture or in maintaining the smooth flow of conversation.

Instructions

Instructions to the client about the discourse task can have a major impact upon verbal performance. For example, if the client is simply asked to tell how to use an American supermarket, he or she may very well assume that the clinician possesses a reasonable level of shared knowledge, and the procedural discourse will probably be considerably abbreviated. In contrast, if the client is told to tell a foreigner how to use an American supermarket, it is probable and appropriate that the discourse behavior will become much more detailed and highly specific in defining components of the situation. As a second example, the client's response to describing a Norman Rockwell picture can and will be strongly influenced by instructions. If the clinician merely says, "Describe this picture as completely as possible," the client may choose to list the picture contents, as opposed to attempting to link or relate events occurring on the picture. However, if the clinician says, "I want you to tell me a story about this picture," all the rules and organizational constraints of story grammar should be evoked. Finally, when a linguistic model is provided, discourse performance in retelling a story will be affected by whether task instructions ask individuals to retell the story "in their own words" or whether the examiner requests fidelity to the linguistic model (e.g., "Follow my wording as closely as possible in retelling the story").

Personal Relevance

Personal relevance is another often-overlooked variable in discourse performance (Bottenberg, Lemme, & Hedberg, 1987; Shadden, 1988). Basically, tasks that address topics within the personal experience of the client can be expected to elicit greater quantities of language and higher quality of performance. Asking an older woman who has never driven to describe how you change a flat tire may not be unreasonable in that she has probably observed this experience, but the task does not tap into any level of personal, experiential relevance. The Cookie Theft picture (Goodglass & Kaplan, 1983) may or may not appear terribly relevant to an older male stroke victim. It should be noted, however, that unpublished data from a picture stimulus comparable to the Cookie Theft picture in number of elements but with older adults depicted revealed no major discourse differences (Shadden, 1988). It might be argued, however, that the Living Room picture used in this study presented stereotypical images that did not appear personally relevant to some older subjects (see Figure 2–1). Describing where you were and what you were doing when John F. Kennedy was assassinated may evoke less personalized responses from a 36-year-old who was six years old at the time than from a 50-year-old. The issue is not whether a personally relevant task is better than a nonrelevant one but rather what the clinician wants to elicit in terms of discourse behaviors.

Option for Exercise of Personal Style

Along with personal relevance, one last variable deserves mention. Discourse behavior can and does reflect individual stylistic differences, at least in non–brain-injured speakers. Little is known about these stylistic differences, yet it is reasonable to assume that some elements of personal discourse style will be maintained in various client groups. It is important to recognize, therefore, that certain tasks will be likely to allow greater freedom to exercise some form of individual style than others. For example, conversational interactions, open-ended story-telling, and recounting of memorable events provide much more opportunity to frame the message in a unique fashion than do more constrained tasks such as the Cat Story or Lady Story retelling (Arizona Battery for Communication Disorders of Dementia; Bayles & Tomoeda, 1991). Whether the exercise or dem-

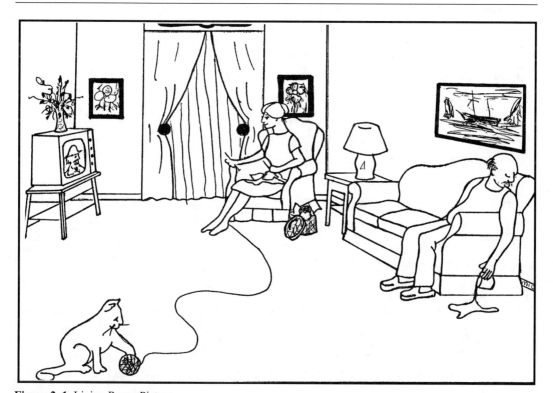

Figure 2–1 Living Room Picture

onstration of individual style is desirable is a matter to be determined by the clinician.

Case Examples

Perhaps the best way of illustrating the manner in which different tasks elicit very different kinds of behaviors in a single client is through examination of a series of discourse transcripts from one client. In Exhibits 2–1 through 2–6, six discourse samples are presented from client L.C., including two picture description tasks (the Living Room picture description task described earlier, Shadden, 1988; see Figure 2–1), with one response being verbal and the other being written; one storytelling task based on sequenced pictures (the Cat Story); two procedural discourse tasks (telling how to make scrambled eggs and telling a foreigner how to use an American supermarket); and a conversational sample. No other information will be provided, so as to avoid biasing the reader with diagnostic labels that might influence perceptions of the client's discourse performance. These samples will be used again later in this chapter and in Chapters 3 and 5 to illustrate selected analyses.

After a reading of these transcripts without any further analysis, certain clinical observations should be apparent. First, L.C. shows pronounced verbal disruption in most tasks, as evidenced by extensive revisions and repetitions and general fragmentation of utterances. Problems appear to be greater in the Living Room picture description task and in conversation than in any other tasks. One suspects that there is a linguistic base to these difficulties; however, a review of L.C.'s performance on the one written discourse task suggests that, with considerable time (23 minutes), basic lexical items are accurately retrieved, although syntactic omissions

Exhibit 2–1 Verbal Living Room Picture Description from Client L.C.

```
    Hum, ah, a woman and ah her husband, looks like, a woman and her ah, husband sitting in a, a room,
a living room, um watching TV. Now the woman was watching TV and also doing some needlework. Um, and
her husband was sitting on the couch, but looks like he was asleep um with a coffee cup in his cup, in
his hand which was pouring on the floor, dripping on the floor, the coffee. And a man and ah the woman
was sitting in a chair and she was not sitting with her husband. Her husband was sitting on a couch. In
between the two, the chair and the couch, there was ah ah a lamp, a table, ah ah there was a table. On
top the table there's a, there was a, a lamp. And above the couch there was a painting of um ships, ah,
a ship, um, shipping on the ocean, I guess, water. Um, and above the chair the woman was sitting, which
the woman was sitting, um, there was a picture behind her, above her chair. It's a painting of a
flower. On the woman's right hand there was a door which a curtain was drawn, drawing, there was a
curtain um hanging on the door, yes, looks like it. And on the other side of the door there's another
painting which is ah is a flower also. Ah, and ah, the, ah, facing the woman there was a, there was a
TV set and it's on top of, the TV's sitting on the table. And on top of the TV, um, no, the TV was
sitting on the table and on top of the TV's a vase of flowers. And a cat was, is playing, cat was
playing in the middle of the floor, and the cat was playing the, the, um the ball of threads in the
middle of the floor. And see, oh, um next to the woman's chair is a sewing, ah, basket. That's all.
```

Exhibit 2–2 Written Living Room Picture Description from Client L.C. (23 Minutes)

In a living room, there's a man, a woman, and a cat. The man is sitting in the couch asleep with his empty coffee cup in his hand. Above the couch is a painting of a ship sailing in the ocean. Next to to the couch is a small end table with a lamp on top of it. On the other side of the is a chair. The man's wife is sitting in the chair doing needlework and watch TV at the same time. Above the chair that she is sitting in is a picture of a flower. On the other side of the chair is a door which has a curtain hanging across it. There is another flower picture on another wall which is matching the first flower painting that is hanging on the other side of the door. A TV is standing across from the woman. On top of the TV has a vase full of flowers. The cat is play the thread ball in the middle of the floor.

Exhibit 2–3 Cat Story Generation from Client L.C.

OK, there was a little girl. She was crying to her dad. She said, "Well, my cat on the tree and I can't get her off the tree." And so her dad said, "Well." And he decided he's gonna get that cat for her. So he start climbing the tree and ah, he climbed to the top on the branch where the cat was and so he swing his, his arms and try to catch the cat. And the cat jump, the cat jump off, jumped off the, um, tree on . . . and, ah, the dad end up hanging on the branch while he was trying to catch the cat. And the girl start crying again and the police, because her dad was hanging on a tree branch with a cloth and the branch caught his, ah, ah, the back of his collar. And the, ah, the fire, the fireman, I guess that's a fireman, and he was trying to rescue him.

Exhibit 2–4 Procedural Discourse Sample on How To Make Scrambled Eggs from Client L.C.

OK. How to make scrambled eggs. Um, break the egg and stir it in a bowl. Break the eggs in a bowl, put all eggs in a bowl and stir it and with a spoon or something. Then you, ah, put, ah, ah, some milk in it, just a little portion of milk. Ah, you start a fire and put in the other pan, heat the pan, and you pour the milk, ah, the liquid egg in the pan. And then you stir it. Don't, don't heat it too hot and stir it and, and until it kinda form to a solid pieces, a small solid pieces, solid pieces. And that's about it. Depends on how you like it. (Clinician: True, that's true. OK.) Then you can put some pepper and salt on it if you want. (Clinician: OK, anything else?) Anything else? You can eat it. (Clinician: I just wanted to be sure you were actually through before I started something.) You can eat it, put it on a bowl and put it on a plate and eat it.

Exhibit 2–5 Procedural Discourse Sample on How To Use an American Supermarket from Client L.C.

What to do. OK, when you walk into walk into the door, walk in the door, and there's a person in the door and give you a shopping cart, and so you push this shopping cart and walk around the store and decide what you want and you just pick whatever you needed and put in the bag, in the cart. And after you selected all the items you needed and go to the, ah, [XXX]* cash register line and and then you just, ah, put all things on the ah table and check all things through the machine. And then they open the sacks, put them in the sacks for you, and sometimes you have to put in sacks by yourself, depends on where you are going. Most time they'll put in the sacks for you. Um, ah, then you just pay them in a check or money, cash. And then push the cart out in the car and put in your trunk. And that's all. (Clinician: OK, then you're ready to go.) Then you're ready to go. Push the cart back or you can put it in, in the little lot, they have a lot where they keep the carts.

*Unintelligible portion of sample.

Exhibit 2–6 Conversational Discourse Sample between Client L.C. and Clinician (C).

L: Well, I was watching something and they said, um, now they I think was in French or Canada. I don't remember which one.

C: In France?

L: France, I think it's France. Maybe it's in Canada. I don't remember which one. Anyway they're building this new building for the third world country because, um, like, oh, I don't know what, but anyway the [XXX]* they build this big building and it's like, ah, it's, um, it's a round building and have little tubes. Well, it's not a tube it's, uh, called a unit.

C: Hmmm.

L: They build this unit. It it has everything in it—like bathroom, you know, bed and living room and everything and just a little cube unit and it's kinda like container shape and [XXX]* put this unit in this building and it's like, ah, oh, maybe 20 years need to change a new one and just take this unit out put a new unit it, it's kinda like . . .

C: Interesting. Like a module, in/out nothing else moves.

L: Nothing else. And then they have, it's like a skeleton and just put everything . . .

C: Now, who's going to stay in those?

L: I don't know . . .

C: You said something about third world countries.

L: That's what they do because it's cheap and they can build so many of them just in no time.

C: So they're doing research in France or Canada and then they'll apply it?

L: They're trying to. Probably in 20 . . .

*Unintelligible utterance.

and inaccuracies are still evident. There also appear to be specific difficulties with reference and with overall cohesion (lexical ties across utterances). The conversational discourse task is most revealing of this unclear, empty speech pattern, whereas the picture description tasks (in which the stimulus items are immediately present to be labeled) evidence the least difficulty in this domain. Level of information clearly varies from task to task, and organization of information, particularly the temporally sequenced information in the procedural discourse tasks, appears inadequate. The client's linguistic and cognitive editing process appears quite evident on the surface of her discourse productions.

Many more observations can be made, but the most important points to consider after reviewing this discourse sample are the following. First, if only one discourse task had been used, the clinical impressions of L.C.'s discourse abilities would have been very incomplete. Only the profile created by cross-task comparisons allows an accurate indication of her difficulty level. Second, without any further analysis, the clinician could use this sample to make some informed decisions about which discourse analyses to pursue and which samples to use as a baseline for the individual analyses. The picture of an individual experiencing a fair level of communicative effort and some breakdown now needs to be confirmed with more formal analyses.

Exhibits 2–7 through 2–11 illustrate N.T.'s discourse range across a series of tasks that include description of a Norman Rockwell picture; the Cat Story telling task; the Rooster Story retelling task; a procedural discourse task (how to replace a burned-out lightbulb); and a brief conversational sample. Again, without further specific analysis, it is clear that discourse performance is highly variable depending upon stimulus and task demands. For example, the procedural discourse task is highly but appropriately elaborated, with complete and grammatically accurate forms and good sequencing of information. The Cat Story also demonstrates fairly complete information organization in a reasonable fashion with considerable detail, although some formulation and/or word retrieval problems may be surmised. The Rooster Story retelling, in contrast, shows pronounced breakdown. N.T. appears to have retained the gist of the story but is experiencing serious linguistic breakdown as seen in awkward wording, fumbling for words, and even comments on the difficulty of the word search. Finally, both Norman Rockwell picture description and conversation show marked verbal fragmentation, empty language, and a possible tendency toward verbosity. These samples from N.T. further illustrate the amount of information that can be gleaned from even the most informal of discourse samplings. The clinical impressions described here require further documentation.

Exhibit 2–7 Norman Rockwell Picture Description from Client N.T.

The . . . um . . . gentleman is . . . um . . . talking supposedly to his wife. I guess she's
. . . ah . . . looks like she's just . . . um . . . got up out for today's morning activities. And on
the back of her chair is a cat and beneath a dog . . . ah . . . looking at . . . ah . . . their child
sitting in his lap . . . ah . . . with the husband yelling about . . . um . . . a political figure in
the paper or something like that, someone who has their picture on a page of the . . . um . . .
newspaper with his arm over a toaster with a piece of toast in it. And he has some breakfast in front
of him while she has some breakfast also with a . . . a cage with a . . . um . . . bird in it. And they
are sitting in front of a . . . a window with sun shining in [XXX]* the morning and it's by Norman
Rockwell.

(Clinician: Okay, anything else about the picture?)

They . . . um . . . um . . . the . . . um . . . there's a pot of something on top of the oven,
but . . . um . . . there was a, has some gas to it and . . . um . . . there's some [XXX]* sitting on
the table but . . . um . . . not a very, doesn't seem to be a very, the segment I see isn't a very
large . . . um . . . segment of the kitchen, I suppose, with . . . ah . . . a . . . looks like a
picture hanging over the oven and a, maybe a window, no . . . a . . . um . . . a door going into
another room that's behind the gentleman. And lady has on some, a pair of slippers which matches
her . . . um . . . goes along with her . . . um . . . the rest of the attire she has on. She's dressed
in a robe . . . ah . . . and a nightgown with . . . um . . . another maybe her . . . um . . . political
supporting person in another paper in her hands. She's very, her expression is one of . . . um
. . . complete . . . um . . . disappointment and . . . ah . . . not really disappointment but . . . ah
. . . ah . . . a since her husband is yelling at her and they are married, she's . . . um . . . taking
the yell with . . . ah . . . and just not really with a bit of a frown on her face because of his . . .
um . . . confrontation to her. And [XXX]* there's a . . . um . . . a lamp that's . . . ah . . . [XXX]*
that's . . . um . . . not on because it's the middle of the morning, I suppose. So, and that . . .
ah . . . that's about everything except . . . um . . . done by Norman Rockwell.

*Unintelligible utterance.

Exhibit 2–8 Cat Story Generation from Client N.T.

One day a little young girl had lost her cat because of the cat running up a tree and . . .
ah . . . sitting on a limb right above . . . ah . . . the distance anyone could reach. So her, looks
like her father or a gentleman walking by saw her crying about the cat. And the gentleman shimmied up
the . . . ah . . . tree. And while he was shimmying up the tree, the cat moved down to the end of the
limb. And so the gentleman crawled the whole way out the limb to the branch where the cat was . . .
ah . . . cat couldn't go further cause there was no more branch and the branch he got there, the cat
had jumped off which caused the . . . the limb had little . . . um . . . piece sticking up. And
whenever the gentleman . . . um . . . was by there, he fell down. And he did not fall the whole way
because the stem that was sticking up out of the branch was . . . um . . . caught. And it kept him from
falling down, but it made him stuck. And so they called the . . . ah . . . fire department. And the
fire department came and with a ladder helped him . . . helped someone to get him down . . . um . . .
get down himself.

Exhibit 2–9 Narrative Rooster Story Retelling from Client N.T.

There were . . . um . . . two roosters in a flock. And then . . . um . . . the . . . um . . . one
rooster [pause] was . . . um . . . the . . . ah . . . strong rooster. And the one and
so . . . um . . . um . . . the process was a . . . does not come to mind. But . . . a . . . the one
rooster . . . um . . . went away in a corner because of his . . . um . . . humility. And a
[XXX]* . . . the rooster can be a humble person. And . . . um . . . and the other rooster thought it
was . . . a . . . a . . . real problem for him and went up and began to . . . um . . . roost and cackle
on top of some . . . ah . . . mound there. And . . . ah . . . an eagle came along and plucked him up
and took him away. And . . . ah . . . the other . . . um . . . rooster was then then
the . . . um . . . head rooster. And he . . . resumed [umed, umed] resumed the position that
the . . . ah . . . um . . . first rooster had . . . ah . . . vanished from.

*Unintelligible utterance.

Exhibit 2–10 Procedural Discourse Sample on How To Change a Lightbulb from Client N.T.

You first walk into the room and turn the light switch on for the light to go on and the light
does not go on. So you turn the light switch back off and then go out get the . . . um . . . lightbulb
and the ladder to climb up to the lightbulb and return then to the room and . . . um . . . set the
ladder under the lightbulb so you can get up. And then you climb up the ladder with the lightbulb in
hand or somewhere you can reach it and . . . um . . . unscrew the lightbulb in the socket. Replace it
with another new lightbulb. Then . . . um . . . um . . . climb back down the ladder . . . um . . . and
then go to the light switch and turn the lightbulb on and return the ladder from where it came from.

Exhibit 2–11 Conversational Discourse Sample between Client N.T. and Clinician (C).

C: Well, I have never known anyone that wrote a book.

N: That's my papa for you.

C: So, he was very interested in the Civil War?

N: U . . . a . . . um . . . lot of the basic . . . ah . . . confrontations that were going around, around, going on around the world. He's . . . ah . . . he was [XXX]* to watch the news every night, every night before he went to bed, every night, always watching the news to find out what's going on this lovely planet we live on.

C: So, he was interested in current events, not just the Civil War?

N: Exactly.

C: Well, this is really interesting. Have you read it, N.T.?

N: Uh, sorry to say, no, I haven't, but maybe so one of these days whenever I can fit that into my . . . should be . . . it should be a priority, but I, I've never really had a chance to read, read the book itself. I read the front and the back. I like the back, it's . . . ah . . . very . . .

C: Well, tell me about your father.

N: Ah, Dad, he was just really . . . um . . . wise and, and very loving, loving person. He was just, cause he owned, he owned the restaurant and . . . ah . . . he also . . . ah . . . he owned many, many other buildings, like he owned a place called the Book Mart Stationery, stationery store where they sold all sorts of . . . ah . . . ah . . . things for the offices and . . . ah . . . like paper and . . . ah . . . pens, and . . . ah . . . filing cabinets and . . . ah . . . just . . . file folders and stuff, and . . . ah . . . then he had . . . ah . . . a, he went to [XXX]* a, he owned . . . ah . . . he was a very wealthy gentleman. He owned a . . . um . . . a gas station which he had rented out to the American oil estab, American Sixty-Six Station or something like that and . . . ah . . . he owned a few houses. He owned, I guess it was about three houses out, out the road outside of town, and he owned . . . um . . . the house we lived in town which was a block off, two blocks away from the restaurant there and . . . ah . . . he owned . . . ah . . . on the . . . ah . . . ah . . . the . . . ah . . . the restaurant was here, across the block and he owned the two, finally the one building on the corner opposite the restaurant he owned and he bought it in 70, 71, one or two, two, two or one, some place around there and then the building beside that also and then the house. He was quite a wealthy . . . ah . . . gentleman. And, of course, he had it upstairs to make money, the reason why he was such . . . ah . . . cause he was able to work quite efficiently all the time with a, a job that would take . . . um take other, take . . . um . . . um . . . because of his knowledge about that, the operation he was able to don one job which took care of a lot of . . . ah . . . at least a couple of jobs of other people. He was just . . . ah . . . a blessing to have around. And it was a privilege to work with good old dad.

C: So, even though he was very busy, he found time for other things such as writing this book.

N: Right, he wrote the book . . . ah . . . yeah he wrote the book, I guess the year I was . . . ah . . . the year I was born, I guess.

C: Let's see, I believe this says 1950.

N: Fifty? Five years old.

C: Yeah, August 3, 1950.

*Unintelligible utterance.

TASK SELECTION AND ADMINISTRATION

Before beginning the process of selecting and administering discourse tasks and preparing sample transcriptions for further analysis, it is useful to review briefly the reasons for using discourse assessment with adult neurogenic populations. As pointed out in Chapter 1, one definition for *discourse* is that it is the basic unit of communication. As such, structured discourse tasks to varying degrees reflect some of the cognitive and linguistic challenges inherent in various real-life communication situations. Formal language tests and other cognitive assessments provide information about specific component skills necessary for effective discourse, but they do not provide any means of quantifying the qualitative disturbances in communication that are observed in clients. This quantification process is one reason for using discourse assessment procedures. By completing selected analyses, the clinician can develop a much more precise characterization of the discourse and communication characteristics of a given client. The data derived from these analyses can serve both as a baseline for subsequent treatment and as a means of determining appropriate treatment goals and procedures. Comparison of discourse performance with other, more formal tests will also yield strong indicators of underlying deficits contributing to observed behaviors. Thus, if the goal is to maximize functional communication in as many situations as possible, discourse presents an appropriate assessment and intervention vehicle.

Given the variety of discourse tasks available to the clinician, the first step in discourse assessment must be determination of the appropriate task array to represent adequately the range of discourse behaviors in a specific client. Ideally, narrative (storytelling), procedural, and conversational discourse samples will be obtained, at the very minimum. These types of tasks at least represent the range of discourse challenges to the linguistic and cognitive systems. For those wishing to take this approach, the Discourse Abilities Profile or DAP (Ripich, 1991; Terrell & Ripich, 1989) may provide a useful framework for preliminary consideration of discourse performance. The DAP is a screening protocol that may be scored on line or with a brief review of tape-recorded discourse samples. It is recommended that the clinician use the same tasks for the DAP across all patients to develop a better database of task performance and to refine and make more reliable on-line rating skills. Ratings of narrative, procedural, and conversational discourse performance on the DAP may provide useful directions for further assessment.

Alternatively, given the wide variability within as well as across types of discourse tasks, it is probably more appropriate to sample first the discourse performance of a given client across a wide range of tasks and then to determine those tasks warranting further analysis. In this approach, two strategies may be used. First, the clinician may want to select tasks not typically used for baseline measures in order to reserve preferred tasks for later testing. Second, the clinician may want all clients to complete a set corpus of discourse tasks that can be recorded and will be available for subsequent selective analysis. The end result is the same. For example, a traumatic brain-injured client may perform adequately on a storytelling task for which sequential pictures are provided, yet may be virtually unable to retell a story when the story is presented auditorily or when there is a time delay between visual stimulus presentation and story retelling. The clinician will have to determine which narrative task or tasks will provide the most useful baseline data both for focusing interventions and for measuring change over time. Another brain-injured client may show extensive verbal fragmentation in both conversation and picture description tasks with no clear story or theme, yet may perform adequately on other narrative or procedural tasks. Again, the clinician must determine which are the most useful baseline tasks and measures. Examples of different arrays of discourse tasks can be found in Nicholas and Brookshire (1993), Shadden et al. (1991), and Cherney and Canter (1993).

TRANSCRIBING THE SAMPLE

At various points in this book, you will be provided with "shortcuts" to analysis of discourse samples. Some of these shortcuts require simple transcription of the sample without any further breakdown. Others are analyses that can be performed on line, without ever engaging in the process of preliminary transcription. These shortcuts are offered as a way of acknowledging the realities of clinical practice. We are keenly aware that most clinicians will not have the time to do a detailed discourse analysis for the majority of their clients, yet may wish to have some broad index of discourse behaviors.

However, in many instances, a more formal record of the discourse sample will be required. Once an audiotape or videotape of the selected discourse samples has been obtained, many desirable analyses will be based upon appropriate transcription and editing of the sample materials. Ideally, the sample is transcribed using a word-processing program on a computer to facilitate subsequent manipulation and editing of the language material. Also, a number of commercially available language sample transcription programs offer a variety of options. These programs include the SALT II (Miller & Chapman, 1992, 1993) and the CLAN program (Child Language Analysis) used in the CHILDES project (MacWhinney, 1991, 1996; Boles, Holland, & Beeson, 1993). Clinicians with access to these programs will find that many of the analyses mentioned in this book can be performed using specific transcription and analysis program features. The procedures that are described here assume only that the reader has access to some word-processing program, computer, or even a typewriter.

In general, the entire sample should be transcribed verbatim, including interjections (*uh, um*) and some notation of unintelligible utterances. Notations about nonverbal behaviors are optional and are generally included only when they shed light on the communicative context and information being shared. Use of the word processor will allow the clinician to enter the sample quickly and then to go back and segment, bracket, line-through, or otherwise modify the transcript for a particular analysis. There is no need initially to worry about punctuation and sentences in particular, since the analyses proposed here avoid the more traditional concept of the sentence in favor of the use of a different index for a complete utterance. Examples of totally unedited transcripts were shown earlier in Exhibits 2–1 through 2–11. The reader should note that there is a strong tendency to punctuate when transcribing a sample. This is neither correct nor incorrect. The samples provided here are in the actual form in which they were first transcribed. The presence of punctuation serves no function other than to reflect, perhaps, the intuitive first response of the person transcribing as to natural breaks in the communication. The same punctuation will be ignored during the T-unit analysis.

T-UNIT SEGMENTATION

Before any further editing or analysis is performed, it is useful to divide the transcript into T-units. A T-unit was described by Hunt (1965, 1970) as a "minimal terminal unit"; it consists of one main clause plus any subordinate clauses or nonclausal structures attached to or embedded in the main clause. Others have labeled this measure a "communication unit" (Loban, 1976). The purpose of the T-unit measure is to segment passages of continuous language into the shortest unit that is grammatically allowed to be punctuated as a sentence. Use of any smaller unit would result in fragments that would lack any independent grammatical form. If one uses the T-unit structure consistently, problems in determining when an utterance begins and ends are virtually eliminated. The analysis will provide some general indices of syntactic complexity. In addition, the clinician will be able to use the T-unit as a common measurement base for various other analyses (e.g., words per T-unit, verbal disruptions per T-unit).

The concept of the T-unit is built around the clause as the main structural element. In Hunt's (1965, 1970) analyses, an independent or main clause must contain (a) a subject nominal, (b) a finite verb or verb phrase, and (c) depending on the verb, certain objects or complements. Modifiers may be added, the verb phrase may be expanded by the addition of auxiliary verb forms, and subordinate clauses may be embedded in or appended to this independent clause.

Subordinate clauses are divided by Hunt (1965, 1970) into three groups, differentiated primarily by the function they serve in the sentence, and secondarily by placement and linking words. These three groups and various "sentence" forms are reviewed here, since their description will aid the clinician in determining where to divide T-units. The three groups are:

1. *Noun Clause*—usually found as a direct object after verbs such as *think, say,* and *ask.* The noun clause can serve the role of subject, object, complement, or appositive.
   Example: "She thought that the man was handsome."
   Introduced by subordinate conjunctions such as *that, whatever, whoever, wherever, who, what, why, when, where, whether.*
2. *Adjective Clause*—always follows the noun that it modifies (although not always immediately). Adjective clauses serve as modifiers of nouns or pronouns.
   Example: "The dog is the one who barks all the time."
   Introduced by subordinate conjunctions such as *who, which,* and *that.*
3. *Adverb Clauses*—are usually movable and can precede, follow, or interrupt the main clauses to which they are attached. Adverb clauses modify verbs, adjectives, adverbs, or the main clauses. They are connectives that express relationships of place, time, manner, cause, direction, condition, or concession.

Examples:
"I'll leave when she arrives."
"When she arrives, I'll leave."
Introduced by subordinate conjunctions such as *after, although, as, as if, as long as, because, before, if, in order that, provided, since, so, so that, though, until, unless, when, where, while.* (Be careful with *so* and *and so*, since they can also be coordinating conjunctions.)

Both simple and complex sentences are considered one T-unit. A simple sentence type contains only one main clause.

Example: "The cats tried to eat the mouse."

A complex sentence is one that contains only one main clause with one or more subordinate clauses.

Examples:
"I like the movie we saw about vampires."
"The man that the truck hit had bought groceries at the store that had a broken window."

In the case of both the simple sentence and the complex sentence types, each sentence is counted as one T-unit.

Compound or compound/complex sentences are considered to be more than one T-unit, since they consist of *more than one main clause.* Compound sentences are joined by coordinating or correlative conjunctions or by conjunctive adverbs.

1. Coordinating conjunctions might be *and, but, or, nor, yet, besides,* or *so.*
2. Correlative conjunctions might be *either . . . or, neither . . . nor, both . . . and,* or *not only . . . but also.*
3. Conjunctive adverbs might be *also, however, then, therefore, accordingly, nevertheless,* or *consequently.*

In the examples below, there are two T-units, separated where the slash mark appears. The "sentences" consist of two main clauses joined by a coordinating conjunction.

Exhibit 2–12 Hunt's (1995, 1970) Guidelines for T-Unit Analysis

---

Definition: A T-unit is one main (independent) clause plus any subordinate clauses or non-clausal structures attached to or embedded in the main clause. A main clause must have a subject and verb and may have optional objects or complements.

1. Read the transcript carefully several times so that you are certain you understand the meaning and intent of what is being said.
2. Look particularly for specific conjunctions that will act as signals to a specific type of clause being used.
   Simple sentences have one main clause only. *Complex sentences* have one main clause and one or more subordinate clauses, which are introduced by various stated or implied subordinate conjunctions, such as *that, whatever, whoever, wherever, who, what, why, when, where, whether, which, after, although, as, as if, as long as, because, before, if, in order that, provided, since, so, so that, though, until, unless, while.*
   Compound sentences consist of two or more main clauses and thus are two or more T-units. They are conjoined by coordinating or correlative conjunctions or by conjunctive adverbs, such as *and, but, or, nor, yet, besides, so, either . . . or, neither . . . nor, both . . . and, not only . . . but also, also, however, then, therefore, accordingly, nevertheless, consequently.*
3. Identify main clauses first; then examine surrounding language to determine which other clausal units are attached to (subordinate to) the main clause. Disregard false starts or revisions, since the final form of the utterance is all that matters. If necessary, edit out extraneous words and revisions before defining T-units. Even if you are dealing with a written discourse sample punctuated by the client, ignore the punctuation and follow the rules defined here.
4. Pencil in rough breaks between T-units, using a slash mark. Read over the transcript again to make certain your segmentation is correct.
5. Underline subordinate clauses within T-units (This can be done later if so desired.)
6. Number T-units.
7. If using a word processor, make a break at the end of each T-unit so that the next T-unit begins on a separate line.

Examples:
"They bought some fruit/ and they ate it all on the way home."
"They bought some fruit for dessert/ but they ate it all before dinner."

According to Hedberg and Stoel-Gammon (1985) and Hedberg and Westby (1993), *minor sentence* types can also be considered T-units, even if they lack a complete main clause, if they fit one of the following categories.

1. *Completive Sentences*—answers to questions, comments on previous statements, or situational comments such as introductions.

Examples:
(Who was it?) "Nancy."
(When are you leaving town?) "Tomorrow."

2. *Exclamatory Sentences*—primary or secondary interjections.
3. *Aphoristic Sentences*—expressions that operate as full sentences.
   Example: "A dime a dozen."

For those not used to thinking in terms of basic English grammar, the above discussion may seem overly complex. In reality, with very little practice, the T-unit breakdown of a discourse sample becomes quite easy. Some rules of

Exhibit 2–13 L.C.'s Cat Story Discourse Sample, Segmented into T-Units Using Slash Marks, Then Separated into Separate Numbered Lines

---

First T-Unit Segmentation with Slash Marks

OK, there was a little girl./[1] She was crying to her dad./[2] She said, "Well, my cat on the tree and I can't get her off the tree."/[3] And so her dad said, "Well."/[4] And he decided he's gonna get that cat for her./[5] So he start climbing the tree/[6] and ah, he he climbed to the top on the branch where the cat was/[7] and so he swing his, his arms and try to catch the cat./[8] And the cat jump, the cat jump off, jumped off the, um, tree on . . ./[9] and, ah, the dad end up hanging on the branch while he was trying to catch the cat./[10] And the girl start crying again and the police, because her dad was hanging on a tree branch with a cloth and the branch caught his, ah, ah, the back of his collar./[11] And the, ah, the fire, the fireman, I guess that's a fireman, and he was trying to rescue him./[12]

Second T-Unit Segmentation: Numbering on Separate Lines

1. OK, there was a little girl.

2. She was crying to her dad.

3. She said, "Well, my cat on the tree and I can't get her off the tree."

4. And so her dad said, "Well."

5. And he decided he's gonna get that cat for her.

6. So he start climbing the tree

7. and ah, he climbed to the top on the branch where the cat was

8. and so he swing his, his arms and try to catch the cat.

9. And the cat jump, the cat jump off, jumped off the, um, tree on . . .

10. and, ah, the dad end up hanging on the branch while he was trying to catch the cat.

11. And the girl start crying again and the police, because her dad was hanging on a tree branch with a cloth and the branch caught his, ah, ah, the back of his collar.

12. And the, ah, the fire, the fireman, I guess that's a fireman, and he was trying to rescue him.

---

thumb to assist you in this process are shown in Exhibit 2–12. In Exhibit 2–13, L.C.'s Cat Story has been broken into T-units using the first-draft transcription and slash marks, followed by further segmentation so that each T-unit is on a different line and is separately numbered.

A word or two of caution is appropriate at this point. Many researchers and clinicians choose not to break conversational discourse samples into T-units. Instead, they prefer to treat each conversational turn as a discrete entity for analysis purposes. Within the conversational turn, pauses can be coded with a series of dots [. . .], or a natural intonational break may be marked with a slash (/). This approach does have one major advantage, in that many of the utterances produced in conversation are fragments rather than complete T-units. According to the Hedberg and Stoel-Gammon (1985) guidelines noted earlier, these fragments can be analyzed as

Exhibit 2–14 L.C.'s Conversational Discourse Sample Segmented into T-Units

```
L:   1.  Well, I was watching something
     2.  and they said, um, now they I think was in French or Canada.
     3.  I don't remember which one.
C: In France?
L:   4.  France, I think it's France.
     5.  Maybe it's in Canada.
     6.  I don't remember which one.
     7.  Anyway they're building this new building for the third world country because, um, like, oh, I
         don't know what, but anyway the [XXX]* they build this big building
     8.  and it's like, ah, it's, um, it's a round building and have little tubes.
     9.  Well, it's not a tube
    10.  it's, uh, called a unit.
C: Hmmm.
L:  11.  They build this unit.
    12.  It it has everything in it—like bathroom, you know, bed and living room and everything and just a
         little cube unit
    13.  and it's kinda like container shape
    14.  and [XXX]* put this unit in this building
    15.  and it's like, ah, oh, maybe 20 years need to change a new one and just take this unit out put a
         new unit it, it's kinda like . . .
C: Interesting. Like a module, in/out nothing else moves.
L: Fragment: Nothing else.
    16.  And then they have, it's like a skeleton and just put everything . . .
C: Now, who's going to stay in those?
L:  17.  I don't know . . .
C: You said something about third world countries.
L:  18.  That's what they do because it's cheap and they can build so many of them just in no time.
C: So they're doing research in France or Canada and then they'll apply it?
L:  19.  They're trying to.
    Fragment: Probably in 20 . . .

    * Unintelligible utterance.
```

"completive sentence" types and considered in a T-unit count, but the procedure is awkward. L.C.'s conversational sample has been broken into T-units for the reader in Exhibit 2–14 to illustrate how conversation would look with this form of editing.

The second word of caution applies to the application of T-unit analyses to procedural dis-

course tasks, particularly some of the simpler ones such as describing how to change a lightbulb or make a sandwich. Not surprisingly, the normal speaker typically frames the procedural discourse as directions to the conversational partner present in the room. As a result, the implied *you* as subject is used frequently, and extended strings of conjoined predicates (typically with *and*) without any stated subject may occur. Less commonly, the speaker will conjoin multiple predicates with a single-subject pronoun such as *he*.

Consider the following sample:

> You usually . . . get a ladder to help you so you can reach it a sturdy ladder then you climb up the ladder make sure the light's not on just so it's not hot then you turn it um turn the bulb on the light and take it out and change it with a new bulb.

This sample is fraught with difficulties in T-unit analysis. In at least three places, it is difficult to know whether to take the stated subject at face value and ignore implied subjects or whether to treat each predicate as being linked separately (as a main clause) to an implied subject. If you follow the logic of the first approach, taking stated subjects as determiners of the segmentation process, the T-unit edited sample would look like this:

> You usually . . . get a ladder to help you so you can reach it a sturdy ladder/
> then you climb up the ladder make sure the light's not on just so it's not hot/
> then you turn it um turn the bulb on the light and take it out and change it with a new bulb.

This approach would credit the speaker with rather long T-units (although complexity would not be high). Intuitively, however, the information is being communicated in a very simple fashion, as one might expect in a procedural discourse task of this type. The alternative would be to develop a rule of thumb for T-unit analysis in procedural discourse only. Specifically, the rule would state that a T-unit break is inserted whenever a new predicate is introduced and the implied subject *you* would be logical. In this scenario, the transcript would look as follows:

> You usually . . . get a ladder to help you so you can reach it a sturdy ladder/
> then you climb up the ladder/
> make sure the light's not on just so it's not hot/

> then you turn it um turn the bulb on the light/
> and take it out/
> and change it with a new bulb.

Neither approach to T-unit analysis for procedural discourse is right or wrong. Each clinician should select the method that is most logical to him or her and should be consistent.

FURTHER EDITING OF THE TRANSCRIPT

For some analyses, it is considered desirable to edit out unwanted, extraneous language material. In some cohesion analyses, for example, it is important to focus on whether the client actually produced a complete cohesive tie, regardless of how he or she got to that point. The clinician may also want a rough indicator of the amount (number of words) of productive language produced after all revisions, false starts and comments are removed. These word counts can be compared across tasks and assessment sessions if a consistent measurement approach is adopted. The number of words left after editing can also be compared with total (unedited) words as a general index of how disrupted and/or difficult it was for the client to produce the amount of information used. Communication rate (the traditional "words per minute") may also be calculated based on the edited and unedited samples to obtain an idea of overall efficiency (see Chapter 5). Finally, both types of word counts can be important as measures of change over time.

Several authors have addressed the manner in which editing of discourse transcripts and determination of word counts should be accomplished. These systems of editing are very similar. The choice of approach will depend on what is intuitively logical to the individual clinician. For example, Strong and Shaver (1991) advocated counting contractions as one word, whereas Hedberg and Westby (1993) and Nicholas and Brookshire (1993) counted them as two or more words. These three different sets of rules are provided in Exhibit 2–15. Note that no procedure for developing word counts includes nonwords in the total count.

Examples of transcripts after editing using Strong and Shaver's (1991) approach are shown in Exhibits 2–16, 2–17, and 2–18 for the Living Room picture description, the Cat Story, and the conversational sample produced by L.C. Instead of using bracketing, the authors indicate the words eliminated by lining them through. The speaking rate for each sample is also shown.

Exhibit 2–15 Options for Editing and Word Counts

Strong and Shaver (1991)

- Comments or asides are bracketed.
- Bracket exact repetitions of words and/or phrases.
- Bracket syntactic or semantic revisions that do not have a complete thought.
- Note: direct quotes, as in "He said, 'I'll do it,' " are not considered separate T-units.
- Bracket unintelligible words and phrases.
- Contractions count for one word.
- Count sentence fragments as legitimate fragments if intonation suggests that a complete thought was intended.

Hedberg and Stoel-Gammon (1985); Hedberg and Westby (1993)

- Place incomplete words, nonessential repetitions, and asides to examiner in brackets.
- Do count "titles" and "conclusions" in stories.

- Count words according to adult equivalents, for example,
  1. Abbreviations are one word.
  2. Contractions are two or more words.
  3. Elided words are two or more words (e.g., *kinda, hafta*).

Nicholas and Brookshire (1993)

- Bracket/line-through beginning and ending types of phrases ("I can't say more," "I'll stop here") if grammatically separate.
- Don't count filler nonwords or unintelligible words.
- Do count filler words and interjections such as *oh, gosh, aha*.
- Do count contractions as two or more words, whether standard or colloquial.
- Do count commentary on task.
- Do count each word in hyphenated words or numbers or proper names.

Exhibit 2–16 Editing for Word Counts in L.C.'s Living Room Picture Description (Verbal)

	Edited/Total Words
1. ~~Hum, ah~~, a woman and ~~ah~~ her husband, ~~looks like, a woman and her ah, husband~~ sitting in a, ~~a room, a~~ living room, ~~um~~ watching TV.	12/22
2. Now the woman was watching TV and also doing some needlework.	11/11
3. ~~Um~~, and her husband was sitting on the couch,	8/8
4. but ~~looks like~~ he was asleep ~~um~~ with a coffee cup ~~in his cup~~, in his hand which was ~~pouring on the floor~~, dripping on the floor, the coffee. {note left "the coffee" at end—appropriate clarification}	19/28
5. And ~~a man and ah~~ the woman was sitting in a chair	8/11
6. and she was not sitting with her husband.	8/8
7. Her husband was sitting on a couch.	7/7
8. In between the two, the chair and the couch, ~~there was ah ah a lamp, a table~~, ~~ah ah~~ there was a table.	13/19
9. On top the table ~~there's a~~, there was a, ~~a~~ lamp.	8/11
10. And above the couch there was a painting of ~~um ships, ah~~, a ship, ~~um~~, ~~shipping~~ on the ocean, ~~I guess, water~~.	14/19
11. ~~Um~~, and above the chair ~~the woman was sitting~~, which the woman was sitting, ~~um~~, there was a picture behind her, ~~above her chair~~.	15/22
12. It's a painting of a flower.	6/6
13. On the woman's right hand ~~there was a door which a curtain was drawn, drawing~~, there was a curtain ~~um~~ hanging on the door, ~~yes, looks like it~~.	13/27
14. And on the other side of the door there's another painting which is ~~ah is~~ a flower also.	16/17
15. ~~Ah, and ah, the, ah~~, facing the woman there was a, ~~there was a~~ TV set	8/13
16. and ~~it's on top of,~~ the TV's sitting on the table. ~~And on top of the TV, um, no, the TV was sitting on the table~~	7/25
17. and on top of the TV's a vase of flowers.	10/10
18. And a cat was, ~~is~~ playing, ~~cat was playing in the middle of the floor, and the cat was playing the, the, um~~ the ball of threads in the middle of the floor.	15/32
19. And ~~see, oh, um~~ next to the woman's chair is a sewing, ~~ah~~, basket. ~~That's all~~.	10/11

Summary: 19 T-units
   Total words = 309
   Edited words = 208
   Edited/total words = 208/309 = 67.3% (productivity level)

   Speaking rate (wpm) = 112.7
   Communication rate (edited wpm) = 75.6

Exhibit 2–17 Editing for Word Counts in L.C.'s Cat Story Generation

	Edited/Total Words
1. ~~OK~~, there was a little girl.	5/6
2. She was crying to her dad.	6/6
3. She said, "Well, my cat on the tree and I can't get her off the tree."	16/16
4. And so her dad said, "Well."	6/6
5. And he decided he's gonna get that cat for her.	10/10
6. So he start climbing the tree	6/6
7. and ~~ah~~, he climbed to the top on the branch where the cat was	13/13
8. and so he swing ~~his~~, his arms and try to catch the cat.	12/13
9. And ~~the cat jump~~, the cat ~~jump off~~, jumped off the, ~~um~~, tree on . . .	8/13
10. and, ~~ah~~, the dad end up hanging on the branch while he was trying to catch the cat.	17/17
11. And the girl start crying again ~~and the police~~, because her dad was hanging on a tree branch with a cloth and the branch caught ~~his, ah, ah~~, the back of his collar.	27/31
12. And ~~the, ah, the fire~~, the fireman, ~~I guess that's a fireman, and he~~ was trying to rescue him.	8/18

Summary: 12 T-units
Total words = 155
Edited words = 134
Edited/total words = 134/155 = 86.5% (productivity level)

Speaking rate (wpm) = 116.25
Communication rate (edited wpm) = 100.5

Exhibit 2–18 Editing for Word Counts in L.C.'s Conversational Discourse Sample

			Edited/Total Words
L:	1.	~~Well~~, I was watching something	4/5
	2.	~~and they said, um, now they~~ I think was in French or Canada.	7/12
	3.	I don't remember which one.	5/5
C:		In France?	
L:	4.	~~France~~, I think it's France.	4/5
	5.	Maybe it's in Canada.	4/4
	6.	I don't remember which one.	5/5
	7.	Anyway they're building this new building for the third world country ~~because, um, like, oh, I don't know what, but anyway the [XXX]* they build this big building~~	11/26
	8.	and ~~it's like, ah, it's, um,~~ it's a round building and have little tubes.	9/12
	9.	Well, it's not a tube	5/5
	10.	it's, ~~uh~~, called a unit.	4/4
C:		Hmmm.	
L:	11.	They build this unit.	4/4
	12.	It ~~it~~ has everything in it–like bathroom, ~~you know~~, bed and living room and everything and just a little cube unit	19/22
	13.	and it's kinda like container shape	6/6
	14.	and [XXX]* put this unit in this building	7/8
	15.	and ~~it's like, ah, oh~~, maybe 20 years need to change a new one and just take this unit out put a new unit in, ~~it's kinda like~~ . . .	21/26
C:		Interesting. Like a module, in/out nothing else moves.	
L:		Fragment: Nothing else. (not counted in later words/T-unit measures)	2/2
	16.	And ~~then they have~~, it's like a skeleton ~~and just put everything~~ . . .	5/12
C:		Now, who's going to stay in those?	
L:	17.	I don't know . . .	3/3
C:		You said something about third world countries.	
L:	18.	That's what they do because it's cheap and they can build so many of them just in no time.	19/19

continues

Exhibit 2–18 continued

Edited/Total Words

C: So they're doing research in France or Canada and then they'll apply it?

L: 19. They're trying to.   3/3

L: Fragment: Probably in 20. (not counted in later words/T-unit measures)   3/3

Summary: 19 T-units
Total words = 191
Edited words = 149
Edited/total words = 149/191 = 78% (productivity level)

Speaking rate and communication rate—not determined because of difficulty of calculating speaking time for L only—could be worked out if desired

*Unintelligible utterance—counted as word in word count but edited out later.

Results of this preliminary process of editing could be tabled or could be expressed as follows:

As part of this evaluation, L.C. was asked to perform three discourse tasks. In the Living Room picture description task, she produced 309 total words at a speaking rate of 113 wpm. After editing to eliminate extraneous, repetitive, nonrelevant language, the remaining word total was 208, with a communication rate of 76 wpm. Percentage of edited to total words was 67%, suggesting a moderately low productivity level. Similarly, in the Cat Story task (based on sequenced cartoon pictures), L.C. produced 155 total words at a speaking rate of 116 wpm. After editing to eliminate extraneous, repetitive, nonrelevant language, the remaining word total was 134, with a communication rate of 101 wpm. Percentage of edited to total words was 87%, suggesting a moderate productivity level. Finally, in conversation, L.C. produced 191 total words. Speaking rate was not calculated, due to difficulty of segmenting speaker time. After editing to eliminate extraneous, repeti-

tive, nonrelevant language, the remaining word total was 149, with a productivity level of 78%.

Note that ranges of response for each of the analysis categories could also have been provided across tasks to eliminate some wordiness, or data could simply have been tabled. The clinician would then presumably make some comparative statements across tasks to determine the manner in which different task challenges affected gross rates of communication and productivity levels. The pattern in this instance is one that provides quantitative support for impressions identified earlier in this chapter.

If the clinician chooses to engage in this type of editing and word count, both the edited and the original T-unit segmented transcripts should be retained. Certain analyses in the following chapter, particularly specific measures of verbal fragmentation, will require an unedited transcript.

The reader may also recall that it was suggested that the T-unit analysis precede the word count editing process. On occasion, however, the clinician may find it easier to do some preliminary editing to clarify what portions of the discourse sample represent genuine main clauses and/or subordinate clauses as opposed to first-draft behaviors that are subsequently revised. An excellent example occurs in L.C.'s verbal description of the Living Room picture (see Exhibit 2–16 for analyses). In T-units 15, 16, and 17, there is an almost bewildering display of repetition and revision behavior. Without editing of extraneous language, it would have been tempting to add at least one other T-unit, as follows (additional T-unit bracketed):

15. Ah, and a, the, ah, facing the woman there was a, there was a TV set
16. And it's on top of, the TV's sitting on the table
[And on top of the TV, um, no the TV was sitting on the table]
17. And on top of the TV's a vase of flowers

The same type of problem is seen in T-unit 13. It might have been tempting to segment this section of the transcript into two T-units, as follows:

13. On the woman's right hand there was a door which a curtain was drawn, drawing, [there was a curtain um hanging on the door, yes, looks like it.]

Only when one edits out repeated and revised information does the final analysis become clear. The editing is shown in this example by strikeover of the deleted items.

CONCLUSION

The discourse sample selection and appropriate transcription and preliminary editing procedures have been reviewed in considerable detail in this chapter. While some of the procedures may appear cumbersome, the reader is reminded that only selected discourse samples will be chosen for extended transcription and analysis. These samples will then serve two important functions. They will serve as a reference point for determination of appropriate treatment goals and procedures (particularly types of task variables), and they will provide baseline data for demonstrating treatment efficacy and for identifying needed changes in treatment focus.

In the Appendixes, a variety of discourse samples have been provided for further practice. For most of these samples, T-units are identified. The reader may want to practice on or review these samples for additional experience with transcript preparation and editing.

REFERENCES

Bayles, K.A., & Tomoeda, C.K. (1991). *Arizona Battery for Communication Disorders of Dementia*. Tucson, AZ: Canyonlands.

Boles, L., Holland, A.L., & Beeson, P. (1993, November). *Conversation analysis: How much talk is enough?* Miniseminar presented at the annual meeting of the American Speech-Language-Hearing Association, Anaheim, CA.

Bottenberg, D., & Lemme, M. (1990). Effect of shared and unshared listener knowledge on narratives of normal and aphasic adults. *Clinical Aphasiology, 19*, 109–116.

Bottenberg, D., Lemme, M., & Hedberg, N. (1987). Effect of story content on narrative discourse of aphasic adults. In R.H. Brookshire (Ed.), *Clinical aphasiology conference proceedings* (pp. 202–209). Minneapolis, MN: BRK.

Brenneise-Sarshad, R., Brookshire, R.H., & Nicholas, L. (1991). Effects of apparent listener knowledge and picture stimuli on aphasic and non-brain-damaged speakers' narrative discourse. *Journal of Speech and Hearing Research, 34*, 168–176.

Cherney, L.R., & Canter, G.J. (1993). Informational content in the discourse of patients with probable Alzheimer's disease and patients with right brain damage. *Clinical Aphasiology, 21*, 123–134.

Correia, L., Brookshire, R.H., & Nicholas, L.E. (1988). The effects of picture content on descriptions by aphasic and non-brain-damaged speakers. *Clinical Aphasiology, 18*, 447–472.

Easterbrook, A., Brown, B.B., & Perera, K. (1982). A comparison of the speech of adult aphasic subjects in spontaneous and structured interactions. *British Journal of Disorders of Communication, 17*, 93–107.

Gerber, S., & Gurland, G.B. (1989). Applied pragmatics in the assessment of aphasia. *Seminars in Speech and Language, 10,* 263–281.

Goodglass, H., & Kaplan, E. (1983). *The Boston Diagnostic Aphasia Examination* (2nd ed.). Boston: Lea & Febiger.

Hedberg, N., & Stoel-Gammon, C. (1985). *Cohesive tie analysis manual.* Unpublished manuscript.

Hedberg, N.L., & Westby, C.E. (1993). *Analyzing storytelling skills: Theory to practice.* Tucson, AZ: Communication Skill Builders.

Hunt, K.W. (1965). *Grammatical structures written at three grade levels.* (Research Rep. No. 3). Champaign, IL: National Council of Teachers of English.

Hunt, K.W. (1970). Syntactic maturity of school children and adults. *Monograph of the Society for Research in Child Development, 35,* 1–78.

Loban, W. (1976). *Language development.* Champaign-Urbana, IL: National Council of Teachers of English.

MacWhinney, B. (1991). *The CHILDES Project: Tools for analyzing talk.* Hillsdale, NJ: Lawrence Erlbaum.

MacWhinney, B. (1996). The CHILDES system. *American Journal of Speech-Language Pathology, 5,* 5–14.

Miller, J.F., & Chapman, R.S. (1992, 1993). *MacSALT: Basic SALT programs.* Madison: University of Wisconsin-Madison, Waisman Center, Language Analysis Laboratory.

Nicholas, L.E., & Brookshire, R.H. (1993). A system for quantifying the informativeness and efficiency of the connected speech of adults with aphasia. *Journal of Speech and Hearing Research, 36,* 338–350.

Potechin, G.C., Nicholas, L.E., & Brookshire, R.H. (1987). Effects of picture stimuli on discourse production in aphasic patients. In R.H. Brookshire (Ed.), *Clinical aphasiology conference proceedings* (pp. 216–220). Minneapolis, MN: BRK.

Ripich, D.N. (1991). Language and communication in dementia. In D.N. Ripich (Ed.), *Handbook of geriatric communication disorders* (pp. 255–291). Austin, TX: Pro-Ed.

Roth, F.P., & Spekman, N.J. (1984a). Assessing the pragmatic abilities of children: Part I. Organizational framework and assessment parameters. *Journal of Speech and Hearing Disorders, 49,* 2–11.

Roth, F.P., & Spekman, N.J. (1984b). Assessing the pragmatic abilities of children: Part II. Guidelines, considerations, and specific evaluation procedures. *Journal of Speech and Hearing Disorders, 49,* 12–17.

Shadden, B.B. (1988). *A comparison of picture description responses to the Cookie Theft picture and an age-relevant alternative picture stimulus.* Unpublished data.

Shadden, B.B., Burnette, R.B., Eikenberry, B.R., & DiBrezzo, R. (1991). All discourse tasks are not created equal. *Clinical Aphasiology, 20,* 327–341.

Strong, C.J., & Shaver, J.P. (1991). Stability of cohesion in the spoken narratives of language-impaired and normally developing school-aged children. *Journal of Speech and Hearing Research, 34,* 95–111.

Terrell, B.Y., & Ripich, D.N. (1989). Discourse competence as a variable in intervention. *Seminars in Speech and Language, 10,* 282–297.

Ulatowska, H.K., & Chapman, S.B. (1989). Discourse considerations for aphasia management. *Seminars in Speech and Language, 10,* 293–314.

Ulatowska, H.K., Doyle, A.W., Freedman-Stern, R., & Macaluso-Haynes, S. (1983). Production of procedural discourse in aphasia. *Brain and Language, 18,* 315–341.

Ulatowska, H.K., Freedman-Stern, R., Doyle, A.W., Macaluso-Haynes, S., & North, A.J. (1983). Production of narrative discourse in aphasia. *Brain and Language, 19,* 306–316.

Ulatowska, H.K., North, A.J., & Macaluso-Haynes, S. (1981). Production of narrative and procedural discourse in aphasia. *Brain and Language, 13,* 345–371.

CHAPTER 3

Sentential/Surface-Level Analyses

Barbara B. Shadden

Once discourse samples have been obtained and transcripts have been prepared, it is possible to begin analyzing the sample data in a highly selective fashion. The first level of analysis is sometimes referred to as the *sentential* or *surface level*. The term *sentential level* is used because many analyses address aspects of language performance that can be considered within the context of the primary segmentation unit (typically, although not always, the T-unit). The term *surface level* implies that we are more interested in basic language units as they evolve across the sample and less interested in the more complex organizational demands of the particular task and/or the manner in which the client links information throughout the discourse sample.

The primary domains of interest at the sentential or surface level are:

1. syntactic length, complexity, diversity, accuracy, and completeness
2. semantic structure, diversity, and accuracy
3. verbal disruptions (regardless of the underlying linguistic and cognitive processes responsible)

Many researchers and clinicians would argue that at least some of these measures are of limited interest in discourse assessment, since the primary purpose of assessment is to examine language in the context of more global indicators of communicative efficiency and effectiveness in connected speech. It is true that syntactic measures, in particular, may have restricted utility or clinical relevance with a number of neurologically impaired populations. However, since the purpose of discourse assessment is to identify and quantify those language and communication domains warranting further intervention, the clinician should be aware of the range of options available for sentential/surface level analysis. A nonfluent aphasic client may require detailed examination of syntactic productions in a range of connected speech tasks in order to target structures and tasks appropriate for expanding the syntactic/morphologic repertoire. Similarly, a traumatically brain-injured client may appear to be evidencing pronounced verbal fragmentation and rather disconnected speech that is primarily cognitive and semantic until syntactic analyses reveal further deficits in organizing language structure and word order for extended communications.

Two caveats are appropriate before presenting specific analysis procedures. First, it is the clinician's responsibility to determine which analyses are relevant to and necessary for the individual client. In this chapter, a variety of sentential/surface-level analysis options will be presented. The vast majority are drawn from research studies, and readers interested in discourse assessment are urged to continue to monitor the professional literature closely for rating scales and analysis procedures that may have particular clinical utility with a given population. Some of the procedures presented here are also drawn from the child language development and disorders literature. Although certain analyses will be highlighted because of their broad clinical applications, the chapter provides a "potpourri" of techniques and relies on clinician judgment for the selection of one or more analyses.

Second, as previously noted, normative data for adult discourse performance remain sparse at present. The data that are available tend to be embedded in descriptions of control group performance in studies of specific neurologically impaired populations. Certainly, more normative data are needed. However, the absence or limited availability of specific, comprehensive norms for adult discourse performance in many of the sentential/surface-level analysis domains should *not* be of significant concern clinically. At all times, the clinician should remember that the primary focus of discourse assessment is to determine discourse performance patterns that provide a baseline for effecting change and that identify behavioral profiles that can be used in developing treatment goals and techniques.

SYNTACTIC LENGTH, COMPLEXITY, DIVERSITY, ACCURACY, AND COMPLETENESS

Hunt's Analysis Procedures

In Hunt's (1965, 1970) early work with T-unit analysis, he developed a series of measures that he felt were most sensitive to the development of syntactic skills in children, beginning with elementary school–aged children and progressing into adulthood. Although most of these measures were applied initially to written discourse samples, the T-unit analysis process has since been used with spoken language samples from normal adults and from a broad range of clinical populations.

Hunt's analyses focused primarily on the length or complexity domains, with complexity limited to examination of subordinate clause embedding and to the type of subordinate clause. Of his various measures, five are reasonable candidates for discourse assessment in adult neurogenic populations, as described in Exhibit 3–1. Most of the basic steps toward developing these measures have been described in Chapter 2 as part of the sample transcription preparation process.

As can be seen in Exhibit 3–1, the analyses that are proposed reflect considerations of length and/or complexity. Words per clause and words per T-unit are length measures; clauses per T-unit as well as proportions of particular types of subordinate clauses are complexity measures. Some clinicians also find it useful to determine percentages of one-, two-, and more-than-two-clause T-units to examine patterns of clause usage. For example, a client may produce predominantly one-clause T-units, but clauses per T-unit may be inflated due to a few overly embedded T-units. Also, other discourse behaviors may covary with syntactic complexity. The clinician may want to compare single-clause and multiclause T-units for accuracy of syntactic or semantic form or for verbal fragmentation and cohesion. Because the T-unit has a standard meaning in all situations, performance of multiple clients or subjects on a given task can be compared. However, given the pronounced degree of task variability described in Chapter 2, more than one discourse sample should be used for an individual client if Hunt's analyses are to be completed.

Examples of three completed transcripts with appropriate calculations are shown in Exhibits 3–2 through 3–4, using the selected transcripts from client L.C. that were provided in Chapter 2. It should be clear that the tasks differ considerably on all measures. The clinician may find it useful to tabulate various computations and measures across tasks to facilitate task comparisons, as shown in Table 3–1. (This table contains additional information from other analyses to be described later.) Cross-task comparisons will be discussed at the end of the chapter as they relate to clinical decision making.

Exhibit 3–1 Hunt's (1965, 1970) T-Unit Analyses of Length and Syntactic Complexity (Items in Brackets Are Optional Steps)

Refer to Chapter 2 for Steps 1 through 3.

1. Divide sample into T-units, and count number of T-units.
2. Count total words.
[3. Count words remaining after the editing described in Chapter 2, called "edited words".]
4. Examine each T-unit for presence and type of subordinate clause(s), and count number of subordinate clauses and number of each type of subordinate clause (noun, adverbial, adjectival—see Chapter 2 for descriptions).
5. Count total number of clauses (independent and subordinate). This is best accomplished by counting the total number of T-units and adding to that the number of subordinate clauses. For example, if there are 20 T-units and 5 additional subordinate clauses, the total number of clauses is 25.
6. Perform the following calculations:
   a. Words per T-unit = total words divided by number of T-units. [Edited words per T-unit = total edited words divided by number of T-units.]
   b. Words per clause = total words divided by total number of clauses. [Edited words per clause = total edited words divided by total number of clauses.]
   c. Clauses per T-unit = total number of clauses (independent and subordinate) divided by total number of T-units.
   d. Percent of one-clause, two-clause, and more-than-two-clause T-units.
   e. Proportion or percentage of each type of subordinate clause in relationship to total number of subordinate clauses: for example, noun clauses/total subordinate clauses, adjectival clauses/total subordinate clauses, and adverbial clauses/total subordinate clauses. So, if there are five subordinate clauses, and three are adjectival, one is noun, and one is adverbial, the percentages would be as follows:
      Adjectival = 60%
      Noun = 20%
      Adverbial = 20%

Although only three of L.C.'s transcripts were analyzed here for demonstration purposes, cross-task differences are highly apparent. Some of these differences are truly task based; others may reflect underlying deficits interfering with language performance. For example, both Living Room picture description tasks (verbal and written) elicited primarily adjectival subordinate clause usage. Given the highly descriptive nature of that task, this pattern of usage appears quite appropriate. However, the two tasks do vary in complexity, as seen by examination of clauses per T-unit. The higher complexity of the written language task may simply suggest that breakdown occurs primarily with verbal formulation. It is interesting to note that L.C. used many more words in the verbal version of this task to communicate essentially the same content as in the written version of the task. However, higher complexity in the written task may also reflect the ability to plan, monitor output, and edit appropriately when given sufficient time. Support for this hypothesis may be found in the fact that it took L.C. 23 minutes to complete this comparatively brief written discourse sample.

Exhibit 3–2 Hunt's (1965, 1970) Analyses Applied to L.C.'s Verbal Living Room Picture Description

1. ~~Hum, ah~~, a woman and ~~ah~~ her husband, ~~looks like, a woman and her ah, husband~~ sitting in a, ~~a room,~~ ~~a~~ living room, ~~um~~ watching TV.

2. Now the woman was watching TV and also doing some needlework.

3. ~~Um~~, and her husband was sitting on the couch,

4. but ~~looks like~~ he was asleep ~~um~~ with a coffee cup ~~in his cup~~, in his hand [which was *Adj.* ~~pouring on the floor~~, dripping on the floor], the coffee. (Note: left "the coffee" at end—appropriate clarification.)

5. And ~~a man and ah~~ the woman was sitting in a chair

6. and she was not sitting with her husband.

7. Her husband was sitting on a couch.

8. In between the two, the chair and the couch, ~~there was ah ah a lamp, a table, ah ah~~ there was a table.

9. On top the table ~~there's a~~, there was a, ~~a~~ lamp.

10. And above the couch there was a painting of ~~um ships, ah~~, a ship, ~~um, shipping~~ on the ocean, ~~I guess, water~~.

11. Um, and above the chair ~~the woman was sitting~~, *Adj.* [which the woman was sitting], ~~um~~, there was a picture behind her, ~~above her chair~~.

12. It's a painting of a flower.

13. On the woman's right hand ~~there was a door which a curtain was drawn, drawing~~, there was a curtain ~~um~~ hanging on the door, ~~yes, looks like it~~.

14. And on the other side of the door there's another painting [which is *Adj.* ~~ah is~~ a flower also].

15. ~~Ah~~, and ~~ah, the, ah~~, facing the woman there was a, ~~there was a~~ TV set

16. and ~~it's on top of~~, the TV's sitting on the table. ~~And on top of the TV, um, no, the TV was sitting on the table~~

continues

Exhibit 3–2 continued

17. and on top of the TV's a vase of flowers.

18. And a cat was, ~~is~~ playing, ~~cat was playing in the middle of the floor, and the cat was playing~~ ~~the, the, um~~ the ball of threads in the middle of the floor.

19. And ~~see, oh, um~~ next to the woman's chair is a sewing, ~~ah,~~ basket. ~~That's all~~.

T-units = 19
Words = 309
Edited words = 208
Total clauses = 22
Words/clause = 14.0
Edited words/clause = 9.5
Clauses/T-unit = 1.16
Subordinate clauses = 3, all adjectival = 100% adjectival

In contrast, in producing the Cat Story narrative discourse, L.C. used predominantly noun and adverbial subordinate clauses, again presumably reflecting the nature of the action-oriented task. However, the story structure of the task, possibly coupled with the available sequenced stimuli, elicited higher syntactic complexity measures. One might conclude that L.C. has the ability to produce more complex syntactic forms when given sufficient structure for the task.

One analysis note is important here. As can be seen in Exhibits 3–2 through 3–4, edited versions of the transcript were used in determining subordinate clause usage. This choice reflects the examiner's decision not to credit L.C. with subordinate clauses that were subsequently reformulated to restate the same point. Use of an edited transcript with the other two samples would have made no difference, However, with the Living Room verbal picture description, at least one additional adjectival subordinate clause would have been identified in T-unit 13. This decision is purely a clinical judgment and

will have no impact on eventual outcomes if the clinician is consistent in applying one criterion to the analysis process.

According to Hunt (1965, 1970), during maturation, single-clause T-units are reduced, and T-units with one or more subordinate clauses are increased. As this reduction occurs, T-unit length increases, virtually doubling from 4th grade to 12th grade (at least in written language). Clause length is the measure most consistently related to chronological and mental age in Hunt's research. There is an increase in noun clauses and adjectival clauses from Grades 4 to 12, with a corresponding decrease in adverbial clause usage. For superior adults in Hunt's (1970) study, 30% of T-units had one clause, 34% had two clauses, and 35.5% had more than two clauses. Average clause length was 11.5 words, and mean number of clauses per T-unit was 1.78. Since these data are based on superior adults and on written samples, alternate samples of normal adults (particularly older adults) can be found in the clinical research literature (Shadden, Burnette, Eikenberry, & DiBrezzo,

Exhibit 3–3 Hunt's (1965, 1970) Analyses Applied to L.C.'s Narrative Cat Story

---

1. O̶K̶, there was a little girl.

2. She was crying to her dad.

                    Noun   **Noun**
3. She said, "[Well, my cat on the tree]ᵃ and [I can't get her off the tree]."ᵃ

4. And so her dad said, "Well."

                              Noun
5. And he decided [he's gonna get that cat for her].

6. So he start climbing the tree

                                        Adj.
7. and a̶h̶, he climbed to the top on the branch [where the cat was]

8. and so he swing h̶i̶s̶, his arms and try to catch the cat.

9. And t̶h̶e̶ ̶c̶a̶t̶ ̶j̶u̶m̶p̶, the cat j̶u̶m̶p̶ ̶o̶f̶f̶, jumped off the, um, tree on . . .

                                            Adv.
10. and, a̶h̶, the dad end up hanging on the branch [while he was trying to catch the cat].

                                        Adv.
11. And the girl start crying again a̶n̶d̶ ̶t̶h̶e̶ ̶p̶o̶l̶i̶c̶e̶, [because her dad was hanging on a tree branch with

                            Adv.
a cloth]ᵇ and [the branch caught h̶i̶s̶,̶ ̶a̶h̶,̶ ̶a̶h̶, the back of his collar].ᵇ

12. And t̶h̶e̶,̶ ̶a̶h̶,̶ ̶t̶h̶e̶ ̶f̶i̶r̶e̶, the fireman, I̶ ̶g̶u̶e̶s̶s̶ ̶t̶h̶a̶t̶'̶s̶ ̶a̶ ̶f̶i̶r̶e̶m̶a̶n̶, a̶n̶d̶ ̶h̶e̶ was trying to rescue him.

T-units = 12
Words = 155
Edited words = 134
Total clauses = 19
Words/clause = 8.1
Edited words/clause = 7
Clauses/T-unit = 1.58
Subordinate clauses = 7   Adjectival = 1 = 14.3%
                                   Noun = 3 = 42.9%
                             Adverbial = 3 = 42.9%

ᵃ Both are object of verb *said*.

ᵇ Separate subordinate clauses explaining *because* in both instances.

1991; Ulatowska, Doyle, Freedman-Stern, & Macaluso-Haynes, 1983; Ulatowska, Freedman-Stern, Doyle, Macaluso-Haynes, & North, 1983; Ulatowska, North, & Macaluso-Haynes, 1981). It is interesting to note that in comparing the "normal" subjects in these two studies across either different or identical discourse tasks, mean performances on such measures as number of clauses, number of T-units, words per T-unit, and clauses per T-unit vary considerably. Clinical judgment, rather than reference to any single normative source, should provide the basis for determining whether performance warrants further treatment.

Exhibit 3–4 Hunt's (1965, 1970) Analyses Applied to L.C.'s Written Living Room Picture Description

---

1. In a living room, there's a man, a woman, and a cat.

2. The man is sitting in the couch asleep with his empty coffee cup in his hand.

3. Above the couch is a painting of a ship sailing in the ocean.

4. Next to ~~to~~ the couch is a small end table with a lamp on top of it.

5. On the other side of the is a chair.

6. The man's wife is sitting in the chair doing needlework and watch TV at the same time.
   Adj.
7. Above the chair [that she is sitting in] is a picture of a flower.
   Adj.
8. On the other side of the chair is a door [which has a curtain hanging across it].
   Adj.
9. There is another flower picture on another wall [which is matching the first flower painting]
   Adj.
   [that is hanging on the other side of the door].

10. A TV is standing across from the woman.

11. On top of the TV has a vase full of flowers.

12. The cat is play the thread ball in the middle of the floor.

T-units = 12
Words = 171
Edited words = 170
Total clauses = 16
Words/clause = 10.7
Edited words/clause = 10.6
Clauses/T-unit = 1.33
Subordinate clauses = 4, all adjectival

Computerized Analyses of Syntactic Length, Form, and Complexity

For those with access to computerized language analysis systems, many length and syntactic structure and complexity measures can be computed by program software once discourse transcripts are entered into the computer in the required fashion. Although virtually all of these programs were designed for analysis of child language samples, they can be adapted for use with adults. For example, the SALT programs (Miller & Chapman, 1992, 1993) provide extensive analyses of many syntactic and morphologic forms, plus considerations of completeness and accuracy, mazes, conversational patterns, length of utterance and turn, type-token ratios, and other user-programmable features. The CLAN (computerized language analysis) program that is part of the CHILDES project (Child Language Data Exchange System, MacWhinney, 1991, 1996) has also been used

Table 3–1 Additional Cross-Task Data Comparisons for Client L.C. at the Sentential/Surface Level

Measure	LR-Vrb	LR-Wrt	Store	Egg	Cat	Conv
Length/Complexity						
Total words	309	171	179	134	155	191
Edited words	208	170	164	109	134	149
T-units	19	12	18	17	12	19
Sub. clause/type	3	4	6	3	7	2
	3 adj	4 adj	3 adv	2 adv	3 noun	1 noun
			1 adj	1 noun	3 adv	1 adv
			2 noun		1 adj	
Words/T-unit	16.3	14.3	9.9	7.9	11.9	10.1
Edited words/T-unit	10.9	14.2	9.1	6.4	11.2	7.8
Words/clause	14	10.7	7.5	6.7	8.1	9.1
Edited words/clause	9.5	10.6	6.8	5.5	7	7.1
Clause/T-unit	1.16	1.33	1.33	1.18	1.58	1.11
Syntactic accuracy and completeness (Shadden)	78.9%	66.7%	55.6%	82.4%	50%	68.4%
Word Retrieval (WR)						
Global (% T-units with problems)	13/19	1/12	6/18	8/17	4/12	7/19
	68.4%	8.3%	33.3%	47.1%	33.3%	36.8%
Total WR instances	35	1	7	10	9	14
Total WR/T-unit	1.84	.08	.39	.58	.75	.74
% Reformulations	16		4	5	5	4
	45.7%		57.1%	50%	55.6%	28.6%
% Repetitions	8	1	3	4	3	5
	22.9%		42.9%	40%	33.3%	35.7%
% Time fillers	5			1		
	14.3%			10%		
% Insertions	5				1	3
	14.3%				11.1%	21.4%
% Empty speech						2
						14.3%
% Substitutions	1					
	2.9%					

Note: LR-Vrb, Living Room picture verbal description task; LR-Wrt, Living Room picture written description task; Store, Going to Store procedural description task; Egg, Making Scrambled Eggs procedural description task; Cat, Cat Story narrative task; Conv, conversational task.

effectively with adult neurogenic populations (Boles, Holland, & Beeson, 1993).

Other Measures of Syntactic Complexity

Shewan and Henderson (1988) have developed their own sentential-level analysis ap-
proach, termed the Shewan Spontaneous Language Analysis (SSLA) system. Language samples based on picture description were used to generate data subsequently analyzed for (a) number of utterances, (b) speaking time, (c) rate, (d) length, (e) melody, (f) articulation, (g) complex sentences, (h) grammatical errors, (i) con-

tent units, (j) paraphasia, (k) repetitions, and (l) communication efficiency. Many of the measures used in this approach parallel the syntactic length and complexity analyses discussed in this chapter.

Child language sample analysis literature also provides clinicians with ideas for other measures that may be of interest. For example, Stickler (1987) suggested consideration of such indices of syntactic complexity as prepositional phrases, infinitive elements, and gerund usage. These are measures that are often considered in some of the computerized language analysis programs. The work of Kemper and colleagues (e.g., Kemper, 1987; Kemper, Kynette, & Norman, 1991; Kynette & Kemper, 1986), among others, also suggests some interest in or value to considering the placement of the dependent or subordinate clauses—specifically whether it is right branching, left branching, or center embedded. Although this type of psycholinguistic analysis may seem overly sophisticated for clinical use, specific clients who will undergo a systematic treatment process of increasing syntactic complexity may benefit from consideration of their current pattern of clause embedding.

Clinicians may find other analyses of interest in specific research articles. For example, Gleason et al. (1980) examined the narrative strategies of normal-speaking and aphasic (Wernicke's and Broca's) subjects. For those who wish to avoid the T-unit analyses discussed here and in Chapter 2 and simply would prefer to examine sentence structure at a less formal level, the measures used by Gleason et al. (1980) may be helpful. Essentially, these researchers examined narrative discourse samples for the presence of

- simple concatenation (use of *and*)
- more complex syntactic relationships
  1. embedding (subordination): (a) temporal conjunction, (b) participle, and (c) relative marker
  2. disjunction (*but, or*)
  3. causal conjunctions (*so, because*)
  4. infinitive verb complements

Measures of syntactic complexity for normal speakers exceeded those of Wernicke's aphasic speakers in all categories, with the aphasic speakers relying excessively on simple concatenation, as compared to the normal speakers, who used fairly high levels of embedding and relativization.

Syntactic Analysis Shortcuts

For the clinician interested in a cursory measure of syntactic accuracy and/or completeness without any further considerations of the nature and degree of complexity, several shortcuts can be suggested. In a 1989 study, Roberts and Wertz developed a T-unit scoring system that was designed to address the issue of *syntactic well-formedness*. Procedures and criteria for this analysis are shown in Exhibit 3–5. The analysis depends on breaking the sample into T-units and then assigning a "+" or a "–" to each T-unit depending on whether it meets the criteria for syntactic well-formedness. An example of one of L.C.'s samples coded in this fashion is shown in Exhibit 3–6. For client L.C., syntactic well-formedness measures hover around the 50-percent level, with the written sample that allows monitoring and editing showing better performance than the other two verbal samples.

Although the syntactic well-formedness measure is not difficult to apply, many of the criteria appear to address issues that overlap with the semantic, informational, and cohesion domains. For example, additions of extralexical elements or awkward topicalization may reflect underlying semantic deficits or perhaps problems in the cognitive organization of the task rather than outright syntactic and morphological difficulties.

As one alternative to this procedure, Shadden (1994) has proposed an analysis that attempts to look at underlying syntactic form, which presumably reflects some degree of basic linguistic competence in this domain. In Shadden's approach, the discourse sample is broken down into T-units, then edited to remove redundancies, revisions, false starts, and so forth (see Ex-

Exhibit 3–5 Syntactic Well-Formedness and Semantic Accuracy

1. Divide discourse sample into T-units.
2. For *syntactic well-formedness*, score each T-unit as a "+" or a "–" on the basis of the following criteria, which define a failure to meet the test of syntactic well-formedness. Assign a minus if there are any of the following:
   a. verb errors
   b. obligatory word omissions
   c. additions of extralexical elements
   d. incompleteness
   e. plural errors
   f. pronoun errors
   g. word order errors
   h. awkward topicalization
3. For *semantic accuracy*, score each T-unit as a "+" or "–" on the basis of the following criteria, which define a failure to meet the test of semantic accuracy. Assign a minus if there are any of the following:
   a. empty or vague vocabulary
   b. given/new information errors
   c. semantic or neologistic paraphasias
   d. inaccurate information
   e. ambiguous or contentless information
   f. inappropriate lexical items
   g. incompleteness
4. Calculate the percentage of T-units with plus scores in either the *syntactic well-formedness* or the *semantic accuracy* domain. For example, if there are 20 T-units and 10 receive a "+" score in syntactic well-formedness, the result would be expressed by saying, "Fifty percent of the T-units evidenced syntactic well-formedness."

Source: Reprinted with permission from J.A. Roberts and R.T. Wertz, Comparison of Spontaneous and Elicited Oral–Expressive Language in Aphasia, *Clinical Aphasiology*, Vol. 18, p. 481, © 1989.

hibit 3–7 for description). The editing process is described in Chapter 2, following guidelines by Strong and Shaver (1991). Each T-unit in the remaining sample is then examined to determine whether it meets basic rules for morphological and syntactic *accuracy* and *completeness*. Examples of this analysis are shown in Exhibits 3–8 through 3–10 for the three samples analyzed according to Hunt's measures. The percentage of T-units receiving a "+" for syntactic accuracy and completeness can be calculated.

The editing process eliminates many of the language units that would have resulted in "–" scores in the Roberts and Wertz (1989) approach. In fact, as a rule of thumb, the more verbally fragmented the sample, the greater the discrepancy between these two measures. However, in Shadden's (1994) approach, the clinician is provided with an index of basic, underlying syntactic forms produced by the client, and the procedure takes little time once preliminary transcript editing has been completed. In effect, an indirect estimate of syntactic/morphologic

competence can be developed. One additional advantage to the Shadden approach is that, with little effort, an additional analysis step can be performed to identify the extent to which the observed syntactic problems are the result of outright word omissions (incompleteness) and/or inaccuracies in syntactic/morphological form (typically the result of noun-verb mismatch, although other such errors are possible). For example, in the Cat Story sample, T-unit 3 shows an omission error, whereas T-units 6 and 8 show inaccuracies because of noun-verb disagreement and tense problems, resulting in inappropriate morphological marking of the verb. For certain clients, this additional step in analyzing omissions versus outright inaccuracies may provide important intervention clues.

In both of these shortcuts, the clinician must be cautious about using overly rigid standards of syntactic accuracy or completeness. For example, in the verbal Living Room picture description task, a "+" was given to edited T-Unit 4, even though it ended with a dangling phrase

Exhibit 3–6 Scoring of Syntactic Well-Formedness and Semantic Accuracy

Syntax	*Semantics*	
+	+	1. OK, there was a little girl.
+	+	2. She was crying to her dad.
−	+	3. She said, "Well, my cat on the tree and I can't get her off the tree."
+	+	4. And so her dad said, "Well."
+	+	5. And he decided he's gonna get that cat for her.
−	+	6. So he start climbing the tree
+	+	7. and ah, he climbed to the top on the branch where the cat was
−	+	8. and so he swing his, his arms and try to catch the cat.
−	−	9. And the cat jump, the cat jump off, jumped off the, um, tree on . . .
−	+	10. and, ah, the dad end up hanging on the branch while he was trying to catch the cat.
−	−	11. And the girl start crying again and the police, because her dad was hanging on a tree branch with a cloth and the branch caught his, ah, ah, the back of his collar.
−	−	12. And the, ah, the fire, the fireman, I guess that's a fireman, and he was trying to rescue him.

Syntactic Well-Formedness = 5/12 T-units = 41.7%
Semantic Accuracy = 9/12 T-units = 75%

Source: Reprinted with permission from J.A. Roberts and R.T. Wertz, Comparison of Spontaneous and Elicited Oral–Expressive Language in Aphasia, *Clinical Aphasiology*, Vol. 18, p. 479–488, © 1989.

Exhibit 3–7 Method for Evaluating Syntactic Accuracy and Completeness (Shadden, 1984)

1. Break sample into T-units.
2. Perform preliminary editing of transcript, using Strong and Shaver (1991) or similar approach described in Chapter 2.
3. Examine the language remaining in each T-unit, and assign a "+" if it meets basic rules of syntactic accuracy and completeness.
4. Calculate percentage of syntactically accurate and complete T-units, and compare across discourse tasks if desired.

Exhibit 3–8 Shadden's Syntactic Analyses Applied to L.C.'s Verbal Living Room Picture Description

- 1. ~~Hum, ah~~, a woman and ~~ah~~ her husband, ~~looks like, a woman and her ah, husband~~ sitting in a, ~~a room, a~~ living room, ~~um~~ watching TV.

+ 2. Now the woman was watching TV and also doing some needlework.

+ 3. ~~Um~~, and her husband was sitting on the couch,

+ 4. but ~~looks like~~ he was asleep ~~um~~ with a coffee cup ~~in his cup~~, in his hand which was ~~pouring on the floor~~, dripping on the floor, the coffee. (Note: left "the coffee" at end—appropriate clarification)

+ 5. And ~~a man and ah~~ the woman was sitting in a chair

+ 6. and she was not sitting with her husband.

+ 7. Her husband was sitting on a couch.

+ 8. In between the two, the chair and the couch, ~~there was ah ah a lamp, a table, ah ah~~ there was a table.

- 9. On top the table ~~there's a~~, there was a, a lamp.

+ 10. And above the couch there was a painting of ~~um ships, ah~~, a ship, ~~um, shipping~~ on the ocean, ~~I guess, water~~.

- 11. Um, and above the chair ~~the woman was sitting~~, which the woman was sitting, ~~um~~, there was a picture behind her, ~~above her chair~~.

+ 12. It's a painting of a flower.

+ 13. On the woman's right hand ~~there was a door which a curtain was drawn, drawing~~, there was a curtain ~~um~~ hanging on the door, ~~yes, looks like it~~.

+ 14. And on the other side of the door there's another painting which is ~~ah is~~ a flower also.

+ 15. ~~Ah~~, and ~~ah, the, ah~~, facing the woman there was a, ~~there was a~~ TV set

+ 16. and ~~it's on top of~~, the TV's sitting on the table. ~~And on top of the TV, um, no, the TV was sitting on the table~~

+ 17. and on top of the TV's a vase of flowers.

- 18. And a cat was, is playing, ~~cat was playing in the middle of the floor, and the cat was playing the, the, um~~ the ball of threads in the middle of the floor.

+ 19. And ~~see, oh, um~~ next to the woman's chair is a sewing, ~~ah~~, basket. ~~That's all~~.

78.9% syntactically accurate and complete T-units
Majority of errors are omissions of obligatory words.

Exhibit 3–9 Shadden's Syntactic Analyses Applied to L.C.'s Narrative Cat Story

+ 1. ~~OK~~, there was a little girl.

+ 2. She was crying to her dad.

− 3. She said, "Well, my cat⌃on the tree and I can't get her off the tree."

+ 4. And so her dad said, "Well."

+ 5. And he decided he's gonna get that cat for her.

− 6. So he start⌃climbing the tree

+ 7. and ~~ah~~, he climbed to the top on the branch where the cat was

− 8. and so he swing ~~his~~, his arms and try to catch the cat.

− 9. And ~~the cat jump~~, the cat ~~jump off~~, jumped off the, um, tree on . .

− 10. and, ~~ah~~, the dad end⌃up hanging on the branch while he was trying to catch the cat.

− 11. And the girl start⌃crying again ~~and the police~~, because her dad was hanging on a tree branch with a cloth and the branch caught ~~his, ah, ah~~, the back of his collar.

+ 12. And ~~the, ah, the fire~~, the fireman, ~~I guess that's a fireman, and he~~ was trying to rescue him.

50% syntactically accurate and complete T-units
2 missing words or phrases
5 examples of morphological errors (verb tense)

("the coffee"). The rationale was that this type of clarification is frequently provided by speakers in connected discourse and does not necessarily reflect an underlying deficit in syntactic form. Similarly, in T-unit 17, the phrasing "on top of the TV's a vase" is technically incorrect, since the form of the copula verb *be* should not be contracted. However, once again, this type of behavior is common in normal connected discourse and was not viewed as a true syntactic problem.

SEMANTIC STRUCTURE, DIVERSITY, AND ACCURACY

Despite the importance of the semantic domain in the discourse performance of many adult neurologically impaired clients, the strong linkage of semantic behaviors to other areas of discourse analysis makes it particularly difficult to tease out purely semantic attributes at the sentential or surface structure level. Semantic structure, diversity, and accuracy are all potentially related to the discourse behaviors that are considered in analyses of information content and efficiency, cohesion, and verbal fragmentation, as well as to other macrostructural and superstructural elements. In essence, what the clinician should be looking for at this level are ways to quantify and analyze semantic properties of connected discourse apart from performance on more formal and standardized tests of word-finding difficulty or general vocabulary limitations (such as the Boston Naming Test;

Exhibit 3–10 Shadden's Syntactic Analyses Applied to L.C.'s Written Living Room Picture Description.

+ 1. In a living room, there's a man, a woman, and a cat.
        ?

+ 2. The man is sitting <u>in</u> the couch asleep with his empty coffee cup in his hand.

+ 3. Above the couch is a painting of a ship sailing in the ocean.

+ 4. Next to ~~to~~ the couch is a small end table with a lamp on top of it.

− 5. On the other side of the is a chair.

− 6. The man's wife is sitting in the chair doing needlework and wa<u>tch</u> TV at the same time.

+ 7. Above the chair that she is sitting in is a picture of a flower.

+ 8. On the other side of the chair is a door which has a curtain hanging across it.

+ 9. There is another flower picture on another wall which is matching the first flower painting
       that is hanging on the other side of the door.

+ 10. A TV is standing across from the woman.

− 11. On top of the TV (has) a vase full of flowers.

− 12. The cat is <u>play</u> the thread ball in the middle of the floor.

66.67% syntactically accurate and complete T-units
2 missing words
3 examples of morphological errors

Kaplan, Goodglass, & Weintraub, 1983). Some possible semantic analysis techniques are described briefly here.

Type-Token Ratio and Related Measures

Templin (1957) has described a procedure—the type-token ratio (TTR)—designed to examine the proportion of different words used to total words used in a language sample. In this context, a *type* is a unique word form, and a *token* is one of potentially many instances of usage of that word form. In essence, the TTR is intended to provide an index of vocabulary diversity. Although developed for children from age 3 to age 8, the procedure has been applied to connected discourse in adults as well (Critchley, 1984; Walker, Roberts, & Hedrick, 1988). Pri-

mary norms remain those provided by Templin (1957). Approximate TTRs of 1:2 (actually between .43 and .47) were obtained for children in the normative sample.

Procedures for completing a TTR analysis for adult discourse samples are provided in Exhibit 3–11. Because the TTR might be presumed to be highly sensitive to specific task differences, it is recommended that the TTR be computed across several discourse tasks to reduce this sensitivity. An example of a completed TTR for client L.C. on the Cat Story is shown in Exhibit 3–12. For this single task, the TTR was .40, slightly below the child norms and below levels reported from studies of control adult samples. The majority of types were verbs (35.5%), followed by nouns (19.4%) and pronouns (14.5%). Across all tokens, the majority of word forms were verbs

Exhibit 3–11 Type-Token Ratio

1. Prepare an analysis sheet as shown in Exhibit 3–12.
2. Go through transcript word by word and assign each word to a part of speech. When a word occurs more than once, an extra tally mark should be placed next to the word on the analysis sheet. Rules for counting words are as follows:
   a. Count subject/predicate contractions as two words (e.g., *we're, that's*).
   b. Count verb/negative contractions as one word (e.g., *don't*).
   c. Each part of a complex verb form with auxiliary elements counts as a separate word (e.g., *has been jumping*).
   d. Count hyphenated and compound nouns as one word.
   e. Count common verbal expressions such as *all right* or *oh gosh* as one word if they are used repeatedly as a unit.
   f. Count articles (*a, an, the*) as single words.
   g. Do not count bound morphemes and noun or verb inflections separately.
3. Tally the separate words in each column. This gives you the number of different *types* of each part of speech. Adding all of these tallies gives the total number of word *types* in the sample.
4. Tally the total number of words in each column. This gives you the number of different *tokens* of each part of speech. Adding all of these tallies gives the total number of *tokens* in the sample (which should equal any other count of total words, with the exception of rules used to address contractions).
5. Divide total number of different words (types) by total number of words (tokens), yielding the type-token ratio (TTR).

Note: This same analysis sheet can also be used for computing other ratios, such as noun/verb or noun/adjective ratios.

(23.2%), followed by nouns (18.1%), pronouns (16.1%), and articles (14.2%).

While the calculation of the TTR may seem excessively cumbersome in most instances, completion of this analysis can yield other measures of interest. For example, Gleason et al. (1980) computed a noun/verb ratio for normal-speaking and aphasic subjects in six different narrative tasks. All tokens in each category were used, with the exception of indefinite noun terms (e.g., *thing*) and copula, modal, and auxiliary verb forms. They found that their normal speaking subjects produced ratios close to 1.0 across all tasks, although there were clearly task differences. In contrast, subjects with Broca's aphasia consistently produced more nouns than verbs, and subjects with Wernicke's aphasia produced more verbs than nouns. In the sample analysis for one task shown in Exhibit 3–12, the ratio of noun/verb tokens was exactly 1.0 (omitting auxiliary, copula, and modal forms as recommended). Thus, this information would not be considered helpful for this particular client. However, for an aphasic client whose treatment was going to target certain word types, the ratio might prove more useful as a baseline measure. Similarly, ratios such as noun/adjective calculations might provide indices of the degree to which a given client was able to use descriptive terms. In other words, discourse analysis at the sentential/surface level continues to focus on providing useful measures for identifying client behavioral patterns that will direct subsequent treatment.

Retherford, Schwartz, and Chapman's Codes for Semantic Roles, Grammatical Categories, and Conversational Devices

To return briefly to the child language sample analysis literature, it is worth noting that, for clients with extremely limited verbal output, it is critical to find some way of characterizing the semantic functions of the limited language that

Exhibit 3–12 Type-Token Ratio for L.C.'s Cat Story

Nouns	Verbs	Adjectives	Adverbs	Prepositions	Pronouns	Conjunction	Neg./Affirm.	Articles	"Wh" Words	Misc.
girl—2	was—6	little	off—3	to—5	there	and—13		a—3		Ok
dad—4	crying—2		up	on—5	she—2	so—3		the—19		well—2
cat—7	said—2		again	off—3	her—5	where				
tree—4	can't			for	my—1	while				
top	get—2			of	I—2	because				
branch—3	decided			with	he—7					
arms	gonna				that—2					
police	start—2				his—4					
cloth	climbing				him					
collar	climbed									
fire	swing									
fireman—2	try									
	catch—2									
	jump—2									
	jumped									
	end									
	hanging—2									
	trying—2									
	caught									
	guess									
	rescue									
	is—2									
12	22	1	3	6	9	5	0	2	0	2
28	36	1	5	16	25	19	0	22	0	3

Type-Token Ratio = 62/155 = .40

Most frequent word type = verbs (35.5% of types), followed by nouns (19.4% of types), and pronouns (14.5% of types).

Most frequent word tokens = verbs (23.2%), followed by nouns (18.1%), pronouns (16.1%), and articles (14.2%).

is being produced. The clinician may want to turn to the types of codes for analyzing mother-child semantic content developed by Retherford, Schwartz, and Chapman (1981; see also Stickler, 1987). In this analysis system, 15 semantic categories are provided, along with five additional grammatical categories, seven conversational devices, and seven communicative routines. The routines are of limited value in adult discourse analysis, since they reflect pragmatic conventions and activities appropriate to young children.

Because of the extensive nature of this system and its limited utility to all but perhaps the nonfluent aphasic population, the 35 codable categories are not provided here. The interested reader is referred to one of the references noted above. Use of this coding system, however, could provide an excellent base for determining pragmatically and semantically oriented treatment goals intended to increase communicative range despite limited language form. In fact, this form of coding can be useful in conducting treatment approaches such as Promoting Aphasic Communicative Effectiveness (PACE) therapy (Davis & Wilcox, 1985), since an idea of the types of semantic functions most and least readily communicated by the client can be determined.

Semantic Accuracy: A Shortcut

Earlier in this chapter, Roberts and Wertz's (1989) plus-minus rating scale for syntactic well-formedness was described. A similar scale was also developed by these authors for coding *semantic accuracy*. Procedures and criteria for this analysis are shown in Exhibit 3–5. As with the syntactic well-formedness scoring, the discourse sample is first segmented into T-units; then each T-unit is assigned a "+" or a "–" depending on whether it meets the stated criteria for semantic accuracy. One of L.C.'s samples coded in this fashion is shown in Exhibit 3–6. Although there appears to be some overlap in criteria between semantic accuracy and syntactic well-formedness, the semantic criteria appear more consistent in reflecting lexical and broader

semantic concerns. The analysis process is relatively simple to complete once the transcript has been prepared appropriately.

Word Choice

Analysis of patterns of word choice is another measurement approach related to vocabulary content and distribution that may be useful with some clients. In many neurological populations, particularly those with aphasia, it has been established that available vocabulary is almost always restricted (e.g., Fillenbaum, Jones, & Wepman, 1961; Howes, 1964; Wachal & Spreen, 1973). Recent investigations have attempted to determine whether common discourse elicitation tasks and stimuli reflect appropriately the everyday language required of adults in real-life conversations (e.g., Doyle, Goda, & Spencer, 1995; Doyle, Thompson, Oleyar, Wambaugh, & Jackson, 1994) and whether different elicitation conditions elicit different patterns of word choice (Brookshire & Nicholas, 1993). Yorkston, Zeches, Farrier, and Uomoto (1993) have also examined "lexical pitch" in traumatically brain-injured patients, a pattern of word retrieval related to word choice.

The concepts of word choice and of lexical pitch and procedures of analysis are borrowed from Hayes (1988, 1989). Patterns of word choice represent graphically the cumulative proportion of word types lying at or below word ranks, from "1," which is most frequent (*the*), to the 10,000th most frequent type. According to Hayes's (1988) research, adult-to-adult conversations are skewed slightly from frequency norms in the *American Heritage* corpus (Carroll, Davies, & Richman, 1971) and from analyses of newspaper texts, suggesting use of more common words and fewer rare words. In normal adult-to-adult conversations, the 75 most commonly used words account for approximately 50% of all words used, with the majority being function words (88%). *Lexical pitch* refers to the level at which discourse is "pitched" to the real or hypothetical audience. Hayes (1988) stated that lexical pitch reflects variations in lexical choice that are dependent on both lexical access and audience effects. The concept is similar to that of a lexical register and to questions about the ability pragmatically to shift lexical register (Yorkston et al., 1993).

In the Brookshire and Nicholas (1993) study, non–brain-damaged adults performed much in accordance with Hayes's adult-to-adult conversation data across all except the procedural discourse tasks (which led to slightly higher proportions of the most frequent words). Somewhat more surprising was the finding that aphasia did not markedly influence word choice patterns, with the exception of overuse of *and* and nonfluent subjects' underuse of other function words.

The analyses in the Brookshire and Nicholas (1993) study were performed using Hayes' (1989) computerized lexical text analysis program, called QLEX, available through the author and described in a technical report from Cornell University. Clinicians who feel that this particular type of analysis might suit their needs can contact the author. Alternatively, discourse samples may be analyzed using a database created by Yorkston et al. (1993), in which all transcript vocabulary was entered into one word-processing file and lists of all the different words produced were generated. (Computerized language sample analysis programs typically yield similar lexical analyses.) Each word was then evaluated by a group of judges as evidencing low lexical pitch, neutral lexical pitch, or high lexical pitch. Word tallies for low-pitched and high-pitched items could be conducted for each sample, and a composite lexical pitch score could be generated.

For the most part, word choice and lexical pitch reflect analyses of real interest in the clinical setting; however, computing these measures may be comparatively impractical (at present) for most clinicians. Semantic measures described earlier in this chapter may suffice. In addition, many other discourse measures tap into semantic issues and, along with standardized tests, may provide a sufficient database and baseline to initiate appropriate treatment.

VERBAL FRAGMENTATION OR DISRUPTION

Verbal fragmentation is one of the most intriguing features of the language output of neurologically impaired clients and thus is also one of the most valuable sentential/surface-level analysis domains. The terms *verbal fragmentation* and *verbal disruption* are used very loosely here to refer to disturbances in the flow of information that result from any one of a number of language and nonlanguage behaviors that impair continuity of language sequencing and information content. In many instances, these fragmentations are related directly to word retrieval deficits, but they may also reflect underlying difficulties with cognitive organization or structuring of task performance, or even with syntactic form. Certainly, verbal fragmentation draws considerable attention to the speaker's language output and, regardless of the cause, is often a behavior that clinicians wish to see modified during the course of treatment.

Verbal fragmentation is present in the discourse of all speakers. The nature and degree of disruption often serve to distinguish normal speakers from those with specific deficits. Indeed, disruption can be discussed in terms of fluency or disfluency; we are all familiar with the literature on normal and stuttering disfluencies and on methods of evaluating disfluent behaviors. Some researchers have actually applied stuttering-related categories of disfluent behavior to the speech of nonstuttering adults. Pindzola, McCloskey, and Moran (1989), for example, used Yairi's (1981) categories of disfluency to examine speech breakdown in normal older adults. Categories used for the study included (a) part-word repetitions, (b) single-syllable–word repetitions, (c) polysyllabic-word repetitions, (d) phrase repetitions, (e) interjections, (f) revisions or incomplete phrases, (g) tense pauses, and (h) dysrhythmic phonation. Others have suggested using pause duration as a major indicator of speech disruption in discourse (Cooper, 1990).

Exhibit 3–13 Verbal Fragmentation Analyses

Glosser et al. (1988)—Verbal Disruptions
1. Mazes—false starts of words or phrases that are subsequently self-corrected and all other verbalizations that are prosodically or syntactically incomplete
   Example: He went to the grocery . . . candy store.
2. Repetitions of one or more contiguous words or parts of words
   Example: She bought a new a new dress.
3. Paraphasias
   Examples:
   The little boy is falling off a *stool.*
   I like your new *earlobe* [for earring].
4. Omission of part of a word, a complete word, or an unspecified group of words required by an existing syntactic frame
   Example: After we go to _____, we can watch the movie.
5. Filler (*well, oh boy, anyway*)
6. Other

Nicholas et al. (1985)—Empty Speech Categories
(Words or phrases that detract from or do not contribute to coherent picture description)
1. Empty phrases—words or phrases used as continuation devices (*and so on, like that*)
2. Indefinite terms—nonspecific nouns such as *thing, junk, stuff*
3. Deictic terms—*here, there, this, that*
4. Pronouns without antecedents
5. Comments on task (*It's hard for me to say that; that's a weird one*)
6. Neologisms—without discernible targets
7. Literal paraphasias—phonologically related to target
8. Unrelated verbal paraphasias (*dog* for *chair*)
9. Semantic paraphasias

10. Verbal/phonological paraphasias—real words related phonologically to target word
11. Repeated words or phrases
12. Personal value judgments about stimulus (*what a dumb move she made*)
13. The word *and* in place of other conjunctions
14. Absence of logical conjunctions—*but, so, or, because*

Brookshire and Nicholas (1995)—Speech Deviations Not Scored as Correct Information Units (CIUs)
• Nonword
  1. Part-word or unintelligible production
  2. Nonword filler such as *um*
• Non-CIU
  1. Inaccurate
  2. False start
  3. Unnecessary exact repetition
  4. Nonspecific or vague language
  5. Filler
  6. *and*
  7. Off task or irrelevant
  8. Uncategorizable productions

Walker et al. (1988)—Interruptive Behavior
1. Interjections—empty word or words, or filled pause, when used as filler or starter
   Examples:
   I want one of those *you know* those chairs.
   Well, see, she didn't mean it.
2. Revisions—any deliberate change in utterance wording
   *Example: Robert went *hopping . . . dancing* with Susan.*
3. Repetitions—exact repetitions of syllables, words, or phrases

Source: Verbal Disruptions and Empty Speech Categories, © American Speech-Language-Hearing Association. Reprinted by permission.

Fragmentation Measures of Interest with Adult Populations

However, since our interest in discourse analysis is primarily related to nonstuttering disfluencies, it is probably more appropriate to turn to the literature on neurogenic and other communicatively disordered populations to identify potential tools for the analysis of verbal fragmentation. Exhibit 3–13 contains four research-derived classifications of behaviors that may be useful in the analysis of verbal disruptions. All of the analysis tools to be discussed in this section presume that the clinician is working with an unedited transcript, in the sense that words and phrases have not been eliminated to provide accurate word counts of productive language (see Chapter 2).

The Glosser, Wiener, and Kaplan (1988) six-part classification is intended to reflect what the authors have termed *verbal fragmentations* in the language of aphasic adults. The orientation toward aphasia can be seen in the inclusion of paraphasias as one category of fragmentation, as well as the inclusion of an omission category. The limited number of categories makes this system easy to apply to a discourse sample, although the maze category is very broad and inclusive. The Nicholas, Obler, Albert, and Helm-Estabrooks (1985) 14-component classification of *empty speech* was also developed for neurologically impaired populations—specifically, individuals with Alzheimer's disease and fluent aphasic adults. In this system, five rating categories reflect some paraphasic breakdown, and a number of other categories tap into the expected empty speech and poor cohesion that might be found in these populations. Both systems appear comprehensive, yet somewhat biased toward particular populations. The Nicholas et al. (1985) classification would be particularly cumbersome in clinical applications unless used in a highly specific manner with individual clients.

Brookshire and Nicholas (1995) developed a classification system for words and nonwords not scored as correct information units (CIUs; see Chapter 5) in a range of discourse samples. The classification was intended to capture *connected speech deviations* in both normal and aphasic (fluent and nonfluent) subjects, and groups were differentiated on the basis of particular performance deviations. This classification may be useful with a broad range of populations. Similarly, in a study of normal elderly people, Walker et al. (1988) examined disruptions in discourse through only three categories of what they termed *interruptive behavior*. The three categories of interjections, revisions, and repetitions are also described in Exhibit 3–13. Unlike the other classification systems consid-

ered so far, this approach focuses almost exclusively on behaviors that disturb the ongoing continuity and flow of the language output of the individual. There is no attempt to quantify other language behaviors that interfere with informativeness or disrupt cohesive linkages. For the clinician looking for a quick analysis tool for identifying levels of disruption in the flow of language, the Walker et al. (1988) approach may be appealing.

If the clinician uses any of these four approaches, there are several data summary options. First, if the pattern of verbal disruptions is the only behavior of clinical interest, the total number of instances of verbally disruptive behavior can be counted, and the proportion or percentage of each type of fragmented behavior can be calculated. Second, the number of words involved in verbal fragmentations can be determined and can then be divided by the total number of words to develop an indicator of how much behavior at the word level is involved in fragmentation. Third, the average instances of verbal fragmentation per T-unit can also be determined, as an index of the extent to which each utterance-level linguistic unit is disrupted. Finally, the percentage of T-units with one or more instances of verbal fragmentation may be calculated. These approaches to data summary are outlined and illustrated in Exhibit 3–14.

Fragmentations Presumed To Reflect Word Retrieval Difficulties

One final analysis option appears to offer the greatest flexibility in analyzing verbal fragmentations in the discourse of adult neurogenic patients. German and Simon (1991) and German (1993) provided a system for classifying behaviors in children and adolescents that were presumed to reflect underlying word retrieval problems. German and Simon (1991) stated quite clearly that the behaviors selected for their classification system were gleaned from literature on both child and adult word-finding characteristics but that no attempt was being made to

Exhibit 3–14 Quantifying Measures of Verbal Disruption or Fragmentation—Options for Data Summary

---

Example for Computation Purposes—Narrative Discourse Task:
Total verbal disruptions (Glosser et al., 1988) = 40
    Maze = 10
    Repetitions = 5
    Paraphasias = 8
    Omissions = 5
    Filler = 4
    Other = 8
Total words = 200
Total words involved in verbal disruptions = 80
Total T-units = 20
Total T-units with instances of verbal disruptions = 15

Option 1: Determine proportion of total verbal disruptions represented by each type of verbal disruption, as follows:
    Maze = 10/40 = .25
    Repetitions = 5/40 = .125
    Paraphasias = 8/40 = .20
    Omissions = 5/40 = .125
    Filler = 4/40 = .10
    Other = 8/40 = .20
Convert to percentages by multiplying by 100 if desired.

Option 2: Determine total number of words involved in all verbal disruptions, and divide by total number of words in sample, as follows:
    80 disrupted words/200 total words = .40 or 40% of all words disrupted

Option 3: Determine average number of verbal fragmentations per T-unit by dividing total verbal disruptions by total T-units, as follows:
    40 verbal disruptions/20 T-units = average of 2 verbal disruptions/T-unit

Option 4: Determine percentage of T-units evidencing verbal fragmentation by dividing verbally disrupted T-units by total T-units, as follows:
    15 disrupted T-units/20 T-units = .75 or 75% of T-units disrupted

---

specify the processes underlying observed discourse behaviors. They suggested that regardless of the underlying process (planning, execution, monitoring, and/or repair), there is evidence to support the idea that the surface-level breakdown occurs as part of the process of word selection.

The German and Simon (1991) system for identifying and summarizing seven specific indices of word retrieval problems is shown in Exhibit 3–15. This system has evidenced consistent utility with a variety of clients in clinical prac-

tice. Modifications can, of course, be made to address the behaviors of a particular client, but the basic behaviors targeted for analysis appear sufficiently comprehensive for baseline assessment and for development and monitoring of treatment.

Basically, German and Simon (1991) proposed developing both global and specific measures of verbal fragmentation (or word retrieval difficulties). After the transcript has been segmented into T-units, each T-unit is examined and notated for occurrences of one or more of

Exhibit 3–15 Indices of Word Retrieval Problems (German, 1993; German and Simon, 1991)

Within each T-unit, note the presence of one or more of the following:
1. Repetitions (REP)— at the word level or above
2. Word reformulations (REF)—essentially revision, where a word or phrase has been changed or replaced with a revised version
3. Empty words (EMP)—words that do not add content or provide greater specificity
4. Insertions (INS)—words or phrases that act as comments on the language process
5. Substitutions (SUB)—word replacing a target word. There are a number of substitution types, including
   a. Semantic—*hammer* for *screwdriver*
   b. Perceptual—*boot* for *boat*
   c. Nonspecific words—*foodstuff* for *hamburger*
   d. Multiple word responses—*morning beverage* for *coffee*
   e. No response—*I want to drink ___ after lunch.*
6. Delays (DEL)—of six seconds or more
7. Time fillers (TF)—filled pause material like *um, uh, ah, er,* when more than three occur in a T-unit

Calculate global measure = percentage of T-units with one or more word-finding problems.

Calculate mean word-finding problems per T-unit = total number of indicators of word retrieval problems divided by number of T-units.

Determine frequency of occurrence of different types of word retrieval indicators:
1. Count up all instances of word retrieval problems.
2. Count up number of instances of each type of word retrieval problem.
3. Calculate frequency of occurrences of each type as follows:

$$\frac{\text{Instances of Specific Type}}{\text{Total Instances of Word Retrieval Problems}} \times 100$$

the seven word-finding characteristics of interest. Exhibits 3–16 and 3–17 show earlier transcripts notated in this fashion. The global word-finding characteristic index, the mean word-finding problems per T-unit, and the frequency of occurrence of word-finding or fragmentation behaviors can be calculated, as illustrated in Exhibits 3–16 and 3–17.

A comparison of word retrieval analyses is seen in Table 3–1, along with other measures. The analysis confirms subjective impressions of marked disruption in discourse but also points to patterns that may later be significant. For example, client L.C. showed considerably more disruption in the verbal picture description task than in the Cat Story task. Both tasks depend upon pictures for visual stimuli. However, the Cat Story pictures are sequenced and simple, providing organization to the flow of the narrative story. In contrast, considerably more information is depicted on the Living Room picture, and there is no intrinsic organization to the task. It appears that the client's discourse breaks down markedly when she is required to deal with complex visual stimuli or when the stimulus does not provide any kind of organizational structure to the cognitive component of the discourse task. Further, across all tasks analyzed for this client, including some not shown here, her most common strategy for dealing with language programming is reformulation, followed closely by repetition.

Exhibit 3–16 Verbal Fragmentation Analysis of L.C.'s Verbal Living Room Picture Description

✓ 1. (Hum, ah,) a woman and (ah) her husband, [INS] looks like, [REP] a woman and her (ah) husband sitting in a, a room, [REF] a living room, (um) watching TV. *plus TF*

2. Now the woman was watching TV and also doing some needlework.

3. (Um,) and her husband was sitting on the couch,

✓ 4. but [INS] looks like he was asleep (um) with a coffee cup in his [SUB] cup, [REF] in his hand which was pouring on the floor, [REF] dripping on the floor, the coffee.

✓ 5. And a man and (ah) [REF] the woman was sitting in a chair

6. and she was not sitting with her husband.

7. Her husband was sitting on a couch.

✓ 8. In between the two, the chair and the couch, there was (ah)(ah) a lamp, [REF] a table, (ah)(ah) [REP] there was a table. *plus TF*

✓ 9. On top the table there's a, [REF] there was a, [REP] a lamp.

✓ 10. And above the couch there was a painting of (um) ships, (ah,) [REF] a ship, (um,) [REF] shipping on the ocean, [INS] I guess, [REF] water. *plus TF*

✓ 11. (Um,) and above the chair the woman was sitting, [REF] which the woman was sitting, (um,) there was a [REF] picture behind her, above her chair.

12. It's a painting of a flower.

✓ 13. On the woman's right hand there was a door which a curtain was drawn, [REF] drawing, there was a curtain (um) [REF] hanging on the door, yes, [INS] looks like it.

✓ 14. And on the other side of the door there's another painting which is (ah) [REP] is a flower also.

✓ 15. (Ah,) and (ah,) the, (ah) facing the woman there was a, [REP] there was a TV set *plus TF*

✓ 16. and it's on top of, [REF] the TV's sitting on the table. And on top of the TV, (um,) no, the TV was [REF] sitting on the table

17. and on top of the TV's a vase of flowers.

✓ 18. And a cat was, [REF] is playing, cat was playing in the middle of the floor, and [REP] the cat was playing the, the, (um) [REP] the ball of threads [REP] in the middle of the floor.

continues

Exhibit 3–16 continued

√ 19. And <u>see,</u> (oh) (um) next to the woman's chair is a sewing, (ah) basket. *plus TF*
   INS

   That's all.

Global Word-Finding Characteristic Index = 13/19 = 68.4%

Total Word Retrieval Instances = 35

Word Retrieval Instances/T-unit = 1.84   % Time Fillers = 5/35 = 14.3%
                                            % Repetitions = 8/35 = 22.9%
                                            % Reformulations = 16/35 = 45.7%
                                            % Substitutions = 1/35 = 2.9%
                                            % Insertions = 5/35 = 14.3%

   Note: Circled words indicate time fillers.

Exhibit 3–17 Verbal Fragmentation Analysis of L.C.'s Narrative Cat Story

1. OK, there was a little girl.

2. She was crying to her dad.

3. She said, "Well, my cat on the tree and I can't get her off the tree."

4. And so her dad said, "Well."

5. And he decided he's gonna get that cat for her.

6. So he start climbing the tree

7. and (ah) he climbed to the top on the branch where the cat was

√ 8. and so he swing his, <u>his</u> arms and try to catch the cat.
      REP

√ 9. And the cat jump, <u>the cat jump</u> off, <u>jumped off</u> the, (um) tree on . . .
      REP   *REF*

10. and, (ah) the dad end up hanging on the branch while he was trying to catch the cat.

√ 11. And the girl start crying again and the police, <u>because her dad was</u> hanging on a tree branch
       REF
    with a cloth and the branch caught his, (ah) (ah) <u>the</u> back of his collar.
                                                      REF

√ 12. And the, (ah) <u>the</u> fire, <u>the fireman</u>, <u>I guess that's a fireman</u>, <u>and he</u> was trying to rescue him.
             REP   *REF*   *INS*   *REF*

Global Word-Finding Characteristic Index = 4/12 = 33.3%

Total Word Retrieval Instances = 9

Word Retrieval Instances/T-unit = 75%   % Time Fillers = 0
                                         % Repetitions = 3/9 = 33.3%
                                         % Reformulations = 5/9 = 55.6%
                                         % Substitutions = 0
                                         % Insertions = 1/9 = 11.1%

   Note: Circled words indicate time fillers.

Exhibit 3–18 Verbal Fragmentation Analysis of Traumatically Brain-Injured Patient's Changing a Lightbulb Procedural Discourse

(*Note:* T-unit convention used—implied subject *you* treated as separate T-unit.)

1. You first walk into the room

2. and turn the light switch on for the light to go on

3. and the light does not go on.

4. So you turn the light switch back off

5. and then go out get the . . . (um) . . . lightbulb and the ladder to climb up to the lightbulb

6. and return then to the room

7. and . . . (um) . . . set the ladder under the lightbulb so you can get up.

8. And then you climb up the ladder with the lightbulb in hand or somewhere you can reach it

9. and . . . (um) . . . unscrew the lightbulb in the socket.

10. Replace it with another new lightbulb.

11. Then . . . (um) . . . (um) . . . climb back down the ladder . . .

12. (um) . . . and then go to the light switch

13. and turn the lightbulb on

14. and return the ladder from where it came from.

Global Word-Finding Characteristics Index = 0% of T-units with word retrieval problems

Note: Circled words indicate time fillers.

The informativeness of the German and Simon (1991) type of analysis can also be demonstrated by considering two analyses performed on discourse samples from a 37-year-old traumatically brain-injured client (see Exhibits 3–18 and 3–19). In the procedural discourse sample (how to change a lightbulb), there are no instances of word-finding difficulties, and there is a fair degree of complexity to the utterances being framed. In contrast, in the Rooster Story retelling, the same client shows global word-finding difficulties on 77.8% of the T-units, an average of 1.67 word retrieval problems per T-unit, and a pattern of heavy use of time fillers and repetitions, followed by reformulations, in an effort to deal with formulation problems. Apparently, the procedural discourse task was sufficiently rote or there was sufficient flexibility in language choice that disruption was minimized. However, when asked to remember and replicate to any degree an auditorially presented story, the client experienced pronounced breakdown in verbal fluency and information continuity, often at the beginning of new thought sequences. Although he eventually captured the basic elements of the story, much of the lan-

Exhibit 3–19 Verbal Fragmentation Analysis of Traumatically Brain-Injured Patient's Narrative Discourse, Retelling the Rooster Story

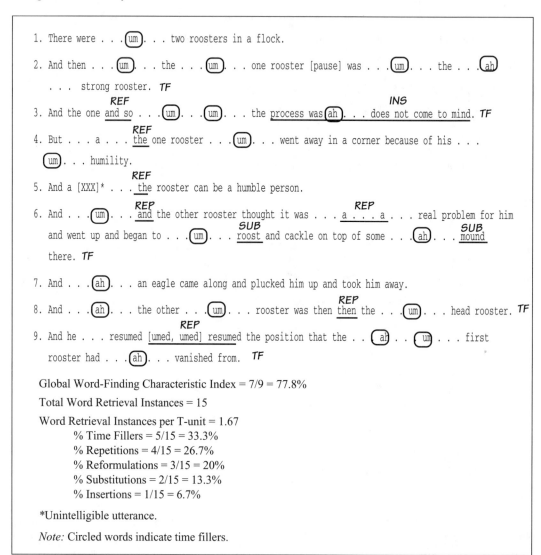

1. There were . . . (um) . . . two roosters in a flock.

2. And then . . . (um) . . . the . . . (um) . . . one rooster [pause] was . . . (um) . . . the . . . (ah)
   . . . strong rooster. *TF*

    REF   *INS*
3. And the one <u>and so</u> . . . (um) . . . (um) . . . the <u>process was</u>(ah) . . . <u>does not come to mind</u>. *TF*

                  REF
4. But . . . a . . . <u>the</u> one rooster . . . (um) . . . went away in a corner because of his . . .
   (um) . . . humility.

                  REF
5. And a [XXX]* . . . <u>the</u> rooster can be a humble person.

          REP   *REP*
6. And . . . (um) . . . <u>and</u> the other rooster thought it was . . . a . . . a . . . real problem for him
                              SUB   *SUB*
   and went up and began to . . . (um) . . . <u>roost</u> and cackle on top of some . . . (ah) . . . <u>mound</u>
   there. *TF*

7. And . . . (ah) . . . an eagle came along and plucked him up and took him away.

                                                    REP
8. And . . . (ah) . . . the other . . . (um) . . . rooster was then <u>then</u> the . . . (um) . . . head rooster. *TF*

            REP
9. And he . . . resumed <u>[umed, umed] resumed</u> the position that the . . . (ah) . . . (um) . . . first
   rooster had . . . (ah) . . . vanished from. *TF*

Global Word-Finding Characteristic Index = 7/9 = 77.8%

Total Word Retrieval Instances = 15

Word Retrieval Instances per T-unit = 1.67
    % Time Fillers = 5/15 = 33.3%
    % Repetitions = 4/15 = 26.7%
    % Reformulations = 3/15 = 20%
    % Substitutions = 2/15 = 13.3%
    % Insertions = 1/15 = 6.7%

*Unintelligible utterance.

Note: Circled words indicate time fillers.

guage deviated inappropriately from the original model.

CLINICAL IMPLICATIONS AND RECOMMENDATIONS

At the beginning of this chapter, it was noted that sentential and/or surface levels of analysis of discourse are considered by some to be of limited interest when contrasted to the data that can be gathered from discourse about the organizational demands of a particular task and the complex interplay between cognition and language in the communicative domain. Nevertheless, many of the analysis procedures demonstrated in this chapter have particular value when dealing with a specific disorder type or individual client. The analyses are most productive and revealing when compared across tasks, as shown in Table

3–1 for client L.C. In this table, additional information has been added for some measures on the basis of analysis of the two procedural discourse tasks and the conversational discourse task whose original samples were presented in Chapter 2. Although many of the entries in Table 3–1 have already been discussed, a few additional comments about clinical implications are appropriate here, since they demonstrate the clinical decision-making process.

The first question one might ask is whether there is a problem with discourse performance as measured at the sentential or surface level of analysis. Even without recourse to "normative" data, the answer should clearly be "yes." Patterns that are most noteworthy include (a) the disparity between total and edited words in several of the tasks (particularly the Living Room verbal picture description and conversation); (b) the clear evidence for problems with syntactic accuracy and completeness, even when all transcripts are first edited to remove initial attempts at correct formulation; (c) apparent evidence of word retrieval deficits or, at the very least, of marked difficulty in organizing and formulating language for particular discourse tasks; (d) consistent recourse to repetition and/or reformulation as strategies in revising messages on line; and (e) patterns that suggest that discourse performance breaks down when the task itself does not provide sufficient guidance in organizing and structuring the language production process.

These patterns not only provide support for the idea that client L.C. has discourse problems at the surface level of production but also suggest directions for further analysis and intervention. Macro- and superstructural analyses, for example, should indicate whether there are basic cognitive organizational deficits, as opposed to a primary language problem. Cohesion analyses may provide a basis for understanding the extreme degree of incoherence evident upon reading the conversational discourse, since syntactic and even word retrieval measures do not sufficiently characterize this sample. Interventions directed at word retrieval, or more generally verbal fragmentation, and at utterance-level syntactic/morphological formulations should be based upon a hierarchy of tasks that hold constant other organizational and linguistic challenges to the language production system while systematically increasing the challenge to the domain of interest. Written discourse may provide a particularly interesting starting point to facilitate the client's awareness of formulation difficulties and error patterns.

Many other specific cross-task comparisons of particular measures can be made. The intent here is simply to illustrate the richness of the clinical data that can be derived from some basic analyses of a variety of discourse samples from one client. Subsequent chapters will expand the clinical options provided by discourse assessment by providing information on analysis procedures in other discourse domains.

In the Appendixes, a variety of discourse samples have been provided for further practice in analyzing at the sentential/surface level.

REFERENCES

Boles, L., Holland, A.L., & Beeson, P. (1993, November). *Conversation analysis: How much talk is enough?* Miniseminar presented at the annual meeting of the American Speech-Language-Hearing Association, Anaheim, CA.

Brookshire, R.H., & Nicholas, L.E. (1993). Word choice in the connected speech of aphasic and non–brain-damaged speakers. *Clinical Aphasiology, 21*, 101–111.

Brookshire, R.H., & Nicholas, L.E. (1995). Performance deviations in the connected speech of adults with no brain damage and adults with aphasia. *American Journal of Speech-Language Pathology, 4*, 118–123.

Carroll, J.B., Davies, P., & Richman, B. (1971). *The American Heritage word frequency book.* New York: Houghton-Mifflin.

Cooper, P.Y. (1990). Discourse production and normal aging: Performance on oral picture description tasks. *Journal of Gerontology, 45*, P210–P214.

Critchley, M. (1984). And all the daughters of musick shall be brought low: Language function in the elderly. *Archives of Neurology, 41*, 1135–1139.

Davis, G.A., & Wilcox, M.J. (1985). *Adult aphasia rehabilitation: Applied pragmatics.* San Diego, CA: College Hill.

Doyle, P.J., Goda, A.J., & Spencer, K.A. (1995). The communicative informativeness and efficiency of connected discourse in adults with aphasia under structured and conversational sampling conditions. *American Journal of Speech-Language Pathology, 4*, 130–134.

Doyle, P.J., Thompson, C.K., Oleyar, K.S., Wambaugh, J.L., & Jackson, A.V. (1994). The effects of setting variables on conversational discourse in normal and aphasic adults. *Clinical Aphasiology, 22*, 135–144.

Fillenbaum, S., Jones, L.V., & Wepman, J.M. (1961). Some linguistic features of speech from aphasic patients. *Language and Speech, 4*, 91–102.

German, D.J. (1993). *Word finding intervention program.* Tucson, AZ: Communication Skill Builders.

German, D.J., & Simon, E. (1991). Analysis of children's word-finding skills in discourse. *Journal of Speech and Hearing Research, 34*, 309–316.

Gleason, J.B., Goodglass, H., Obler, L., Green, E., Hyde, M.R., & Weintraub, S. (1980). Narrative strategies of aphasic and normal-speaking subjects. *Journal of Speech and Hearing Research, 23*, 370–382.

Glosser, G., Wiener, M., & Kaplan, E. (1988). Variations in aphasic language behaviors. *Journal of Speech and Hearing Disorders, 53*, 115–124.

Hayes, D.P. (1988). Speaking and writing: Distinct patterns of word choice. *Journal of Memory and Language, 27*, 572–585.

Hayes, D.P. (1989). *Guide to lexical analysis of texts* (Tech. Rep. Ser. 89–96). Ithaca, NY: Cornell University, Department of Sociology.

Howes, D. (1964). Application of the word-frequency concept to aphasia. In A.V.S. de Reuck & M. O'Conner (Eds.), *CIBA Foundation Symposium on Disorders of Language.* Boston: Little, Brown.

Hunt, K.W. (1965). *Grammatical structures written at three grade levels* (Research Rep. No. 3). Champaign, IL: National Council of Teachers of English.

Hunt, K.W. (1970). Syntactic maturity of school children and adults. *Monograph of the Society for Research in Child Development, 35*, 1–78.

Kaplan, E., Goodglass, H., & Weintraub, S. (1983). *The Boston Naming Test.* Philadelphia: Lea & Febiger.

Kemper, S. (1987). Life-span changes in syntactic complexity. *Journal of Gerontology, 42*, 323–328.

Kemper, S., Kynette, D., & Norman, S. (1991). Age differences in spoken language. In R. West & J. Sinnott (Eds.), *Everyday memory and aging* (pp 321–352). New York: Springer-Verlag.

Kynette, D., & Kemper, S. (1986). Aging and the loss of grammatical forms: A cross-sectional study of language performance. *Language and Communication, 6*, 65–72.

MacWhinney, B. (1991). *The CHILDES Project: Tools for analyzing talk.* Hillsdale, NJ: Lawrence Erlbaum.

MacWhinney, B. (1996). The CHILDES system. *American Journal of Speech-Language Pathology, 5*, 5–14.

Miller, J.F., & Chapman, R.S. (1992, 1993). *MacSALT: Basic SALT programs.* Madison University of Wisconsin-Madison, Waisman Center, Language Analysis Laboratory.

Nicholas, M., Obler, L.K., Albert, M.L., & Helm-Estabrooks, N. (1985). Empty speech in Alzheimer's disease and fluent aphasia. *Journal of Speech and Hearing Research, 28*, 405–410.

Pindzola, R.B., McCloskey, L., & Moran, M.J. (1989, November). *Communicative fluency in aged persons.* Paper presented at the annual meeting of the American Speech-Language-Hearing Association, St. Louis, MO.

Retherford, K., Schwartz, B., & Chapman, R. (1981). Semantic roles in mother and child speech: Who tunes into whom? *Journal of Child Language, 3*, 81–98.

Roberts, J.A., & Wertz, R.T. (1989). Comparison of spontaneous and elicited oral-expressive language in aphasia. *Clinical Aphasiology, 18*, 479–488.

Shadden, B.B. (1994, May). *Sentential/surface level analysis.* Paper presented at the Conference on Managing Discourse Problems in the Neurologically Impaired Adult: A Practical Approach, Rehabilitation Institute of Chicago, Chicago.

Shadden, B.B., Burnette, R.B., Eikenberry, B.R., & DiBrezzo, R. (1991). All discourse tasks are not created equal. *Clinical Aphasiology, 20*, 327–341.

Shewan, C.M., & Henderson, V.L. (1988). Analysis of spontaneous language in the older normal population. *Journal of Communication Disorders, 21*, 139–154.

Stickler, K.R. (1987). *Guide to analysis of language transcripts.* Eau Claire, WI: Thinking Publications.

Strong, C.J., & Shaver, J.P. (1991). Stability of cohesion in the spoken narratives of language-impaired and normally developing school-aged children. *Journal of Speech and Hearing Research, 34*, 95–111.

Templin, M. (1957). *Certain language skills in children: Their development and relationships.* Minneapolis: University of Minnesota Press.

Ulatowska, H.K., Doyle, A.W., Freedman-Stern, R., & Macaluso-Haynes, S. (1983). Production of procedural discourse in aphasia. *Brain and Language, 18*, 315–341.

Ulatowska, H.K., Freedman-Stern, R., Doyle, A.W., Macaluso-Haynes, S., & North, A.J. (1983). Production of narrative discourse in aphasia. *Brain and Language, 19*, 306–316.

Ulatowska, H.K., North, A.J., & Macaluso-Haynes, S. (1981). Production of narrative and procedural discourse in aphasia. *Brain and Language, 13*, 345–371.

Wachal, R.S., & Spreen, O. (1973). Some measures of lexical diversity in aphasic and normal language performance. *Language and Speech, 16*, 169–181.

Walker, V.G., Roberts, P.M., & Hedrick, D.L. (1988). Linguistic analyses of the discourse narratives of young and aged women. *Folia Phoniatrica, 40*, 58–64.

Yairi, E. (1981). Disfluencies of normally speaking two-year-old children. *Journal of Speech and Hearing Research, 24*, 490–495.

Yorkston, K.M., Zeches, J., Farrier, L., & Uomoto, J. (1993). Lexical pitch as a measure of word choice in narratives of traumatically brain injured and control subjects. *Clinical Aphasiology, 21*, 165–172.

CHAPTER 4

Cohesion Analyses

Betty Z. Liles and Carl A. Coelho

Cohesion is defined as structural coherence among parts of a text (Halliday & Hasan, 1976). Sentences are conjoined by various kinds of meaning relations described as *cohesive ties*. The kinds of ties vary, depending on the nature of the text (i.e., communicative function), as well as the style and ability of the speaker. A speaker's relative frequency of the use of the various categories of cohesive ties is referred to as *cohesive style* (Liles, Coelho, Duffy, & Zalagens, 1989). Each of the different types of discourse (e.g., procedural, descriptive, story narratives) is distinct and therefore requires a different pattern of cohesive use that is consistent with the underlying structural rules needed for the creation of a cohesive text. Speakers normally shift their patterns of cohesive use across types of discourse; they may also modify cohesive use in response to differences in the context in which the text is being created. Cohesional analyses have been useful in the characterization of language-impaired individuals' narrative texts in terms of their ability to organize content (Coelho, Liles, & Duffy, 1991, 1995; Liles, 1985, 1993; Liles et al., 1989; Mentis & Prutting, 1987). In general, brain-injured adults have performed less adequately than their noninjured peers.

For researchers and clinicians to apply reliably a procedure used to describe text coherence, a fairly rigorous structure of procedural "rules" was devised. These procedures evolved as a result of a rather long and arduous process of observing the frequency of particular instances of cohesive use in the verbal narratives of children and adults. In addition, the ability and inability of various examiners to agree on specific judgments was central to the usefulness of the analysis. The question of reliability was a formidable one, since Halliday and Hasan's (1976) description of cohesive use across a variety of categories is broad and, in some cases, overlapping. This chapter reviews and illustrates a modified version of Halliday and Hasan's cohesion analyses.

There are three major tasks or steps involved in the cohesion analysis. The first is the identification of words that are used as cohesive ties; the second is the classification of those ties as linguistically structured categories of cohesion use; and the third is the determination of the "adequacy" of the tie's cohesive function in a particular text.

The first task, the identification of words used as cohesive ties, is obviously the most critical. If cohesive ties are not reliably identified, analysis of linguistic function and adequacy will not represent a faithful description of the individual's performance. To ensure reliability, Halliday and Hasan's (1976) definition of a cohesive element must be rather vigorously applied. Consistent with Halliday and Hasan's criterion that a tie's interpretation is dependent on other textual referents, no item is described as "cohesive" unless its use reliably requires the listener to go outside the sentence for a correct and complete interpretation of the meaning.

The second task in the procedure is the classification of ties as explicit linguistic structures that alert the listener to look elsewhere in the text for the related meaning. The assertion here is that a speaker's use of a particular linguistic form cues the listener to expect that the information resides outside the sentence. It is through the use of these linguistic structures that a speaker or writer realizes cohesive organization and often displays various styles of language use.

According to Halliday and Hasan (1976), each instance of a cohesive tie can be classified according to one of the following linguistic categories of meaning relations:

- reference (personal, demonstrative, or comparative)
- substitution
- ellipsis
- conjunction (additive, adversative, causal, or temporal)
- lexical (reiteration, collocation)

Definitions of these types of cohesive ties are presented in Exhibit 4–1. Specific guidelines for identification of cohesive ties and for handling confusing or ambiguous items will be presented later in this chapter. Cohesion by ellipsis and cohesion by substitution are not discussed extensively within this chapter because of their extremely low frequency of occurrence in the narrative samples from children and adults we have collected over the past several years (this is consistent with the observations of Mentis and Prutting, 1987). The remaining categories presented by Halliday and Hasan (1976) are included.

The third and final task in the procedure pertains to the "adequacy" of the subjects' use of cohesion. Since speakers cannot be expected to be perfect in the realization of their narrative organization, procedures have been developed to describe how an individual might depart from complete clarity and accuracy in indicating the meaning relation between the cohesive items. This procedure describes only to what extent the subjects are successful at presenting the listener with "complete" (i.e., unambiguous or non-erroneous) semantic relationships. Speakers' departures from the text are categorized as complete, incomplete, or errors. Each of these categories of cohesive adequacy is defined in Exhibit 4–1 and discussed at length toward the end of the chapter.

INTEREXAMINER RELIABILITY

Interexaminer reliability measures for all of the procedures described in this chapter have been presented in previous publications (Liles, 1985; Liles et al., 1989). Using the analyses of 150 narratives of children and approximately 100 adults, we obtained reliability measures for sentence distribution, identification of cohesive elements, classification of cohesive markers, and the adequacy of cohesive tying. All reliability measures obtained have been high, thus demonstrating the reliability of these procedures developed for the measurement and description of cohesion within a text.

DISTRIBUTION OF NARRATIVES INTO T-UNITS

The procedures for the distribution of narrative utterances into T-units have been described at length in Chapter 2. However, a few points are important to review.

There is surprisingly little disagreement in T-unit redistribution if the original story is known to the transcribers. The major source of disagreement pertains to the T-unit segmentation of utterance "chains" joined by the conjunctions *and* or *and then*. Reliability can be increased by applying Lee's (1974) procedure. That is, when a narrative contains a "chain" of utterances conjoined by the same conjunction, distribute as separate sentences if an independent structural unit (i.e., subject and predicate)

Exhibit 4–1 Definition of Cohesion Markers and Cohesive Adequacy

A word is identified as a *cohesive marker* if its meaning cannot be adequately interpreted by the listener and if the listener must "search" outside of that sentence for the completed meaning. In addition, a word may be judged as a cohesive element if it is used as a linguistic marker that leads the listener to expect that its interpretation is outside the sentence (e.g., definite articles).

Cohesive Marker Types

- **Reference**

  The information to be retrieved is the identity of the thing or class of things being referred to in the preceding (*anaphora*) or following text (*cataphora*).

  1. Personal

     Personal pronouns, possessive determiners, and possessive pronouns that represent a single system of persons, referring to the identity of relevant persons, objects, and events (e.g., *he, mine, it, one*).
     Example:
     Tom is an engineer. *He* works in Ohio.

  2. Demonstrative

     A form of verbal pointing, identifying the referent by location in place or time (e.g., *this, that, there, those*).
     Example:
     Sally is at home. You can call her *there*.

- **Conjunction**

  Specification of the way that sentence meaning (i.e., content) that has gone before is to cohere with content of the sentence to follow. The following types of conjunctive cohesion are listed from most to least complex.

  1. Causal

     Sentence meanings that cohere via the expression of a relationship that specifies result, reason, and purpose (e.g., *because, for this reason, to this end, otherwise*).
     Example:
     I didn't hear about it. *Otherwise*, I would have come immediately.

  2. Adversative

     Sentence meanings that cohere via the expression of a relation that is contrary to expectation (e.g., *yet, though, only, but, instead*).
     Example:
     The three of us worked for hours. *Yet* we hardly made a dent in the whole job.

  3. Temporal

     Sentence meanings that cohere via the expression of a relation that specifies time (e.g., *simultaneously, then, afterward, subsequently*).
     Example:
     We warmed ourselves by the fire. *Then* we made some coffee.

continues

Exhibit 4–1 continued

4. Additive	Sentence meanings that cohere simply by denoting added information, similarity of meaning, alternative meanings, and de-emphatic afterthought (e.g., *and, furthermore, likewise, by contrast, incidentally*). *Example:* Bill worked all night. *And* his typing kept the rest of us awake.
• **Lexical**	Lexical cohesion is achieved by selection of vocabulary. Lexical cohesion may take the form of *reiteration* (i.e., where both the cohesive item and that to which it refers have a common referent) or *collocation* (i.e., where cohesion is achieved through association of lexical items that regularly co-occur).
1. Reiteration –Same word	*Example:* We went to the house on the beach. It was a huge *house*.
–Synonym	*Example:* He's a fine boy. He's one of the smartest *lads* I know.
–Superordinate	*Example:* You can have the carrots. I have all the *vegetables* I need.
–General word	*Example:* I gave Tom our tickets. The *idiot* lost them all.
2. Collocation	*Example:* I told her to call the doctor. She was very *ill*.
• **Ellipsis**	*Ellipsis* refers to sentences or clauses whose structure is such as to presuppose some preceding item, which then serves as the source of the missing information. Ellipsis is simply "substitution by zero." Ellipsis consists of three categories:
1. Nominal	*Example:* What kind of car are you looking for? *Ford* (car).
2. Verbal	*Example:* Who's coming along? *We are* (coming).
3. Clausal	*Example:* Has he finished the basement? *He has* (finished the basement).
• **Substitution**	In substitution, the cohesive link is established through the use of a substitute linguistic item of the same grammatical class as the item necessary for interpretation. The substitute item has the same structural function as that for which it is substituted.

continues

Exhibit 4–1 continued

1. Nominal	*one, ones; same*
	Example: I need a drink of water. Would you get me *one*?
2. Verbal	*do*
	Example: I have no idea what all those fancy words mean, and I don't think you *do* either.
3. Clausal	so, not
	Example:
	Then they didn't win?
	Unfortunately *not*.

Cohesive Adequacy

- Complete tie
A tie is complete if the information referred to by the cohesive tie is easily found and defined with no ambiguity.
Example:
The boy was very thirsty. *He* drank a glass of water.

- Incomplete tie
A tie is judged to be incomplete if the information referred to by the cohesive marker is not provided in the text.
Example:
The kids walked home from school. They stopped at *her* home for a snack.

- Erroneous tie
A tie is judged to be an error if the listener is guided to ambiguous information.
Example:
Dave and Joe went to the supermarket. *He* bought a bag of apples.

follows each conjunction. In cases of examiner disagreement, pause times and intonation cues from the audio recordings are used as the criteria for the determination of sentence boundaries. After the redistribution of utterances into T-units, list by number.

Corrections, Repetitions, and Asides

Repetitions and asides to the listener are bracketed and not analyzed at the sentence level.

Example: Freddie [uh, yeah, Freddie] went home [I'm not really sure].

When a portion of a sentence is corrected or revised, bracket the portion that was changed, and analyze only the corrected portion of the sentence if needed for within-sentence grammatical use.

Example: Freddie took the [wagon—uh] horse to his uncle.

These repetitions, asides, and remarks, as well as corrections, are retained in the text (although not analyzed at the sentence level) because in some instances they contain information that may be an element in a cohesive tie in a later sentence. Since Halliday and Hasan's (1976) description of cohesion is a semantic analysis, retaining such information is appropriate and does not violate the analysis or render a "sentence" a "nonsentence." See Chapter 2 for examples of T-unit distributions.

IDENTIFICATION OF WORDS MARKED AS COHESIVE

Once the sentences have been distributed, the next step is the identification of words that mark the use of cohesive elements. It is important that the examiner be familiar with the original or "target" story that is being retold. In this procedure, the "contract" between the examiner and the client is that the client is to tell the examiner the narrative text that he or she has just heard or seen. The client therefore should be intent on producing as faithful a replication of the original as he or she is capable of. Under these circumstances, the reliability of the procedure is greatly enhanced. To maximize reliability and to reduce the time required in the analysis, the following steps should be followed:

1. Read the entire narrative to get an overall sense of the speaker's text.
2. Read each T-unit separately as a *complete unit* before identifying those words that mark cohesion.

At this stage in the analysis, the examiner views each sentence as isolated from the text. From this perspective, the examiner judges a word to be a cohesive element or not under the following conditions.

Uninterpretable Meaning within the T-Unit

A particular word is a cohesive marker if its meaning cannot be fully understood by the listener without going outside the T-unit.

Example: Two men had patiently awaited a *sign.*

It would be natural in this situation for the reader to ask, "What sign?" or "Sign for what?" and then to look outside the T-unit to recover the information. The assumption here is that the speaker is presupposing information shared with the recipient.

Structural Linguistic Cues Serving as Cohesive Markers

A word is a cohesive marker if it has a structural function marking presupposed information (e.g., definite articles versus indefinite articles). See Exhibit 4–1 for a listing of structural markers that may lead the listener to "expect" that the information is outside the T-unit as well as definitions. The following examples may serve to establish some conventions for classifying ties that appear ambiguous.

Conjunctions

When two or more conjunctions (e.g., *and then* or *and so then*) are conjoined in a sentence, code only one of the conjunctions as a cohesive item. Select the conjunction that is the most complex according to the following hierarchy: (a) causal, (b) adversative, (c) temporal, and (d) additive. The hierarchy is based on developmental acquisition and the assumption that the more complex use is the meaning being marked by the speaker.

Reference: Demonstrative and Comparative

When both a demonstrative and a comparative reference are used (e.g., *the other*), code only as one cohesive item (comparative) rather than as two items (demonstrative and comparative).

Reference: Personal and Demonstrative

If two or more references (i.e., either personal or demonstrative) are judged to be cohesive in the same sentence, code all markers, even though they refer to a common referent.

Example: *He* took *his* comic books home.

While the sentence structure indicates that *his* refers within the sentence to *he*, there is no lexical support within the sentence to provide the listener with the information needed to know to whom *his* refers. Therefore, *he* and *his* are both identified as cohesive markers.

This rule seems contradictory to the convention of identifying words as cohesive markers only if they refer outside the sentence. The modification was made to increase reliability across scorers. In our experience, some sentences were ambiguous regarding coreference. By identifying all personal reference items that do not refer within the sentence to explicit referents, reliability is substantially improved, particularly for language-impaired individuals' texts.

Relationships within the Sentence

Do not judge an item as a cohesive marker if the information referred to is recoverable within the sentence.

Example: Some boys took *their* car home.

The personal reference *their* refers to *boys*; therefore, the information is recoverable within the sentence.

Example: There was *this* scientist that had a hideout. In *these* mountains where there was this radar tower to blow up metal things that fly in the air.

In the example above, the information referred to by the use of *this* and *these* as selective demonstrative references (i.e., in contrast to nonselective) is recovered within the sentence. Thus, the examiner would not identify *this* or *these* as a cohesive marker (i.e., information recoverable outside the sentence). The next example demonstrates a cohesive and a noncohesive marker in the same sentence.

Example: One of the boys went home.

The demonstrative reference *the* marks which or what *boys*, and serves as a cue to the reader that the information is recoverable outside the sentence; therefore, it is cohesive. However, *one of* refers within the sentence to *boys* and is not a cohesive marker. The analysis of *the* often presents some ambiguity. Halliday and Hasan (1976, p. 70) described *the* as "nonselective" (as opposed to *this, that, these*, and *those*, which are selective). In this procedure, we are, in special cases, describing *the* as selective. That is, the use of *the* in some cases points to the selection of specific references important to the text's meaning.

Text Influence on Judgment

Although the examiner should view each sentence as independent from the text when initially identifying cohesive markers, there are instances when the total text must be considered. For example, in the sentence "*Marie didn't want to go on the hike,*" the listener may need more information about *Marie* to comprehend the text. In this particular text, the reader would ask, "Who is Marie?"

Thus, the decision as to whether a particular item is identified as a cohesive marker is based on the extent to which adequate interpretation of the information is "text dependent." As texts vary, specific items may vary in their cohesive function. The examiner therefore may be required to change perspective during the analysis.

Text Influence on Demonstrative Reference

While *the* is a "selective" demonstrative reference, it may also be used in combination with words to express a unit of meaning: for example, "the road," "the radio," "the newspaper." It may be difficult to determine when the speaker intends to use *the* as a selective demonstrative reference or as a nonselective functor. To make this judgment, the examiner must take the text into consideration. For example, if the speaker used "the road" and the examiner judges that reference to a particular road is important within the text, he or she may judge that the speaker intended *the* to be used as a selective reference and may further identify it as a cohesive marker. The following rule will facilitate this judgment: if in doubt about the use of *the* because of the above reasons, do not code *the* as a selective demonstrative reference if *a* or *some* can be substituted without producing a crucial change in the meaning of the text.

THE CLASSIFICATION OF COHESIVE MARKERS

After the cohesive markers within each sentence have been identified according to the rules presented above, the T-unit should be reread from a different perspective. The markers that have been identified as cohesive are now viewed as a part of the text.

Since each cohesion marker must (or should) be "tied" to the information recoverable elsewhere in the text, the examiner locates the sentence containing the tied information. The sentence number and item are noted (see Exhibit 4–2 for an example of an analyzed text).

On the basis of the type of relationship evidenced by the tie, the examiner then classifies the cohesive marker. The listing in this chapter of cohesive markers by linguistic categories has been derived from Halliday and Hasan's (1976) description. However, consistent with their model of cohesion, identification and classification of specific markers are dependent on their use in the text. The listing supplied here should be used only as a probable guide to the identification of cohesive markers in a text. Some markers have been specified in terms of our procedure and should not necessarily be interpreted as Halliday and Hasan's.

The referent for a cohesive item may not be in sentences immediately preceding or following the sentence containing the item being analyzed. Indeed, speakers may refer back to any number of sentences and often do. Some of the unimpaired children produced 15 or 20 sentences be-

tween an original referent and its eventual "tie." In scanning for tied information, include a fair number of sentences, keeping in mind the total text. As stated previously, the examiner should always read the entire text before the analysis is initiated. These steps (i.e., classifying the cohesive marker) will be completed more accurately and quickly if the examiner has resisted the temptation to analyze the text sentence by sentence without prior knowledge of the total narrative.

Cohesion by Reference

Referential cohesive ties assume *exact identity* of the marker with the noun or phrase or context that it references. Following is a listing of referential linguistic markers that ordinarily cue the reader to recover information outside the sentence and are therefore coded as cohesive.

Personal

Code first-person personal pronouns (*I, you, we, us*) that are within quotes and refer to the speaker of the quote if he or she has been named in the text.

> *Example:* Mary isn't home. Her note says, "*I* will be home at six."

Code third-person personal pronouns (*he, her, his, hers, him, them, it*, and also *one* when *one* is used as a generalized human; see Halliday & Hasan, 1976, p. 46).

> *Examples:*
> I found the book. *It* was on the table.
> John's hat is not here. *His* hat is at the house.

There are some special instances:

> *Example:* When *this* balloon came out, he shot it down.

Code *this* (i.e., as demonstrative reference, see the second example under "Relationships within the Sentence") but not *it* because *it* is defined by the structure of the sentence and the referent (i.e., *balloon*) is recoverable within the sentence.

Demonstrative

Code all the following determiners: *this, that, these, those.*

Examples:
We went home. *That* was fun.
We went home on weekends. *Those* were some of the best moments.

Code *the* except in the following types of instances:

Example: The boy wearing a red sweater choked.

Do not code *the* because the determiner is defined completely within the sentence by *boy wearing a red sweater.*

Example: The newspaper was on a chair.

Do not code *the* if *a* or *some* can be substituted without producing a crucial change in the meaning of the text.

Example: A newspaper was on a chair.

Comparative

Code items that express comparisons between items in the text, such as

- Identity: *same, equal, identical,* etc.
  Example: I have an *equal* number of clock hours.
- Similarity: *such, similar, likewise,* etc.
  Example: Your dress pattern is *similar.*
- Difference: *other, differently, unlike,* etc.
  Example: What *other* did you bring me?

Do not code as cohesive comparisons that are explained within the sentence.

Examples:
They gave *similar* excuses.
You have the *same* teacher that I do.

Code words that make particular comparisons such as numerations: *more, fewer, less, as many as,* etc.

Example: She has *more* endurance.

Code epithets *better, so, as, more,* and comparative adjectives or adverbs.

Example: Your painting is just *as* beautiful.

Do not code comparatives as cohesive when the referent is within the sentence.

Example: The movie was *so* exciting.

Cohesion by Conjunction

Additive

Code markers as additive if they (a) conjoin two consecutive sentences that describe events that have occurred simultaneously.

Example: He looked in the bushes. *And* she searched in the grass.

or (b), that indicate sequential information without intervening events or time lapse.

Example: He turned the corner. *And* he saw a skunk.

The following is a listing of several additive markers:

- Additive: *and, and also,* etc.
- Negative: *nor, and . . . not, neither,* etc.
- Alternative: *or, else,* etc.
- Afterthought: *incidentally, oh yes and,* etc.
- Similar: *in the same way, similarly,* etc.
- Dissimilar: *on the other hand, conversely,* etc.
- Expository: *I mean, that is,* etc.
- Exemplificatory: *for example, like, thus,* etc.

In addition, Halliday and Hasan (1976) presented the following as additive conjunctions:

- *now:* cohesive when meaning the opening of a new stage in the communication
- *of course:* indicating that something is obvious
- *well:* what follows is a response to what has preceded

- *anyway:* brushing aside the preceding sentence
- *surely:* it demands an answer and is cataphoric
- *after all:* what has been said is reasonable given what preceded it

Adversative

Code the following markers as adversative (i.e., indicating something contrary to expectation):

- Simple: *yet, though*, etc.
- *But*
- Emphatic: *however, despite*, etc.
- Avowal: *in fact, actually*, etc.
- Correction: *instead, rather*, etc.
- Correction of wording: *at least, I mean*, etc.
- Dismissal: *in any case, whatever*, etc.

Causal

Code the following types of markers as causal:

- Simple: *and so, so, therefore* etc.
- Emphatic: *consequently, because of this*
- Reason: *it follows, for this reason*
- Result: *in consequence, so*
- Purpose: *with this intention, so*
- Reversed polarity: *otherwise*
- With respect to: *with regard to this*

Temporal

Code the following types of markers as temporal:

- Sequential: *and then, after that*
- Simultaneous: *just then, simultaneously*
- Preceding: *earlier, before that*
- Immediate: *at once, just then*
- Interrupted: *soon, later*
- Repetitive: *next time, again*
- Conclusive: *finally, at last*
- Temporal: *then, next*
- Here and now: *up to now, from now on*
- Summary: *to sum up, anyhow*

Interpretation of Conjunctive Cohesion

Comparison of cohesion by conjunction and reference shows substantial differences between the two. Words used as reference cohesion do what their name implies: they make specific references to people, places, and events that are presented elsewhere in the text. In contrast, conjunctive cohesive markers typically refer to content presented immediately (i.e., preceding or following the marker) and refer to total propositional meaning contained within the T-unit rather than specific referents.

This distinction has clinical implications, for the misuse of conjunctive cohesion may indicate a difference in management approaches when compared with misuse of cohesive reference (Liles, 1987).

Lexical Cohesion

Recall that an item is defined as cohesive only when it cues the reader or listener that the information is recoverable outside the sentence. Application of Halliday and Hasan's (1976) description of lexical cohesion, however, often violated this rule and resulted in poor reliability across examiners.

Example: The children bought *balloons.* Then the *balloons* popped.

The use of *balloons* in the second sentence is an obvious example of lexical reiteration, as Halliday and Hasan proposed, but its use does not necessarily require the reader to look outside the sentence for additional information, or at least this judgment proved to be unreliable. By our definition, the word *balloon* would not be identified as a cohesive marker. The demonstrative reference *the*, however, does cue the listener that more information is recoverable outside the sentence and is coded as a selective demonstrative reference pointing back to the immediate sentence. As this example indicates, the descriptions of lexical cohesion obtained by use of our procedures may not be consistent with Halliday and Hasan's intentions for describing lexical cohesion as they do.

Exhibit 4–2 Sample Narrative with Sentences Distributed into T-units, Numbered, and Analyzed

1. Well, there were three main people, Homer, Louie and Freddie.

2. [And they] and Louie and Freddie were over at Homer's house.

3. And they started reading.

4. They read a comic, Super Duper.

5. And they got into a conversation about it.

6. Then Louie and Freddie had to go home.

7. And [he, and Louie called, I mean] Freddie called Homer and said that there was a movie on [Friday, uh] Saturday and [then–they–] that Super Duper was gonna be there.

8. So that Saturday they went.

9. And they saw Super Duper.

10. [They were going–] that night they were going home.

11. And they saw Super Duper speeding down the road in his car.

12. And he went off the road around the corner.

13. And then [he–] they wondered what happened to him.

14. So they went over and looked.

15. And [they ducked–] they ducked into some weeds.

16. And they were seeing if Super Duper was gonna lift the car with one hand.

17. But he got caught in some barbed wire.

18. And they left.

19. And they went and helped him out.

20. They didn't ask him, but they wondered why he didn't lift the car with one hand.

21. So [they brought–] they pulled the car out with [the horse–] the horse.

22. And they brought him home.

23. And his father fixed the car.

24. And Super Duper gave them some comics.

25. And he left.

continues

Exhibit 4–2 continued

SUBJ ID _____ TASK_____ SCORED BY _____ DATE_____

T-U #	Item (Word)	COHESIVE MARKER TYPE							COHESIVE ADEQUACY				
1	THERE	Rp	(Rd)	Lex	Ca	Ct	Ccau	Cadv	Comp	(Inc)	Inc-T	Error	Error-T
2	AND	Rp	Rd	Lex	(Ca)	Ct	Ccau	Cadv	(Comp)	Inc	Inc-T	Error	Error-T
	LOUIE	Rp	Rd	(Lex)	Ca	Ct	Ccau	Cadv	(Comp)	Inc	Inc-T	Error	Error-T
	FREDDIE	Rp	Rd	(Lex)	Ca	Ct	Ccau	Cadv	(Comp)	Inc	Inc-T	Error	Error-T
	HOMER'S	Rp	Rd	(Lex)	Ca	Ct	Ccau	Cadv	(Comp)	Inc	Inc-T	Error	Error-T
3	AND	Rp	Rd	Lex	(Ca)	Ct	Ccau	Cadv	(Comp)	Inc	Inc-T	Error	Error-T
	THEY	(Rp)	Rd	Lex	Ca	Ct	Ccau	Cadv	(Comp)	Inc	Inc-T	Error	Error-T
4	THEY	(Rp)	Rd	Lex	Ca	Ct	Ccau	Cadv	(Comp)	Inc	Inc-T	Error	Error-T
5	AND	Rp	Rd	Lex	(Ca)	Ct	Ccau	Cadv	(Comp)	Inc	Inc-T	Error	Error-T
	THEY	(Rp)	Rd	Lex	Ca	Ct	Ccau	Cadv	(Comp)	Inc	Inc-T	Error	Error-T
	IT	(Rp)	Rd	Lex	Ca	Ct	Ccau	Cadv	(Comp)	Inc	Inc-T	Error	Error-T
6	THEN	Rp	Rd	Lex	Ca	(Ct)	Ccau	Cadv	(Comp)	Inc	Inc-T	Error	Error-T
	LOUIE	Rp	Rd	(Lex)	Ca	Ct	Ccau	Cadv	(Comp)	Inc	Inc-T	Error	Error-T
	FREDDIE	Rp	Rd	(Lex)	Ca	Ct	Ccau	Cadv	(Comp)	Inc	Inc-T	Error	Error-T
7	AND	Rp	Rd	Lex	(Ca)	Ct	Ccau	Cadv	(Comp)	Inc	Inc-T	Error	Error-T
	FREDDIE	Rp	Rd	(Lex)	Ca	Ct	Ccau	Cadv	(Comp)	Inc	Inc-T	Error	Error-T
	HOMER	Rp	Rd	(Lex)	Ca	Ct	Ccau	Cadv	(Comp)	Inc	Inc-T	Error	Error-T
	SUPER DUPER	Rp	Rd	(Lex)	Ca	Ct	Ccau	Cadv	(Comp)	Inc	Inc-T	Error	Error-T
8	SO	Rp	Rd	Lex	Ca	Ct	(Ccau)	Cadv	(Comp)	Inc	Inc-T	Error	Error-T
	THAT	Rp	(Rd)	Lex	Ca	Ct	Ccau	Cadv	(Comp)	Inc	Inc-T	Error	Error-T
	THEY	(Rp)	Rd	Lex	Ca	Ct	Ccau	Cadv	(Comp)	Inc	Inc-T	Error	Error-T
	WENT	Rp	Rd	(Lex)	Ca	Ct	Ccau	Cadv	(Comp)	Inc	Inc-T	Error	Error-T
9	AND	Rp	Rd	Lex	(Ca)	Ct	Ccau	Cadv	(Comp)	Inc	Inc-T	Error	Error-T
	THEY	(Rp)	Rd	Lex	Ca	Ct	Ccau	Cadv	(Comp)	Inc	Inc-T	Error	Error-T
	SUPER DUPER	Rp	Rd	(Lex)	Ca	Ct	Ccau	Cadv	(Comp)	Inc	Inc-T	Error	Error-T

continues

Exhibit 4–2 continued

T-U #	Item (Word)	COHESIVE MARKER TYPE							COHESIVE ADEQUACY				
10	THAT	Rp	(Rd)	Lex	Ca	Ct	Ccau	Cadv	(Comp)	Inc	Inc-T	Error	Error-T
	THEY	(Rp)	Rd	Lex	Ca	Ct	Ccau	Cadv	(Comp)	Inc	Inc-T	Error	Error-T
11	AND	Rp	Rd	Lex	(Ca)	Ct	Ccau	Cadv	(Comp)	Inc	Inc-T	Error	Error-T
	THEY	(Rp)	Rd	Lex	Ca	Ct	Ccau	Cadv	(Comp)	Inc	Inc-T	Error	Error-T
	SUPER DUPER	Rp	Rd	(Lex)	Ca	Ct	Ccau	Cadv	(Comp)	Inc	Inc-T	Error	Error-T
12	AND	Rp	Rd	Lex	(Ca)	Ct	Ccau	Cadv	(Comp)	Inc	Inc-T	Error	Error-T
	HE	(Rp)	Rd	Lex	Ca	Ct	Ccau	Cadv	(Comp)	Inc	Inc-T	Error	Error-T
13	AND THEN	Rp	Rd	Lex	Ca	(Ct)	Ccau	Cadv	(Comp)	Inc	Inc-T	Error	Error-T
	THEY	(Rp)	Rd	Lex	Ca	Ct	Ccau	Cadv	(Comp)	Inc	Inc-T	Error	Error-T
	HAPPENED	Rp	Rd	(Lex)	Ca	Ct	Ccau	Cadv	(Comp)	Inc	Inc-T	Error	Error-T
	HIM	(Rp)	Rd	Lex	Ca	Ct	Ccau	Cadv	(Comp)	Inc	Inc-T	Error	Error-T
14	SO	Rp	Rd	Lex	Ca	Ct	(Ccau)	Cadv	(Comp)	Inc	Inc-T	Error	Error-T
	THEY	(Rp)	Rd	Lex	Ca	Ct	Ccau	Cadv	(Comp)	Inc	Inc-T	Error	Error-T
	OVER	Rp	Rd	(Lex)	Ca	Ct	Ccau	Cadv	(Comp)	Inc	Inc-T	Error	Error-T
15	AND	Rp	Rd	Lex	(Ca)	Ct	Ccau	Cadv	(Comp)	Inc	Inc-T	Error	Error-T
	THEY	(Rp)	Rd	Lex	Ca	Ct	Ccau	Cadv	(Comp)	Inc	Inc-T	Error	Error-T
16	AND	Rp	Rd	Lex	(Ca)	Ct	Ccau	Cadv	(Comp)	Inc	Inc-T	Error	Error-T
	THEY	(Rp)	Rd	Lex	Ca	Ct	Ccau	Cadv	(Comp)	Inc	Inc-T	Error	Error-T
	SEEING	Rp	Rd	(Lex)	Ca	Ct	Ccau	Cadv	(Comp)	Inc	Inc-T	Error	Error-T
	SUPER DUPER	Rp	Rd	(Lex)	Ca	Ct	Ccau	Cadv	(Comp)	Inc	Inc-T	Error	Error-T
	THE (CAR)	Rp	(Rd)	Lex	Ca	Ct	Ccau	Cadv	(Comp)	Inc	Inc-T	Error	Error-T
17	BUT	Rp	Rd	Lex	Ca	Ct	Ccau	(Cadv)	(Comp)	Inc	Inc-T	Error	Error-T
	HE	(Rp)	Rd	Lex	Ca	Ct	Ccau	Cadv	(Comp)	Inc	Inc-T	Error	Error-T
18	AND	Rp	Rd	Lex	(Ca)	Ct	Ccau	Cadv	(Comp)	Inc	Inc-T	Error	Error-T
	THEY	(Rp)	Rd	Lex	Ca	Ct	Ccau	Cadv	(Comp)	Inc	Inc-T	Error	Error-T
	LEFT	Rp	Rd	(Lex)	Ca	Ct	Ccau	Cadv	Comp	(Inc)	Inc-T	Error	Error-T

continues

Exhibit 4–2 continued

T-U #	Item (Word)	COHESIVE MARKER TYPE	COHESIVE ADEQUACY
19	AND	Rp Rd Lex **(Ca)** Ct Ccau Cadv	**(Comp)** Inc Inc-T Error Error-T
	THEY	**(Rp)** Rd Lex Ca Ct Ccau Cadv	**(Comp)** Inc Inc-T Error Error-T
	HELPED	Rp Rd **(Lex)** Ca Ct Ccau Cadv	**(Comp)** Inc Inc-T Error Error-T
	HIM	**(Rp)** Rd Lex Ca Ct Ccau Cadv	**(Comp)** Inc Inc-T Error Error-T
	OUT	Rp Rd **(Lex)** Ca Ct Ccau Cadv	**(Comp)** Inc Inc-T Error Error-T
20	THEY	**(Rp)** Rd Lex Ca Ct Ccau Cadv	**(Comp)** Inc Inc-T Error Error-T
	HIM	**(Rp)** Rd Lex Ca Ct Ccau Cadv	**(Comp)** Inc Inc-T Error Error-T
	THEY	**(Rp)** Rd Lex Ca Ct Ccau Cadv	**(Comp)** Inc Inc-T Error Error-T
	HE	**(Rp)** Rd Lex Ca Ct Ccau Cadv	**(Comp)** Inc Inc-T Error Error-T
	THE (CAR)	Rp **(Rd)** Lex Ca Ct Ccau Cadv	**(Comp)** Inc Inc-T Error Error-T
21	SO	Rp Rd Lex Ca Ct **(Ccau)** Cadv	**(Comp)** Inc Inc-T Error Error-T
	THEY	**(Rp)** Rd Lex Ca Ct Ccau Cadv	**(Comp)** Inc Inc-T Error Error-T
	THE (CAR)	Rp **(Rd)** Lex Ca Ct Ccau Cadv	**(Comp)** Inc Inc-T Error Error-T
	OUT	Rp Rd **(Lex)** Ca Ct Ccau Cadv	**(Comp)** Inc Inc-T Error Error-T
	THE (HORSE)	Rp **(Rd)** Lex Ca Ct Ccau Cadv	Comp **(Inc)** Inc-T Error Error-T
22	AND	Rp Rd Lex **(Ca)** Ct Ccau Cadv	**(Comp)** Inc Inc-T Error Error-T
	THEY	**(Rp)** Rd Lex Ca Ct Ccau Cadv	**(Comp)** Inc Inc-T Error Error-T
	BROUGHT	Rp Rd **(Lex)** Ca Ct Ccau Cadv	**(Comp)** Inc Inc-T Error Error-T
	HIM	**(Rp)** Rd Lex Ca Ct Ccau Cadv	**(Comp)** Inc Inc-T Error Error-T
23	AND	Rp Rd Lex **(Ca)** Ct Ccau Cadv	**(Comp)** Inc Inc-T Error Error-T
	HIS	**(Rp)** Rd Lex Ca Ct Ccau Cadv	Comp Inc Inc-T **(Error)** Error-T
	THE	Rp **(Rd)** Lex Ca Ct Ccau Cadv	**(Comp)** Inc Inc-T Error Error-T
24	AND	Rp Rd Lex **(Ca)** Ct Ccau Cadv	**(Comp)** Inc Inc-T Error Error-T
	SUPER DUPER	Rp Rd **(Lex)** Ca Ct Ccau Cadv	**(Comp)** Inc Inc-T Error Error-T
	THEM	**(Rp)** Rd Lex Ca Ct Ccau Cadv	**(Comp)** Inc Inc-T Error Error-T
25	AND	Rp Rd Lex **(Ca)** Ct Ccau Cadv	**(Comp)** Inc Inc-T Error Error-T
	HE	**(Rp)** Rd Lex Ca Ct Ccau Cadv	**(Comp)** Inc Inc-T Error Error-T

The application of our definition of a cohesive marker has resulted in the reduced incidence of distinctions made within the lexical category (i.e., repetition and reiteration; see Exhibit 4–1). It was not found to be practical to attempt to make these distinctions reliably. Therefore, all instances of lexical cohesion have been combined into a single category in our procedure.

ASSESSING THE ADEQUACY OF TIES ACROSS SENTENCES

Thus far, we have described the identification of the cohesive markers in the text and their linguistic classification. The third and final major step is the description of how well these markers have met the criterion for "adequate" cohesion (i.e., the cohesion that the listener might expect the speaker to provide in a well-organized, ideal or perfect narrative). See Exhibit 4–1 for definitions of complete, incomplete, and erroneous ties.

Adequate Tying

If the referent for the item is easily found and defined with no ambiguity, judge the item as "complete" (C).

Less-Than-Adequate Tying Attempts

If the attempted tie is not adequate (i.e., not "complete") and if it deviates from a clear, unambiguous relationship between cohesive marker and text, it may be classified in one of the following four ways: "incomplete" (Inc), "error" (E), "incomplete-tie" (Inc-T), or "error-tie" (E-T).

Incomplete (Inc)

To be classified as incomplete, the cohesive marker must refer to information that is not provided in the text.

> *Example:* Two boys went to see a movie. They saw *his* car parked in front.

In this example, the speaker had not provided the information (i.e., whose car) but used the personal reference *his*, cueing the reader to recover the information outside the sentence. The personal reference *his* would be judged as incomplete (Inc). The use of an incomplete reference is interpreted to mean that while the speaker is referring to something (and thus may "remember" the person or event), he or she is not sufficiently semantically organized to include this information in narrative production. Examples of incomplete tying attempts for each type of cohesion are provided in Exhibit 4–3.

Error

In addition to incomplete tying attempts, cohesive "errors" can also be produced by the speaker. These "erroneous" attempts at tying (E) are distinct from incomplete attempts in the following ways.

An item is judged as a cohesive error if the listener or reader is guided to ambiguous information.

> *Example:* Homer and Freddie went to the movie. *He* enjoyed it very much.

An item is also judged as an error if the referent leads the reader to wrong information. Naturally, the examiner must know the text to make this judgment.

Conjunctions are a special case of errors. Since one cannot reliably judge them as incomplete, all conjunctions that are not completely adequate are judged to be errors. Accordingly, if the ideas or messages presented in the two conjoined sentences are unrelated or are joined by an inappropriate conjunction, judge the conjunction as an "erroneous" marker (E).

> *Example:* Homer and Freddie went to the movie. *But* he enjoyed it very much.

Given the content of the sentences, the use of the conjunction *but* is inappropriate and leads the recipient to misinterpret the meaning relations between the sentences.

Exhibit 4–3 Examples of Incomplete Tying Attempts for Each Type of Cohesion

---

- *Reference*
  1. Personal reference

     Example: Two boys went to see a movie. They saw *his* car parked in front.

  2. Demonstrative reference

     Example: Two boys read some comics. Then they saw *the* movie.

     The reader would not know what movie was being referred to.

  3. Comparative reference

     Example: They played horseshoes. The *other* boy went home.

     The reader does not know who went home.

- *Conjunctions*

  Conjunctions are not judged as incomplete. Such judgments are not reliable across examiners. This rule is consistent with the rationale that this procedure describes rather than explains. Judging a conjunction as incomplete implies that the speaker omitted information between sentences and leads the examiner to "guess" about what the speaker is thinking. Under these circumstances, interscorer reliability is reduced substantially.

- *Lexical*
  1. Proper names: Proper names may be judged incomplete if the character is not properly introduced in the text.

     Example: Super Duper drove by fast.

     If the speaker has not indicated the role of Super Duper in the text, the item is judged as incomplete. This is another instance of how this procedure deviates from Halliday and Hasan's (1976) description. They do not view proper names as part of the cohesive description.

  2. Other lexical items referring to persons or events left unsaid.

     Example: The boys were reading. Homer said, "He always does the same *thing*."

     In this case, *thing* is referring to the action done by the character being read about. Since the actions were not described in the text, *thing* would be judged as an incomplete (Inc) lexical marker.

Cohesive markers tied to previous items (Inc-T) (E-T). In addition to initially incomplete and erroneous tying attempts, there are cohesive ties that continue these initially inadequate attempts. That is, the speaker does not repair the damage to the text that has been introduced by the omission of information or by ambiguous or wrong information. Thus, the incomplete is left incomplete, and the error is continued. In these cases, the cohesive form is intact: that is, the listener can follow the referents sentence by sentence, but the initial attempt is not corrected. Thus, in addition to the inadequate cohesive attempts scored as incomplete (Inc) and error (E), there are incomplete ties (Inc-T) and error-ties (E-T). The following description will clarify these latter two types of inadequate tying.

Incomplete-Tie (Inc-T) is a cohesive marker tied to items previously judged as incomplete. In this case there is adequate cohesion but a continued lack of information.

> *Example:* They saw *Super Duper's* car. *He* went fast.

In the first sentence, *Super Duper* was judged as an incomplete lexical marker since there is no introduction in the text. In the second sentence, *he* is tied to *Super Duper*. While we know that *he* refers to *Super Duper*, we still do not know who *Super Duper* is. Therefore, we judge *he* as an incomplete-tie (Inc-T) rather than just incomplete (Inc). Additional examples follow.

> *Example: The* boys went to a movie. *They* enjoyed it.

In this case, *they* refers to *boys*. In the first sentence, *the* (demonstrative reference) is judged incomplete since the reader does not know who *the boys* are. In the second sentence, the personal reference *they* refers to *boys*, but the reader still does not know who *the boys* are. *They* is judged to be an incomplete-tie (Inc-T), rather than as complete (C) or incomplete (Inc).

Another instance of the incomplete tie is reference to more than one referent, with one being complete and the other being incomplete.

> *Example:* A large German Shepherd jumped at *him*. Then *they* were hit by a car.

Him is judged as incomplete, *They* refers to both *German Shepherd* and *him*. Therefore, the personal reference *they* directs the reader to more than one referent. If, as in the preceding sentence, one referent has been judged as complete (*German Shepherd* did not require the listener to go outside the sentence) but the other has been judged as incomplete (*him*), the plural reference *they* is an incomplete-tie (Inc-T) rather than an incomplete (Inc). That is, the reader knows who or what is being referred to, but some information is still unknown.

Error-Tie (E-T) is a cohesive marker tied to items previously judged as errors. In this case, there is adequate cohesive form but a continuation of the initial error. For example:

> *Example:* Homer and Freddie went to the movie.
> *He* enjoyed it very much.
> Afterwards, *he* drove home in the wagon.

The error in the second sentence results in the reader's not knowing which boy enjoyed the movie. The confusion is continued into the third sentence: that is, the reader still does not know which boy drove home in the wagon. To the extent that this confusion continues in the text, the reader may remain in a quandary, even though the cohesive form, sentence by sentence, is adequate. *He* is an error-tie (E-T).

SCORING COHESION

Once the analysis of cohesion has been completed for a given text or discourse sample, the examiner may choose to compile some numbers to further objectify the indices of an individual's cohesion skills. Examples of such tallies are

- number of cohesive ties divided by the number of "complete" ties
- percentage of error ties
- percentage of incomplete ties

Any number of such scores may be derived once the basic analysis has been completed, and which "score" is eventually used to report an individual's performance will depend on what the examiner finds useful.

CONCLUSION

We have found these procedures to be useful and reliable in quantifying the language-impaired individual's ability to organize a cohesive text. We would caution that the procedures have not been standardized on nonimpaired individuals but rather have always been used as a research tool with a control group or as a criterion-based assessment over time. Because of the pragmatic nature of textual cohesion, it is doubtful that this ability can be predicted across all texts regardless of content or elicitation method. For this reason, the most appropriate clinical application would be in the assessment and management of clients over a fairly substantial time period.

In the Appendixes, a variety of discourse samples have been provided for further practice. For many of these samples, cohesion analyses have been completed. The reader may want to practice on copies of the blank cohesion analysis form provided in Appendix 4–A, or review these samples for additional experience with cohesion analyses.

REFERENCES

Coelho, C.A., Liles, B.Z., & Duffy, R.J. (1991). Discourse analysis with closed head injured adults: Evidence for differing patterns of deficits. *Archives of Physical Medicine and Rehabilitation, 72*, 465–468.

Coelho, C.A., Liles, B.Z., & Duffy, R. (1995). Impairment of discourse abilities and executive function in traumatically brain injured adults. *Brain Injury, 5*, 471–477.

Halliday, M.A.K., & Hasan, R. (1976). *Cohesion in English.* London: Longman.

Lee, L. (1974) *Developmental sentence analysis.* Evanston, IL: Northwestern University Press.

Liles, B.Z. (1985). Narrative ability in normal and language disordered children. *Journal of Speech and Hearing Research, 28*, 123–133.

Liles, B.Z. (1987). Episode organization and cohesive conjunctives in narratives of children with and without language disorder. *Journal of Speech and Hearing Research, 30*, 185–196.

Liles, B.Z. (1993). Narrative discourse in children with language disorders and children with normal language: A critical review of the literature. *Journal of Speech and Hearing Research, 36*, 869–882.

Liles, B.Z., Coelho, C.A., Duffy, R.J., & Zalagens, M.R. (1989). Effects of elicitation procedures on the narratives of normal and closed head-injured adults. *Journal of Speech and Hearing Disorders, 54,* 356–366.

Mentis, M., & Prutting, C.A. (1987). Cohesion in the discourse of normal and head-injured adults. *Journal of Speech and Hearing Research, 30*, 88–98.

Sample Cohesion Form

SUBJ ID _____TASK_____ SCORED BY _____ DATE_____   Page_____

T-U # Item (Word)	COHESIVE MARKER TYPE							COHESIVE ADEQUACY				
	Rp	Rd	Lex	Ca	Ct	Ccau	Cadv	Comp	Inc	Inc-T	Error	Error-T
	Rp	Rd	Lex	Ca	Ct	Ccau	Cadv	Comp	Inc	Inc-T	Error	Error-T
	Rp	Rd	Lex	Ca	Ct	Ccau	Cadv	Comp	Inc	Inc-T	Error	Error-T
	Rp	Rd	Lex	Ca	Ct	Ccau	Cadv	Comp	Inc	Inc-T	Error	Error-T
	Rp	Rd	Lex	Ca	Ct	Ccau	Cadv	Comp	Inc	Inc-T	Error	Error-T
	Rp	Rd	Lex	Ca	Ct	Ccau	Cadv	Comp	Inc	Inc-T	Error	Error-T
	Rp	Rd	Lex	Ca	Ct	Ccau	Cadv	Comp	Inc	Inc-T	Error	Error-T
	Rp	Rd	Lex	Ca	Ct	Ccau	Cadv	Comp	Inc	Inc-T	Error	Error-T
	Rp	Rd	Lex	Ca	Ct	Ccau	Cadv	Comp	Inc	Inc-T	Error	Error-T
	Rp	Rd	Lex	Ca	Ct	Ccau	Cadv	Comp	Inc	Inc-T	Error	Error-T
	Rp	Rd	Lex	Ca	Ct	Ccau	Cadv	Comp	Inc	Inc-T	Error	Error-T
	Rp	Rd	Lex	Ca	Ct	Ccau	Cadv	Comp	Inc	Inc-T	Error	Error-T
	Rp	Rd	Lex	Ca	Ct	Ccau	Cadv	Comp	Inc	Inc-T	Error	Error-T
	Rp	Rd	Lex	Ca	Ct	Ccau	Cadv	Comp	Inc	Inc-T	Error	Error-T
	Rp	Rd	Lex	Ca	Ct	Ccau	Cadv	Comp	Inc	Inc-T	Error	Error-T
	Rp	Rd	Lex	Ca	Ct	Ccau	Cadv	Comp	Inc	Inc-T	Error	Error-T
	Rp	Rd	Lex	Ca	Ct	Ccau	Cadv	Comp	Inc	Inc-T	Error	Error-T
	Rp	Rd	Lex	Ca	Ct	Ccau	Cadv	Comp	Inc	Inc-T	Error	Error-T
	Rp	Rd	Lex	Ca	Ct	Ccau	Cadv	Comp	Inc	Inc-T	Error	Error-T
	Rp	Rd	Lex	Ca	Ct	Ccau	Cadv	Comp	Inc	Inc-T	Error	Error-T
	Rp	Rd	Lex	Ca	Ct	Ccau	Cadv	Comp	Inc	Inc-T	Error	Error-T
	Rp	Rd	Lex	Ca	Ct	Ccau	Cadv	Comp	Inc	Inc-T	Error	Error-T

CHAPTER 5

Information Analyses

Barbara B. Shadden

It can be and has been argued that the amount of information communicated and the efficiency of communication of information are among the most important indices of successful discourse production. Most definitions of information and/or informativeness relate to units of analysis that are relevant, truthful, nonredundant, and/or reflective of plausible inference. While the idea of communication as being characterized by transmission of information is comparatively old, the concept of measuring this transmission process is much newer. Since the late 1970s, a proliferation of research and clinical approaches to information measurement has followed seminal work regarding content units (Myers, 1979; Yorkston & Beukelman, 1980), thematic units (Gleason et al., 1980), and propositions (Ulatowska, North, & Macaluso-Haynes, 1981). This chapter will provide an overview of some of the literature approaches to measurement of information content and efficiency in discourse. However, the clinician should first be made aware of some of the theoretical and practical analysis issues involved in this process.

MEASUREMENT OF INFORMATION: THEORETICAL ISSUES AND PRACTICAL DIFFERENCES

Aspects of Information

Measurement of informativeness in discourse production has focused on three main aspects of the process of information dissemination. First, some approaches have addressed primarily the *amount of information* that is being communicated. In this context, there is an implied assumption that certain elements of information in a particular task are necessary and/or appropriate in relationship to normal discourse behavior. However, more recently, there have been attempts to break away from task-dependent information indices toward measures that tally informativeness at a more basic and universal level (e.g., correct information units [CIUs]; Nicholas & Brookshire, 1993a, described later in this chapter).

Second, in recognition of the tendency of many neurologically impaired patients to produce information that is not necessary or appropriate but is distinctive to a particular disorder, some researchers and clinicians have advocated information analysis systems that address not only amount but also *quality of information* being communicated. A number of analysis procedures described in this chapter consider information that is defined by descriptors such as *irrelevant, redundant, off topic,* and *overly personalized.* The concept of quality of information is particularly useful in characterizing certain clinical populations whose discourse behaviors are qualitatively different but whose characteristics elude clear definition with traditional linguistically based measures.

Third, for neurogenic populations, *efficiency* or *conciseness* of information behaviors is a critical issue. The right-brain–damaged patient who manages to produce most essential information eventually but who succeeds in this process only after production of many qualitatively nonfocused comments can be described as lacking efficiency in the formulation and delivery of the discourse message. Clear definition of the nature of the nonessential information produced may provide useful directions for treatment. Similarly, the aphasic individual who shows some reduction in information content (with respect to quantity) may evidence an even greater deficit in efficiency, given the delays, errors, and general effortfulness of productions.

Measurement Approaches

Given these three broad domains that can be considered in measuring the informativeness of a discourse sample, it is not surprising that various information analysis systems differ from each other on a variety of dimensions. Some of the more important differences across approaches are noted here.

• Information analysis systems can be categorized as having *a priori* or *a posteriori measurement approaches*. The simplest way of measuring information content, at least with respect to information that is deemed somehow essential or relevant to the task, is to define a priori the information elements that should be present (and that are present in a sufficient number of non–brain-damaged speakers). This type of approach allows the individual client to be compared to some normative expectations and also permits cross-client and even cross-disorder comparisons. The disadvantages of the a priori approach are related to the fact that the measure is irretrievably linked to the specific task. Thus, novel discourse tasks and spontaneously generated behaviors are less readily measured for information content. Examples of a priori information content measures are content units (Yorkston & Beukelman, 1980) and essential content units (Nicholas, Obler, Albert, & Helm-Estabrooks, 1985) for the Cookie Theft picture description;

essential steps in a procedural discourse task (Ulatowska, Doyle, Freedman-Stern, & Macaluso-Haynes, 1983); and essential units agreed upon a priori in a story-retelling task (Bayles & Tomoeda, 1991). In contrast, a posteriori measures seek to define a measurement unit and analysis approach that can be applied to a wide range of tasks and behaviors and used to develop computed measures that have meaning across those tasks. The primary recent example of an a posteriori measurement approach is the CIU, as defined by Nicholas and Brookshire (1993a). Elements of Cherney and Canter's (1993) Informational Content Analysis may also be used in an a posteriori fashion. A priori and a posteriori systems, therefore, differ not only in unit of analysis but also in their utility in a variety of discourse contexts.

• *Unit of analysis.* As implied in the previous statements, the *unit of analysis* is one of the most common sources of variance across information analysis approaches. Terms used to define the unit of measurement include *content units* (Myers, 1979; Yorkston & Beukelman, 1980); *essential information units* (Cherney & Canter, 1993; Hier, Hagenlocker, & Shindler, 1985; Nicholas et al., 1985); *propositions* (Ulatowska et al., 1981); *essential and optional steps* (Terrell & Ripich, 1989; Ulatowska et al., 1981; Ulatowska, Doyle et al., 1983); *main concepts* (Nicholas & Brookshire, 1993b, 1995); *target lexemes* and *thematic units* (Gleason et al., 1980); *unscorable* or *nonessential content* (Tompkins et al., 1993; Trupe & Hillis, 1985); *CIUs* (Nicholas & Brookshire, 1993a); and the *entire utterance* (Arbuckle, Gold, Frank, & Motard, 1989). All of these terms will be defined further in this chapter. As can be seen, however, there is considerable variation, and the clinician will have to make appropriate judgments concerning the nature and level of analysis that are appropriate to a given client and or useful in the particular clinical context.

• *Level of analysis.* Although the term *level of analysis* may not be totally appropriate, it is used here to clarify the distinction between systems that serve as simple checklists and counts of information (i.e., the information unit is either present or absent) and systems that further score or describe the remaining discourse sample information that does not qualify as "essential": in other words, whether the system addresses only quantity of information in the form of a checklist or similar device or whether it in some fashion attempts to code and define other qualitative aspects of the communication. This coding of qualitative information can actually be applied to predetermined information units. For example, Myers (1979) took the Yorkston and Beukelman (1980) list of content units for the Cookie Theft picture and further subdivided them into those that were literal versus those that were interpretative, from the perspective of the stimulus and the client. Qualitative analysis can also be applied to discourse content remaining after essential information units of some kind have been accounted for. Systems used by Tompkins et al. (1993), Trupe and Hillis (1985), and Cherney and Canter (1993) are included among those that examine all content in the discourse task.

• *Efficiency.* Finally, information analysis systems differ from each other with respect to whether they attempt to quantify *efficiency* of information communication and how they quantify this element. Approaches taken include measures of information over time, measures of number of language units (words/syllables) per information unit (or the reverse), various rating scales, and global coding of utterance and sample categories. Both considerations of efficiency and of quality relate as much to the informativeness of the message as to the information presented.

Given the considerable diversity in approaches to characterizing information content in discourse productions, a broad sampling of techniques will be presented in this chapter. The methods of analysis presented here have all been derived from the clinical and research literature, and practitioners are encouraged to remain current with the professional literature in order to identify new possibilities for analysis as these emerge in individual studies. In essence, as in the preceding chapters, the clinician is being provided with an eclectic "bag of tricks" from which to select approaches suitable to a given client or specified clinical population. Several recommendations can be made to assist the clinician in using informational analysis effectively, as shown in Exhibit 5–1.

To guide the reader through the intricate maze of information analysis, the next section will illustrate the manner in which measurement of information specifically related to the Cookie Theft picture has evolved over time. Following sections will address additional a priori information content analyses applied to other discourse tasks, followed by a detailed description of a more global approach to Informational Content Analysis. The basic elements of Nicholas and Brookshire's (1993a) correct information unit (CIU) approach will next be outlined as an alternative to the more a priori approaches. The chapter will conclude with a discussion of measures of efficiency of communicating information, and with an exploration of clinical implications.

THE COOKIE THEFT PICTURE

In both the earlier and revised versions of the Boston Diagnostic Aphasia Examination (BDAE; Goodglass & Kaplan, 1972, 1983), the use of the Cookie Theft picture (Goodglass & Kaplan, 1983) to elicit a spontaneous speech sample represented a marked innovation over earlier aphasia test batteries. Responses to this task were scored via a series of subjective rating scales that formed an integral component in the classification of type of aphasia on this test. Not surprisingly, when interest in further analysis of discourse samples emerged in the late 1970s and early 1980s, responses to the Cookie Theft picture description task were an obvious target for researchers and clinicians, since the language material was readily available in many clinical settings. In some respects, this extended focus

Exhibit 5–1 Guidelines in Selecting and Applying Information Analyses to Discourse Samples

1. Be consistent in selecting baseline tasks for subsequent analysis. Using the same discourse tasks repeatedly will assist the clinician to develop a sense for problems in informativeness and will guide decisions about specific analyses.
2. Use multiple discourse tasks as a baseline, even if all tasks are not subjected to specific analysis.
3. Consider the behaviors observed during baseline discourse elicitation and determine subsequent analyses based on preliminary clinical impressions.*
4. Whatever analysis procedures are selected, be certain to include some index of quantity, quality, and informativeness.
5. Be willing to consider developing your own set of a priori information units for a favorite task or stimulus. Also, be creative in considering formulating rating skills that capture aspects of the information behavior of individual clients if none of the procedures in this chapter appear to address a critical aspect of communication.

*Some clinicians will prefer to stay with selected measures and tasks used across all clients in order to become more familiar with and facile at applying the specific analysis procedures and categories. For the more complex and qualitative measures, this is a reasonable clinical strategy. For example, the clinician may wish to administer routinely the Cookie Theft picture description task, and may score content units in a consistent fashion every time this is administered.

upon this particular task is ironic, since picture description is probably one of the least interesting discourse task formats. Picture description demands little formal organization of verbal responses and provides a constant and unvarying visual stimulus. Tracing the progression of informational analyses of responses to this task, however, provides an excellent introduction to the methodology of information analysis. It is assumed that the reader is familiar with the Cookie Theft picture.

Content Unit Analysis

In 1980, Yorkston and Beukelman set out to determine "an objective, reliable, and clinically useful method of sampling and analyzing verbal output of moderate and mildly aphasic speakers" (p. 28). The picture description task involving the BDAE Cookie Theft picture was administered using standard procedures. Words and syllables were counted, and measures of speaking rate were calculated based on syllables per

minute. The marked innovation in this study was the introduction of the idea of content units. A content unit was defined as "a grouping of information that was always expressed as a unit by normal speakers" (Yorkston & Beukelman, 1980, p. 30), and acceptable content units were identified as those mentioned by 78 normal speakers subdivided into a normal adult group aged 19 to 49 years and a normal geriatric group aged 58 to 93 years. Each subject transcript was examined for occurrences of each content unit on this a priori list (see Exhibit 5–2). Major measures of interest were content units, syllables per minute, and content units per minute. The latter two measures were construed as indices of efficiency of communication. The authors reported that number of content units varied inversely (and thus appropriately) with severity of aphasia, although there was some overlap between mild aphasia and normal speakers. More importantly, the two efficiency measures served to distinguish mild aphasic speakers from normal speakers.

Exhibit 5–2 Content Units for Cookie Theft Picture

Mark a line through the actual content units produced by the client. Count each unit only once, even if it is repeated. Do separate tally of interpretive content units only (those marked with asterisk; Myers, 1979). Record numbers below, along with other relevant information.

two	little	*mother	*in kitchen
children	girl	woman (lady)	(indoors)
little	*sister	children behind	*general disaster
boy	standing	standing	statement
*brother	by boy	by sink	lawn
standing	reaching up	*washing (doing)	sidewalk
on stool	*asking for cookie	dishes	house next door
*wobbling (off balance)	finger to mouth	*drying	open window
three-legged	*saying shhh (keep	faucet on	curtains
*falling over	him quiet)	*full blast	
on the floor	*trying to help (not	*ignoring	
*hurt himself	trying to help)	(daydreaming)	
reaching up	*laughing	water	
*taking (stealing)		overflowing	
cookies		onto floor	
*for himself		*feet getting wet	
*for his sister		dirty dishes left	
*from the jar		puddle	
on the high shelf			
in the cupboard			
with the open door			
*handing to sister			

TOTAL NUMBER OF CONTENT UNITS (CUs): _____

NUMBER OF INTERPRETIVE CUs: _____

NUMBER OF WORDS: _____

TIME TO COMPLETE SAMPLE: _____ seconds

WORDS/MIN. _____   SYLLABLES/MIN. _____

CUs/MIN. = Total CUs/No. of Seconds × 60: _____

WORDS/CU: _____

INTERP. CUs/TOTAL CUs × 100: _____

CU Norms—Mean (Standard Deviation) (from Yorkston & Beukelman, 1980)

	CUs	CUs/min.
Adults (aged 19–49 years, mean 31 years)	18 (4.7)	41.9 (13.2)
Older adults (aged 59–93 years, mean 73 years)	14.7 (3.6)	33.7 (13.5)

In Myers' (1979) study, the interpretive content index for normal subjects averaged 49, with a range of 31 to 66.

Source: © American Speech-Language-Hearing Association. Reprinted by permission.

In addition to the normative list of content units in Exhibit 5–2, some of the more useful measures to be derived from this analysis are summarized, along with norms. Words per minute and content units per minute have been added as measures, since they are consistent with other analyses discussed in this chapter. Examples of two Cookie Theft picture responses from one subject (E.B.) with a cerebral tumor are shown in Exhibit 5–3. The samples represent responses from the first session of therapy, and from a session approximately one month later. The Cookie Theft content unit analyses (along with some additional measures) are shown in Exhibits 5–4 and 5–5. As can be seen, at the first testing, this client (aged 54 years) fell at the very bottom end of the appropriate range for number of content units, but considerably below age-appropriate norms in content units per minute. By

the second testing, number of content units fell right at the mean for an age-appropriate control group, and content units per minute had increased, although performance was nowhere near the normative levels expected. The analyses of the Cookie Theft picture description paralleled clinical impressions of improved information communication (more complete information and fewer word retrieval problems) over the course of one month of treatment, with a continuation of effortful speech-language output and reduced speaking rate.

Further Interpretations of Information Content

As soon as the first list of appropriate content units was developed, questions about the quality of information were raised. Myers (1979) reana-

---

Exhibit 5–3 Cookie Theft Picture Descriptions—Client E.B.

Time 1

Well the first thing I notice the sink is running over in floor and the woman seems oblivious of it–doesn't even seem to notice. A window open towards the outside. She washing or drying dishes but something not in order about those dishes. I don't know what that–oh, its just a towel. The children are going to try to get a cookie but the stool is about to fall over and they don't seem to notice that either. I don't, I don't really see anything else.

Time 2 (1 Month Later)

The mother, the mother is washing the dishes and the sink is running over in floor making a terrible mess and she doesn't even seem to be aware of it. I don't know why she dry the dishes, she doesn't have a drainer or anything. And the children, they're sneaking cookies out of the cookie jar, the boy standing on the stool about to fall off and I don't know if girl says "shh" or tell the mother "no, no, he doing it" or whether she saying that she want a cookie to eat. And that's all.

Exhibit 5–4 Content Units for Cookie Theft Picture—Client E.B. (Time 1)

Mark a line through the actual content units produced by the client. Count each unit only once, even if it is repeated. Do separate tally of interpretative content units only (those marked with an asterisk; Myers, 1979). Record numbers below, along with other relevant information.

two	little	*mother	*in kitchen
~~children~~	girl	~~woman~~ (lady)	(indoors)
little	*sister	children behind	~~*general disaster~~
boy	standing	standing	~~statement~~
*brother	by boy	~~by sink~~	lawn
standing	reaching up	*washing (doing)	sidewalk
~~on stool~~	*asking for cookie	~~dishes~~	house next door
*wobbling (off balance)	finger to mouth	*drying	~~open window~~
three-legged	*saying shhh (keep	faucet on	curtains
~~*falling over~~	him quiet)	*full blast	
on the floor	*trying to help (not	*ignoring	
*hurt himself	trying to help)	(daydreaming)	
reaching up	*laughing	water	
*taking (stealing)		~~overflowing~~	
~~cookies~~		~~onto floor~~	
*for himself		*feet getting wet	
*for his sister		dirty dishes left	
*from the jar		puddle	
on the high shelf			
in the cupboard			
with the open door			
*handing to sister			

TOTAL NUMBER OF CONTENT UNITS (CUs): 15

NUMBER OF INTERPRETIVE CUs: 6

NUMBER OF WORDS: 88

TIME TO COMPLETE SAMPLE: 49 seconds

CUs/MIN. = Total CUs/No. of Seconds × 60: 17.1

WORDS/MIN. 107.8   SYLLABLES/MIN. 145.7

WORDS/CU: 5.9

INTERP. CUs/TOTAL CUs × 100 = 40%

CU Norms—Mean (Standard Deviation) (from Yorkston & Beukelman, 1980)

	CUs	CUs/min.
Adults (aged 19–49 years, mean 31 years)	18 (4.7)	41.9 (13.2)
Older adults (aged 59–93 years, mean 73 years)	14.7 (3.6)	33.7 (13.5)

In Myers' (1979) study, the interpretive content index for normal subjects averaged 49, with a range of 31 to 66.

Source: © American Speech-Language-Hearing Association. Reprinted by permission.

Exhibit 5–5 Content Units for Cookie Theft Picture—Client E.B. (Time 2)

Mark a line through the actual content units produced by the client. Count each unit only once, even if it is repeated. Do separate tally of interpretive content units only (those marked with asterisk; Myers, 1979). Record numbers below, along with other relevant information.

two	little	~~*mother~~	*in kitchen
~~children~~	~~girl~~	woman (lady)	(indoors)
little	*sister	children behind	~~*general disaster~~
~~boy~~	standing	standing	~~statement~~
*brother	by boy	~~by sink~~	lawn
~~standing~~	reaching up	~~*washing~~ (doing)	sidewalk
~~on stool~~	~~*asking for cookie~~	~~dishes~~	house next door
*wobbling (off balance)	finger to mouth	*drying	open window
three-legged	~~*saying shhh~~ (keep	faucet on	curtains
~~*falling over~~	him quiet)	*full blast	
on the floor	*trying to help (not	~~*ignoring~~	
*hurt himself	trying to help)	(daydreaming)	
reaching up	*laughing	water	
~~*taking (stealing)~~		~~overflowing~~	
~~cookies~~		~~onto floor~~	
*for himself		*feet getting wet	
*for his sister		dirty dishes left	
~~*from the jar~~		puddle	
on the high shelf			
in the cupboard			
with the open door			
*handing to sister			

TOTAL NUMBER OF CONTENT UNITS (CUs): <u>20</u>

NUMBER OF INTERPRETIVE CUs: <u>10</u>

NUMBER OF WORDS: <u>97</u>

TIME TO COMPLETE SAMPLE: <u>56</u> seconds

CUs/MIN. = Total CUs/No. of Seconds × 60: <u>21.4</u>

WORDS/MIN. <u>103.9</u>   SYLLABLES/MIN. <u>133.9</u>

WORDS/CU: <u>4.85</u>

INTERP. CUs/TOTAL CUs × 100 = <u>50%</u>

CU Norms—Mean (Standard Deviation) (from Yorkston & Beukelman, 1980)

	CUs	*CUs/min.*
Adults (aged 19–49 years, mean 31 years)	18 (4.7)	41.9 (13.2)
Older adults (aged 59–93 years, mean 73 years)	14.7 (3.6)	33.7 (13.5)

In Myers' (1979) study, the interpretive content index for normal subjects averaged 49, with a range of 31 to 66.

Source: © American Speech-Language-Hearing Association. Reprinted by permission.

lyzed the Yorkston and Beukelman (1980) list of content units in order to develop separate coding for units that were viewed as "literal" (meaning clear in isolation, separate from context) or "interpretive" (meaningful only in the context of events in the picture). Myers' intent was to develop a way to further sensitize this analysis to the communicative deficits shown by right-hemisphere patients. Data on normal performance averages and ranges were reported and are summarized on the bottom of Exhibit 5–2, which can also serve as a scoring sheet for this process. The two samples for client E.B. are also analyzed for literal and interpretive content units on Exhibits 5–4 and 5–5. Both initial and final samples showed interpretive content indices within the range of normal subject performance in Myers' study, suggesting appropriate context sensitivity in responding to information available in the picture stimulus.

Other researchers followed closely upon the work of these earlier researchers with the Cookie Theft picture. Many analyses attempted to examine the content of material not included in the content unit lists originally developed. The purpose of these examinations was to characterize other aspects of communication in specific patient populations, including right-hemisphere, traumatically brain-injured, and dementia patients. For example, Trupe and Hillis (1985)

looked at information conveyed in response to the Cookie Theft picture description task and one other task. For content not included in the Yorkston and Beukelman (1980) list, they developed three additional coding categories, which provided an a posteriori means of analysis. These categories are shown in Exhibit 5–6. On the basis of these codes and counts of numbers of a priori content units, they were able to develop five general descriptors of the general communication efficiency of a particular client's verbal output. These descriptors will be explained later in this chapter in the section "Efficiency or Conciseness of Information Communicated."

In a similar fashion, Tompkins et al. (1993) attempted to characterize more precisely the discourse of right-hemisphere–damaged patients by coding "unscorable content" from Cookie Theft picture descriptions in one of three categories: overpersonalization, excessive detail, and value judgments. These coding categories are explained in greater detail in Exhibit 5–6. A final method of analyzing the qualitative aspects of information provided for the Cookie Theft picture is provided in Cherney's (1990) information content analysis and will be discussed later. In all of these examples of ways to consider information units *not* present on any a priori list, the intent is to develop a clinical statement about the

---

Exhibit 5–6 Coding of Unscorable Content on Cookie Theft Picture

Trupe and Hillis (1985)

1. Bizarre or unrelated content
2. Inaccurate but related content
3. Digressive, tangential, unnecessary data

Tompkins et al. (1993)

1. Overpersonalization—in some fashion integrating narrator into story structure or description of events. *Example*: "My mother always dressed nicely like that."

2. Excessive detail—inappropriate focus on tangential or minor elements of stimulus, or use of intensifying descriptors. *Example*: "This picture would be clearer with color, instead of line drawings."

3. Value judgments—judgments of assumed or interpreted intentions, or value judgments of an action. *Example*: "If children were brought up better today, this kind of thing wouldn't happen."

pattern of behaviors, as well as to provide a basis for measuring change over time.

The number of content units developed by Yorkston and Beukelman (1980) for the Cookie Theft picture is extensive. Some authors have pointed out that additional appropriate content units may be needed in some instances, and it has been noted that regional differences may need to be accounted for (Tompkins et al., 1993). More importantly, there was felt to be a need to reduce the longer list to those elements that might be considered "essential information." One such list of eight elements has been developed by Nicholas et al. (1985) and is shown in Exhibit 5–7. An analysis of the presence or absence of these eight elements in the two Cookie Theft picture descriptions by E.B. is shown in Exhibit 5–8. As can be seen, in the initial task performance, E.B. produced seven out of eight essential information elements, or 87.5% success. By Time 2, one month later, she had produced all eight essential information elements. This apparent improvement, although slight, paralleled counts of the Yorkston and Beukelman (1980) content units from Time 1 to Time 2 and represents a rather simple checklist approach to information analysis.

OTHER APPROACHES TO CODING ESSENTIAL UNITS OF INFORMATION

The idea of focusing on some form of a priori–determined essential information units has been approached from a variety of different perspectives by other researchers and clinicians for other tasks. For example, in an attempt to investigate narrative story retelling in aphasic subjects, Gleason et al. (1980) developed a series of sequenced cartoon pictures that provide visual support to a story read by the examiner. For each story, two basic types of information unit were identified a priori by the examiners through consensus agreement and analysis of control group performance. *Target lexemes* were contentive words produced by at least 90% of the normal control group. *Thematic units* were longer elements of connected speech that represented content that was thematically related and central to the story. An example of a story coded for these elements is provided below (target lexemes are in italics, and slashes separate thematic units).

> After her *mother cleaned* up her *room*, / the little girl *couldn't find* her *shoes*, / so she *asked* her mother where she had *put* them.

This idea of some type of main concept being identified a priori for picture description, storytelling tasks, and even procedural discourse tasks has appeared in a number of other studies (see Bayles & Tomoeda, 1991; Hier et al., 1985; Joanette, Goulet, Ska, & Nespoulous, 1986; Nicholas & Brookshire, 1993b, 1995; Ulatowska, Doyle et al., 1983; Ulatowska, Freedman-Stern, Doyle, Macaluso-Haynes, & North, 1983). Ulatowska and colleagues

---

Exhibit 5–7 Essential Information for Cookie Theft Picture Description

1. woman/mother/lady	5. stealing cookies
2. washing/wiping dishes	6. stool tipping/boy falling
3. sink/water overflowing	7. girl/sister
4. boy/kids	8. mother oblivious/not paying attention

Source: © American Speech-Language-Hearing Association. Reprinted by permission.

Exhibit 5–8 Essential Information Analysis of E.B.'s Cookie Theft Picture Descriptions

---

Time 1

                             3   **1**   **8**

Well the first thing I notice the sink is running over in floor and the woman seems oblivious of

                                               2

it–doesn't even seem to notice. A window open towards the outside. She washing or drying

dishes but something not in order about those dishes. I don't know what that–oh, its just a

             4   **5**   **6**

towel. The children are going to try to get a cookie but the stool is about to fall over and they

don't seem to notice that either. I don't, I don't really see anything else.

Time 2 (1 Month Later)

                 1   **2**   **3**

The mother, the mother is washing the dishes and the sink is running over in floor making a

                             8

terrible mess and she doesn't even seem to be aware of it. I don't know why she dry the dishes,

                                   4   **5**

she doesn't have a drainer or anything. And the children, they're sneaking cookies out of the

                         6   **7**

cookie jar, the boy standing on the stool about to fall off and I don't know if girl says "shh" or

tell the mother "no, no, he doing it" or whether she saying that she want a cookie to eat. And

that's all.

Essential Information

Essential Units	Time 1	Time 2
1. woman/mother/lady	X	X
2. washing/wiping dishes	X	X
3. sink/water overflowing	X	X
4. boy/kids	X	X
5. stealing cookies	X	X
6. stool tipping/boy falling	X	X
7. girl/sister		X
8. mother oblivious/not paying attention	X	X
	7/8	8/8

Source: "Essential Information" © American Speech-Language-Hearing Association. Reprinted by permission.

(Ulatowska et al., 1981; Ulatowska, Freedman-Stern, et al., 1983) have worked extensively with the idea of *propositions*. They view the proposition as the most basic unit of information and define it as an idea unit consisting of one predicate and one or more arguments associated with that predicate. This concept of a proposition is particularly useful when dealing with macro-

and superstructural elements of discourse. For example, the Cat Story task from which a sample is provided in Chapters 2 and 3 can be broken down into 15 a priori propositions. A given client's discourse performance on this task can be measured against these propositions as an index of sheer quantity of information. It is also possible to analyze propositions in an a posteriori fashion, following the approach described by Kintsch and van Dijk (1978).

Ulatowska, Doyle et al. (1983) also popularized the use of procedural discourse tasks in assessment. The idea of analyzing a procedural discourse sample for the presence of essential steps determined a priori taps into the idea of recording in a checklist fashion the presence or absence of essential information that should be included in a procedure. Examples of essential steps in four procedural discourse tasks are presented in Exhibit 5–9. Two procedural discourse samples from different clients are shown in Exhibits 5–10 and 5–11, coded for the presence of these essential steps. Once essential steps have been coded, the clinician may wish to proceed with some analysis of optional steps that have also been addressed. The inclusion of optional steps provides a means of looking at elaborative information content and may also be evaluated qualitatively for appropriateness of information.

In story-retelling tasks, essential information units can readily be identified in an a priori fashion. One available story-retelling tasks involves the story about the lady and the lost wallet used in the Arizona Battery for Communication Disorders of Dementia (Bayles & Tomoeda, 1991). A sample of this task from a traumatically brain-injured patient is shown in Exhibit 5–12, along with scoring sequence and information units. As can be seen, this client produced all but one of the major events to be scored and produced those elements in the correct order. In fact, the one element omitted—"She could not pay for her groceries"—might be considered by some to be implied in the statement that her "wallet wasn't there." However, if one examines the 17 informational units deemed appropriate for completeness of retelling, only 10 of the 17 were produced in the sample (59%). Thus, there appears to be a problem in the overall amount of information, even though the basic elements of the story are present.

Similar lists of essential or main information elements can be and have been generated for other tasks. For example, Cherney and Canter (1993) used information from the Verbal Description subtest of the Illinois Test of Psycholinguistic Abilities (Kirk, 1968) to create a list of 33 essential information units for de-

---

Exhibit 5–9 Procedural Discourse Tasks—Essential Steps

Changing a Lightbulb
1. Get something to stand on/climb up.
2. Unscrew old bulb.
3. Screw in new bulb.
4. Turn on electricity to test bulb.

Making a Sandwich
1. Get bread.
2. Get filling ingredients.
3. Put ingredients on bread.
4. Put bread on top/put it together.

Making Scrambled Eggs
1. Get eggs.
2. Break eggs.
3. Mix eggs/bowl.
4. Put eggs in skillet.
5. Cook eggs (mix/fold).
6. Remove eggs from heat/serve/eat eggs.

Shopping in an American Supermarket
1. Get a cart.
2. Go through store (in any fashion).
3. Check out/pay.

Source: Reprinted with permission from H.K. Ulatowska et al., Production of Procedural Discourse in Aphasia, *Brain and Language*, Vol. 18, pp. 315–341, © 1983, Academic Press.

Exhibit 5–10 Procedural Discourse Steps for Changing a Lightbulb (Traumatically Brain-Injured Client)

You first walk into the room and turn the light switch on for the light to go on and the light does not go on. So you turn the light switch back off and then go out <u>get</u> the . . . um . . . lightbulb
(1)
and <u>the ladder to climb up to the lightbulb</u> and return then to the room and . . . um . . . set the
(1)
ladder under the lightbulb so you can get up. And then you <u>climb up</u> the ladder with the lightbulb in
(2) **(3)**
hand or somewhere you can reach it and . . . um . . . <u>unscrew the lightbulb in the socket</u>. <u>Replace it</u>
<u>with another new lightbulb</u>. Then . . . um . . . um . . . climb back down the ladder . . . um . . . and
(4)
then <u>go to the light switch and turn the lightbulb on</u> and return the ladder from where it came from.

Summary: All four essential steps are present. Further analysis would reveal a variety of optional steps that are appropriate to the task but essentially elaborative.

Exhibit 5–11 Procedural Discourse—Steps for Making Scrambled Eggs (Client L.C.)

(2) **(2)** **(2 & 3 continued)**
OK. How to make scrambled eggs. Um, <u>break the egg</u> and <u>stir it in a bowl</u>. <u>Break the eggs in a bowl,</u>
<u>put all eggs in a bowl and stir it and with a spoon or something.</u> Then you, ah, put, ah, ah, some milk
in it, just a little portion of milk. Ah, you start a fire and put in the other pan, heat the pan,
(4) **(all 5)**
and <u>you pour the milk, ah, the liquid egg in the pan.</u> And <u>then you stir it. Don't, don't heat it too</u>
<u>hot and stir it and, and until it kinda form to a solid pieces, a small solid pieces, solid pieces</u>. And
that's about it. Depends on how you like it. (Clinician: True, that's true. OK.) Then you can put some
(6)
pepper and salt on it if you want. (Clinician: OK, anything else?) Anything else? <u>You can eat it.</u>
(Clinician: I just wanted to be sure you were actually through before I started something.) <u>You can eat</u>
more (6)
<u>it, put it on a bowl and put it on a plate and eat it.</u>

Summary: The client produced five out of six essential steps, although there was a fair bit of redundancy and self-editing (which would have been eliminated if preliminary editing for word counts had been done first). The sequence is correct, although her repetitions force her back a step on several occasions. Some elaboration in the form of optional steps is present (e.g., the manner in which the eggs should be cooked, the pepper and salt, the possible ways of serving).

Exhibit 5-12 Lady Story Retelling by Traumatically Brain-Injured Client, with Scoring

Sample

> There was a lady who was shopping. She lost her wallet. When she was going to pay for the goods she found out that her wallet wasn't there . . . that it dropped on the floor. Then she went home and she received a telephone call . . . someone that someone saying they found her wallet.

Sequence of Major Events

She was shopping	+
She lost her wallet	+
She could not pay for her groceries	____
She went home	+
Her wallet was found	+

Information Units

Lady (woman)	+
Was shopping (at the store; went shopping; went to the grocery story)	+
Her wallet (billfold; coin purse)	+
Wallet fell (dropped; lost; lost her purse)	+
Out of her purse (handbag; pocketbook)	____
She did not see it fall (she didn't know it)	____
At the checkout counter (when she went to pay; at the cashiers)	+
No way to pay (she had no money; she didn't have her wallet)	+
Put the groceries away (put the groceries back)	____
Went home to her house (she went back to her house)	+
As she opened the door (when she got home; just as she got inside)	____
Phone rang (she got a call)	+
Little (young)	____
Girl (lass)	____
Told her (said; reported)	+
She found wallet (coin purse; billfold)	+
Lady relieved (happy; delighted; grateful)	____ **10/17**

Source: Reprinted with permission from K.A. Bayles and C.K. Tomoeda, *Arizona Battery for Communication Disorders in Dementia*, Response Record Form pp. 5 & 13, © 1991, Canyonlands Publishing.

scriptions of a nail, button, envelope, and marble. As mentioned earlier, clinicians can and should feel comfortable developing their own a priori lists of essential information elements for specific tasks if none are available in the testing or research literature. However, mechanisms for developing such lists vary from one publication to the next.

In many studies, the manner of selection of critical information elements and of determination of scoring methods has been noted by Nicholas and Brookshire (1993b, 1995) to be somewhat problematic. Not only is it sometimes difficult to replicate procedures, but also the accuracy and completeness with which main concepts are produced are not always considered. In response to these concerns, Nicholas and Brookshire (1993a) developed a systematic procedure for identifying and scoring *main concepts* in discourse. Tasks involved two single picture descriptions, two picture sequence descriptions, and two requests for procedural information. The main-concepts measure was intended to capture the essence or gist of a stimulus or topic.

Discourse samples were first obtained from 20 non–brain-damaged adults and 15 aphasic adults. Ten speech-language pathologists were then provided with rules for writing main-concept statements and, after training, were asked to write lists of main concepts for each task. Those concept statements that were written in a similar form by 7 out of 10 judges were assigned to the main-concept list for that task. The transcripts of the non–brain-damaged adults were reviewed by two scorers, who bracketed the presence of identified main concepts and assigned each concept on the master list to one of five scores or codes: AC—accurate, complete; AI—accurate, incomplete; IN—inaccurate, complete; II—inaccurate, incomplete; and AB—absent.

Main concepts that were present in some form in the transcripts of 14 out of 20 non–brain-damaged subjects were placed on the final list of concept statements for each task. Main concepts typically took the form of a complete statement, such as "The woman (mother) is after the dog" (Nicholas & Brookshire, 1993b, p. 92). Qualitative scoring for main concepts is described in greater detail in Exhibit 5–13.

This systematic approach to developing main-concepts statements for given tasks may be useful to clinicians wishing to develop their own protocols. In addition, Nicholas and Brookshire (1993b) advocated using several of the above descriptive categories to capture qualitative differences between clinical populations in terms of the manner in which they communicate specific main concepts.

Nicholas and Brookshire (1993b, 1995) reported that presence or absence of main concepts did not consistently discriminate aphasic from non–brain-damaged subjects as a single measure. However, best discrimination of subject groups related to accuracy and completeness, with the combined measure of AI plus IN being most useful. Initial assessment of sensitivity of these measures to change over time suggests that improvement in patient performance is associated with increases in the percentage of accurate and complete (AC) main concepts over time.

INFORMATIONAL CONTENT ANALYSIS

Most of these approaches still lend themselves to checklists for analysis, although the scoring of accuracy and completeness in the Nicholas and Brookshire (1993b) main concepts framework adds significant qualitative information. Cherney and Canter (1993) described a system of *Informational Content Analysis* that provides measures of the individual client's ability to convey a variety of types of information. The system is basically an expansion and systematization of the work developed by others. A variety of tasks were used by these authors, including picture description, object description, procedural discourse, and narrative discourse (story retelling). Discourse samples were analyzed according to the following system of information units, and data were combined across measures to obtain quantitative and qualitative profiles of normal, right-hemisphere–damaged, and demented subjects.

Two broad types of *Information Units*, with various subclassifications, are identified in the Cherney and Canter (1993) approach (see Exhibit 5–14). The first type of information involves what they referred to as *Content-Loaded Information Units*. These are elements of information that are truly content laden with respect to the task or stimulus and are further accurate and relevant with respect to the information

Exhibit 5–13 Scoring of Main Concepts (Nicholas and Brookshire, 1993b, 1995)

- AC—accurate, complete: All essential main-concept information is accurate and complete.
- AI—accurate, incomplete: Part of the main-concept information is accurate, but one or more essential elements are missing.
- IN—inaccurate: Part of the essential main-concept information is inaccurate. If other information is missing, it can be noted, but it is not a reliable measure.
- AB—absent: No essential information for the main concept is provided.

communicated. There are two subcategories within this classification. *Essential Information*, as explained in Exhibit 5–14, involves information units determined a priori to be essential to communicating the essence of the discourse tasks. As originally developed by Cherney (1990), these units were derived from the work of previous researchers, but it is possible to use other tasks and a priori designations of critical elements. *Elaborative Units* add relevant information beyond the baseline minimum essential to the task. In most instances, the presence of elaboration is determined by examining the transcript after the task has been completed, and preferably after essential information has been coded.

The second type of information units coded in this system would be *Nonmeaningful Information Units*. Again, there are subtypes of information within this classification: (a) Irrelevant, (b) Redundant, (c) Incorrect, and (d) Off Topic. The relationship to previous systems is apparent in that the nonmeaningful information units provide strong qualitative information about the nature of the discourse and assist in differential diagnosis by examining the inclusion of discourse material not directly germane to the task or stimulus.

In most systems that include analyses based purely on sample content, as opposed to or in addition to information units determined a priori, the most difficult component of the infor-

mation analysis is defining in a consistent fashion the unit of measurement. Although there are no direct guidelines for scoring the nonessential information units, most clinicians will find it surprisingly easy to define intuitively what such a unit should be. Most of the time, the unit resembles the "proposition" defined earlier, at least in the sense that it is an idea unit. However, a prepositional phrase may be viewed as introducing specific codable information, or a noun phrase, particularly when inaccurate, may need to be scored separately. As with many of the analyses discussed in this text, the primary concern is intrajudge reliability. In other words, if the clinician works long enough with a specific system of analysis, particularly using the same discourse elicitation tasks over time, consistency in application of the system evolves, and there is sufficient reliability for comparisons of baseline to mid- and post-treatment measures.

In Informational Content Analysis, the pattern of distribution of information categories is at least as interesting as the actual numbers (percentages or proportions) of each type of measure. Normative pilot data from the Cherney and Canter (1993) study may be used if clinicians are interested in examining the particular percentages of information units within certain categories. However, analysis of the pattern of meaningful versus nonmeaningful information communication is more useful with most clients because it provides a focus for sub-

Exhibit 5–14 Informational Content Analysis (Cherney, 1990; Cherney & Canter, 1993)

Content-Loaded Information Units—Contain Relevant, Nonredundant, Correct Information

1. Essential—relevant information consistent with major details selected a priori for each task.
2. Elaborative—additional relevant information beyond that established a priori.

Non–Meaningful Information Units

1. Irrelevant—information units that are related to the topic but inconsistent with task requirements.
    a. Descriptions of items irrelevant to task—e.g., style of curtains in Cookie Theft picture.
    b. Interpretations and judgments—"It's not common to find someone willing to return a wallet."
    c. Personal comments—"I once had a cat who got stuck in a tree."
    d. Comments about task or to examiner—"What's your best guess?" or "I can't imagine telling people how to make scrambled eggs."
2. Redundant—information units not adding new information but repeating in some fashion previously provided information. *Example:* "The water is overflowing from the sink. *The water is spilling over from the sink.*"
3. Off Topic—Digressions that are unrelated to the topic or task. *Example:* in the story-retelling task about the lost wallet, "This reminds me of what I forgot to buy at the drugstore."
4. Incorrect—Information units that are intended to be accurate in the context of the stimulus or tasks, but that are inconsistent with object or picture stimulus, not included in original story, or not part of performance of a procedure. *Example:* regarding the Cookie Theft picture, "*The man* is getting ready to wash the dishes."

Efficiency Ratio = Number of Essential Units of Information / Total Words $\times$ 100

---

sequent treatment or a basis for identifying change over time.

Examples of Cherney and Canter's (1993) Informational Content Analysis are provided in Exhibit 5–15 for client E.B., whose samples have already been subjected to other analyses. A review of previous examples suggests that E.B. showed an increase in total content units and in essential content units from Time 1 to Time 2 testing but that her overall ratio of literal to interpretive elements was within normal limits. Both samples evidenced some restrictions in the efficiency of communication of information when primarily time-based measures were used. If these same samples are subjected to Informational Content Analysis, the picture of a fair de-

gree of content-laden information remains. However, further information is added that may be relevant to clinical intervention decisions. For example, the proportion of E.B.'s information units that are content laden remains roughly comparable across the two testing intervals, although she produces more total information units in the second session. In fact, with respect to basic information, E.B.'s performance falls within normative ranges from Cherney and Canter's (1993) research. For this predominantly aphasic and verbally apraxic patient, all measures continue to point to the further need for close examination of efficiency (see the next section).

In Exhibit 5–16, there is a sample of a procedural discourse task from a traumatically brain-

Exhibit 5–15 Informational Content Analyses Applied to Cookie Theft Picture Description by E.B.

Time 1

```
                                    ESS                              ESS         ESS
   Well the first thing I notice [the sink is running over in floor] and the [woman] [seems oblivious
         RED                              ELAB                         ESS
of it]-[doesn't even seem to notice]. [A window open towards the outside]. [She washing or drying
              IRR                                 IRR                        ELAB
dishes] [but something not in order about those dishes]. [I don't know what that]-oh, [its just a
        ESS                    ESS                                ESS
towel.] [The children] [are going to try to get a cookie] but [the stool is about to fall over] and
            IRR (?)ᵃ
[they don't seem to notice that either.] I don't, I don't really see anything else.
```

ᵃ Questionable observation, scored as irrelevant because interpretation and judgment are involved.

Summary: A total of 13 information units were produced in this sample, including 7 of the 8 a priori essential (ESS) units and an additional 2 elaborative (ELAB) units, leading to a total of 9 content-laden units, or 69% of the total information units. The remaining information units were either irrelevant (IRR) or redundant (RED).

Time 2 (1 Month Later)

```
      ESS          RED            ESS                       ESS               ELAB
   [The mother,] [the mother] [is washing the dishes] and [the sink is running over] [in floor]
      ELAB                            ESS                            IRR
[making a terrible mess] and [she doesn't even seem to be aware of it]. [I don't know why she dry the
              IRR                              ESS               ESS
dishes,] [she doesn't have a drainer or anything]. And [the children], [they're sneaking cookies] [out
      ELAB                    ESS                       ELAB          ESS
of the cookie jar], [the boy standing on the stool about to fall off] and [I don't know if [girl] says
                  INC (???)ᵃ                              IRR (?)ᵇ
"shh"] or [tell the mother "no, no, he doing it"] or [whether she saying that she want a cookie to

eat]. And that's all.
```

ᵃ No real evidence for this statement (unlike previous one, which might be inferential); could also be scored as irrelevant.

ᵇ Scored as irrelevant, but some might score as elaborative because of inference.

Summary: A total of 17 information units were produced in this sample, including all 8 of the essential (ESS) units and an additional 4 elaborative (ELAB) units, yielding 12/17 or 70.6% content-laden information units. The remaining 5 (29.4%) of the information units were divided among redundant (RED) units, incorrect (INC) units, and/or irrelevant (IRR) units.

Note: Essential information was determined a priori from Nicholas et al. (1985) (see Exhibit 5–7 earlier in this chapter).

injured patient. It is interesting to note that this client also evidences a fairly high level of content information units, and that the irrelevancies present in the sample related to carrying the designated task "too far" with respect to providing information about serving the sandwich to a presumed guest. In fact, the entire first (unscored) portion of the sample is a run-on irrelevancy, since the task directions appear to have been misunderstood. Although this section of the discourse task was not scored here with respect to Informational Content Analysis, it is quite probable that this type of inappropriate task response characterizes the patient's performance in other domains. The clinician should keep in mind that procedural discourse is typically one of the easier discourse forms for neurologically impaired clients to organize.

Data from Informational Content Analysis can be reported and discussed in a variety of ways, as noted in the preceding paragraphs. Measures of interest include the number/percentage of essential units of information produced (in relationship to the essential units defined a priori), the percentage or proportion of each type of information unit to total information units, and indicators of efficiency. The efficiency ratio used by Cherney and Canter (1993) is calculated by dividing the number of essential units of information by the total words and multiplying by 100 (measure adapted from Hier et al., 1985). A summary table can be used to report these measures for diverse samples; it also includes means and range of performance for normal older subjects found in the original study. A blank sample form is provided in Exhibit 5–17.

CORRECT INFORMATION UNITS

As noted at the beginning of this chapter, most approaches to information analysis in discourse production are linked in some fashion to task-dependent units of information determined in an a priori fashion. Even Cherney and Canter's (1993) Informational Content Analysis contains

elements of predetermined information units. In response to some of the constraints identified with these approaches, Nicholas and Brookshire (1993a) have developed a rule-based information scoring system for "quantifying the informativeness of connected speech elicited with a variety of stimuli" (p. 339). The system is called *Correct Information Unit* (CIU) analysis.

The CIU is defined as a word that is "intelligible in context, accurate in relation to the picture(s) or topic, and relevant to and informative about the content of the picture(s) or topic" (Nicholas and Brookshire, 1993a, p. 348). It should be noted that grammatical correctness is not a factor in scoring, since informativeness is not necessarily affected by inaccuracies in this domain. Exhibit 5–18 describes the specific analysis procedures used in the CIU approach. Uniformity of scoring is achieved by specifying a series of analysis steps that can be applied to all samples. For example, introductory or closing comments are routinely excluded, and preliminary word counts follow a process of elimination of unintelligible elements or nonwords. Further elimination of words from the CIU count is accomplished both by reference to the specific definition of the CIU and through a detailed list of criteria for word exclusion.

Two samples from client L.C. are analyzed using the CIU procedures, as shown in Exhibits 5–19 and 5–20. Large X's mark words eliminated for the preliminary word count. Diagonal slashes mark words subsequently eliminated because they did not meet the criteria for CIUs. On the bottom of each sheet, five measures recommended for calculation are provided, along with a time measure for each task. The number of words and number of CIUs are useful primarily in calculations, since one could compare the Nicholas and Brookshire (1993a) normative data for these measures only if one used identical tasks. Only words per minute, CIUs per minute, and percentage of CIUs can be compared across tasks. It is possible, and sometimes desirable, to combine measures across tasks to derive an overall index of informativeness, in terms of both amount

Exhibit 5–16 Informational Content Analysis of "Making a Sandwich" Procedural Discourse (Traumatically Brain-Injured Patient)

Tell me how you go about making a sandwich.

Yes.

How do you make a sandwich?

First one has to decide what type of sandwich you want to have it then if he's going to have it alone or invite other people he has to prepare the table for other people if there are more people coming they have to make a larger quantity and set up the place for the other people who come then when that person comes he sort of serve them the meal then have a nice conversation with that persons and afterwards maybe invite the person to go in the living room and rest.

Note: There is a major problem with this introductory section, since the client appears to have misunderstood the task. If the content were coded here, the reference to the decision about type of sandwich would be considered elaborative, but the rest would be irrelevant, weighting the entire analysis in that domain. It is probably more appropriate to consider only the section after the task request was restated, as transcribed below. Remember that essential units are determined a priori.

Okay, but how would you actually make the sandwich?

                        ELAB   **ESS-1**

  Yes, well [you go to the refrigerator or the cabinet] then [I'd get the bread] let's see [and the

ESS-2   **ELAB**   **ELAB**

mayonnaise] then [I'd go to the side where I make the sandwich]. [I put the bread apart on the cutting

                        ESS-3[a]   **ESS-3**[a]

block] maybe then [put the mayonnaise or the butter on the bread] then [put the meat on top of it] and

                 ESS-3[a]   **ESS-4**

[a piece of lettuce or something on top of the meat] then [put the sandwich the top piece of bread over

                ELAB   **ELAB**   **IRR**   **IRR**

the other bottom piece] then [cut it] and [put it on the plate] and [put a napkin] and [serve it] [with

RED

a napkin] to the person.

[a] All part of one a priori essential unit and counted as one unit in scoring of information units.

Summary: Total of 12 information units (not counting multiple instances of one essential (ESS) unit). All 4 essential units are represented and there are an additional 5 elaborative (ELAB) units, yielding 9/12 content-laden units or 75%. The remaining 25% of information units are either redundant (RED) or irrelevant (IRR) to the described task.

---

of information and efficiency with which information is communicated.

In their preliminary research addressing the reliability, session-to-session stability, and sensitivity of CIU analyses, Nicholas and Brookshire (1993a) used 20 non–brain-damaged adults and 20 adults with aphasia as subjects. Ten connected speech samples were obtained, including single pictures, picture sequences, requests for personal information, and requests for

Exhibit 5–17 Blank Analysis Form for Informational Content Analysis on Multiple Tasks.

Task and Client	% Essential Units to Total Essential	Meaningful Units			Nonmeaningful Units			Efficiency
		% Essential/ Total Units	% Elaborative/ Total Units	% Irrelevant/ Total Units	% Redundant/ Total Units	% Inaccurate/ Total Units	% Off Topic/ Total Units	
All Tasks Combined								
Normative Data from Cherney & Canter (1993)		40 to 78 Mean = 54	10 to 33 Mean = 20.5	7 to 38 Mean = 22.4	0 to 6 Mean = 3	0 to 1 Mean = 0.2	0	4.42 to 13.64 Mean = 8.75

Exhibit 5–18 Correct Information Units—A System for Quantifying the Informativeness of Connected Speech Elicited with a Variety of Stimuli

Specific procedures for Correct Information Unit (CIU) scoring and counting of words are provided in Nicholas and Brookshire (1993a). Only the broad outlines of the approach are described below.

1. First, delete any statements that precede or follow the actual discourse task verbal performance. In other words, one should eliminate comments that suggest a beginning or an ending to the task process and that are grammatically discrete. It is suggested that a line be drawn through these items. They will not be used in any further word counts.

2. Next, count actual words. The primary criterion for counting words is that the words must be intelligible in context to a listener familiar with the picture stimulus or topic. No judgment is made at this point about accuracy, relevance, or informativeness. The main items to be eliminated are nonword fillers and unintelligible words or word fragments. It is suggested that a red X be used to cross out words that will not be considered in the word count. (Rules for word counts are provided in Chapter 2.)

3. Count CIUs. The definition of the CIU is "words that are *intelligible* in context, *accurate* in relation to the picture(s) or topic, and *relevant* to and *informative* about the content of the picture(s) or topic" (Nicholas & Brookshire, 1993a, p. 348). Grammatical correctness is *not* an issue in this CIU count. Only words remaining after Step 2 above can be considered for inclusion as CIUs. (Again, the reader is referred to the article cited here for specific guidelines.)
   Words excluded from CIU counts should be marked by a diagonal penciled slash. Examples of items to be excluded are
   • words that are inaccurate in portraying the picture(s) or topic
   • attempts to correct word or sound errors, except for final version (if it meets CIU criteria)
   • revisions, dead ends, and other incomplete items
   • repetitions of information that do not add significantly to the communication
   • first examples of pronouns when the referent is ambiguous
   • nonspecific, empty terms without clear referent
   • conjunctive words and phrases if used to continue flow of discourse rather than to provide specific meaningful connections
   • qualifying words or phrases that suggest ambiguity when the picture(s) or topics should be clear
   • word and phrase fillers, interjections, and tag questions that serve no informative function
   • the conjunction *and*
   • comments about the task itself
   • comments about the client's performance on task and/or personal and inappropriate statements

4. Measures that can be obtained include
   • number of words
   • number of CIUs
   • words/minute*
   • CIUs/minute*
   • percentage of CIUs in relationship to total words*

*Items can be compared readily across all types of discourse tasks.

continues

Exhibit 5–18 continues

Nicholas and Brookshire (1993a) have provided some normative data as a reference point for others performing CIU analyses. Since actual counts of number of words and number of CIUs in their study relate to a specific set of discourse samples, only the more readily generalizable measures are provided here. Data provided are taken from the Time 1 sampling of normal subjects.

Measure	M	SD	Range	Cutoff Score[a]
Words per minute	166	22	105–198	131
% of CIUs	86	6	72–93	76
CIUs per minute	143	19	92–175	111

[a]Cutoff scores for "normal performance" were established by using two standard deviations below group mean for a given session.

Source: © American Speech-Language-Hearing Association. Reprinted by permission.

Exhibit 5–19 CIU Analysis of L.C.'s Narrative Cat Story

OK, there was a little girl. She was crying to her dad. She said, "Well, my cat on the tree and I can't get her off the tree." And so her dad said, "Well." And he decided he's gonna get that cat for her. So he start climbing the tree and so he climbed to the top on the branch where the cat was and so he swing his, his arms and try to catch the cat. And the cat jump, the cat jump off, jumped off the, tree on . . . and, the dad end up hanging on the branch while he was trying to catch the cat. And the girl start crying again and the police, because her dad was hanging on a tree branch with a cloth and the branch caught his, the back of his collar. And the, the fire, the fireman, I guess that's a fireman, and he was trying to rescue him.

Words	158
Time (sec.)	80
CIUs	124
Words/min.	118.5
% CIUs	78.4
CIUs/min.	93

Exhibit 5–20 CIU Analysis of L.C.'s Procedural Discourse on How To Use an American Supermarket

What to do. OK, when you walk into walk into the door, walk in the door, and there's[2] a person in the door and give you a shopping cart, and so you push this shopping cart and walk around the store and decide what you want and you just pick whatever you needed and put in the bag, in the cart. And after you selected all the items you needed and go to the, uh, [XXX]* cash register line and and then you just, uh, put all things on the uh table and check all things through the machine. And then they open the sacks, put them in the sacks for you, and sometimes you have to put in sacks by yourself, depends on where you are going. Most time they'll[2] put in the sacks for you. Uh, uh then you just pay them in a check or money, cash. And then push the cart out in the car and put in your trunk. And that's all.

⟵—————— *Repeat*

(Clinician: OK, then you're ready to go.) Then you're ready to go. Push the cart back or you can put it in, in the little lot, they have a lot where they keep the carts.

*Unintelligible utterance.

Words	180
Time (sec.)	88
CIUs	145
Words/min.	122.7
% CIUs	80.6
CIUs/min.	98.9

procedural information. Results of various data analyses suggest that informativeness of connected discourse can be scored reliably. In addition, session-to-session stability was high, particularly for the three calculated measures of words per minute, CIUs per minute, and percentage of CIUs, with the first session demonstrating sufficient stability to warrant use as a baseline performance index. Discriminative power of the CIU measures, particularly the three calculated measures just listed, was good in differentiating connected speech of non–brain-damaged from aphasic adults. The most consistent discriminator was CIUs per minute. However, words per minute and percentage of CIUs were identified as contributing important information about rate and informativeness of performance, yielding a composite index of efficiency. Normative data from Session 1 for the non–brain-damaged adults are provided in Exhibit 5–18 for CIUs per minute, words per minute, and percentage of CIUs, along with indicators of cutoff scores for normal performance (see Nicholas and Brookshire, 1993a, for comparable data for other sessions).

CIU analyses for client L.C. on two discourse measures are shown at the bottom of Exhibits 5–19 and 5–20. Measures can be compared to the Nicholas and Brookshire norms. Results might be reported as follows.

Correct information unit analysis was performed on two discourse samples from L.C. The first sample was a procedural discourse task, and the second was a narrative storytelling task based on sequenced cartoon pictures. The Supermarket procedural task and Cat Story narrative discourse were roughly comparable in words per minute, CIUs per minute, and percentage of CIUs. Although many of L.C.'s scores fell within the lowest part of the normal range for non–brain-damaged subjects in the Nicholas and Brookshire (1993a) research, scores for all tasks and for combined tasks fell below the cutoff scores established for normal performance on efficiency measures (words per minute and CIUs per minute). The percentage of CIUs scores fell above the cutoff score for normal performance. These results are interpreted as suggesting that L.C. is experiencing greater difficulty with rate of communicating information than with general informativeness, as evidenced by below-normal scores in efficiency measures that are rate dependent.

In their preliminary research with CIU analysis, Brookshire and Nicholas (1993) evaluated the degree to which the discourse samples used in their work were representative of word choice patterns seen in normal adult-to-adult conversations. The procedures used for this evaluation are those described by Hayes (1988, 1989) and noted briefly in Chapter 3. In general, Brookshire and Nicholas (1993) reported that word choice patterns for non–brain-damaged subjects in the discourse study paralleled those used in adult-to-adult conversation apart from a greater reliance on the five most common word types (particularly *and*).

After the initiation of research with the CIU analysis procedures, Nicholas and Brookshire (1993b) recognized that the CIU system does not provide any mechanism for assigning a value to the relative importance or centrality of information being communicated, only the overall informativeness. Using main concepts for given tasks to identify essential information is the approach that they have developed to capture these additional critical data. Main concepts were described earlier in this chapter. They represent a priori information chunks. Nicholas and Brookshire (1993a, 1993b) recommended combining CIU analyses with main-concept scoring to develop an appropriate profile of information production in connected discourse.

EFFICIENCY OR CONCISENESS OF INFORMATION COMMUNICATED

At the beginning of this chapter, it was stated that approaches to examining informativeness in discourse have focused on (a) amount of information, (b) quality of information, and (c) efficiency of information communication. Although the preceding sections have emphasized the quantity and quality of information, many of the analyses suggested here have also addressed some version of the concept of efficiency or conciseness. In essence, *efficiency* implies consideration of either length or time of sample in relationship to the information communicated. For many clients, some measure of efficiency will be essential to capture the quality of their spontaneous communications.

Quantity or Rate of Information Output

Some authors advocate simple measures of speaking rate as an important variable reflecting the speed with which language information is communicated (Cherney, 1990; Yorkston & Beukelman, 1980). Measures of overall speaking rate may be particularly significant in distinguishing between clinical populations when rate determinations are coupled with other indicators of information content.

Examples of previously mentioned efficiency measures that specifically relate information content to overall quantity or rate of output are Yorkston and Beukelman's (1980) measure of content units per minute, Gleason et al.'s (1980) measure of overall language output (words/story), Nicholas and Brookshire's (1993a) measures of CIUs per minute and percentage of CIUs, and Cherney and Canter's (1993) efficiency ratio.

Arbuckle et al. (1989) suggested a variant upon some of these measures. Specifically, they recommended exploring the number of content elements (e.g., content units in response to the Cookie Theft picture) produced during the first 50 words of the discourse response as compared with the entire sample. This type of analysis provides an index of whether the person is producing most of his or her critical information in a focused fashion early in the discourse sample, regardless of the length of the sample that continues after this point. Clients with varying linguistic strategies for communication of information could be distinguished in this fashion (see Exhibit 5–21).

Verbosity and Related Measures

Some clinicians and researchers have developed various forms of rating scales to capture more general perceptions of verbosity or taciturnity in speech output. For example, Gold, Andres, Arbuckle, and Schwartzman (1988) have explored the dimension of verbosity by focusing on what they term "off-target verbosity." Off-target verbosity is distinguished from simple talkativeness by its failure to maintain focus on the precipitating stimulus. As a result, the individual producing off-target verbosity may initially respond appropriately to an external stimulus, only to digress further and further through a series of loosely associated recollections into speech output that becomes primarily irrelevant to the conversational context. This concept of off-target verbosity is important both in defining language output and subgroups within the normally aging population and in characterizing certain clinical populations.

In the Gold et al. (1988) approach, interview responses are first scored for *item verbosity*, defined as the number of interview responses in which the subject went off target. Off-target item responses are then scored for *extent verbosity*, using a 5-point Likert scale reflecting the degree of digression from the target topic (see Exhibit 5–21). (In subsequent research, a 9-point Likert scale was used.) Gold et al. (1988) reported being able to reliably distinguish three subgroups of talkers in an older population: (a) extended talkers, (b) controlled talkers, and (c) nontalkers. This concept of rating extent verbosity could be applied readily to the conversational output of certain clinical populations, particularly traumatically brain-injured and right-hemisphere–damaged clients.

Trupe and Hillis (1985) used their data analysis of Cookie Theft picture description responses from right-brain–damaged stroke patients to identify five categories of speakers: those with (a) irrelevant speech, (b) paucity of speech, (c) digressive speech, (d) normal speech, and (e) verbose speech (see Exhibit 5–21). The categories combined consideration of amount of information (total content units) communicated along with efficiency of information communication (syllables per content unit). Categories are described in greater detail in Table 5–1. Clinicians may find this system useful in attaching a descriptive label to picture description output of neurologically impaired patients. The category terms could also be useful in reflecting change over time. For example, if a right-hemisphere–damaged stroke patient shifts over time from the verbose to the normal speech categories, this change may be viewed as clinically significant.

Clinicians are strongly encouraged to consider development of their own rating scales to capture qualitative aspects of information communication that are linked to efficiency of communication. Such scales may be particularly useful in documenting change over time.

Exhibit 5–21 Quantity or Rate of Information Output

Verbosity

(Arbuckle et al., 1989; Gold et al., 1988)

Interview Context

Item Verbosity—number of items on which client goes off target

Extent Verbosity—extent to which client goes off target (on 5-point or 9-point Likert scale)

Constrained Task Context (picture stimuli such as Cookie Theft)
1. Rate patient for item and extent verbosity.
2. Count number of content units (Nicholas et al., 1985) and total words; then calculate words per content unit.
3. Count number of content units in first 50 words.

General Communication Efficiency Classification

(Trupe & Hillis, 1985)

1. **Irrelevant Speech**—few content units and poor efficiency
2. **Paucity of Speech**—few content units and normal efficiency
3. **Digressive Speech**—normal content units and poor efficiency
4. **Normal Speech**—normal content units and normal efficiency
5. **Verbose Speech**—high content units and normal efficiency

---

CLINICAL IMPLICATIONS AND SUMMARY

As noted at the beginning of this chapter, the amount and quality of information communicated and the efficiency with which it is communicated are some of the most important measures to be obtained from discourse analysis. Some of the issues involved in assessment of information content were addressed earlier. Because approaches to analysis vary so extensively, the clinician may find him- or herself overwhelmed at this point. A brief review of the guidelines in Exhibit 5–1 may help refocus the reader.

In Table 5–2, many of the measures described in this chapter are identified in summary fashion, with notation as to the name of the measure; the task(s) to which it can be applied; the a priori or a posteriori nature of the information unit; the extent to which it addresses quantitative, qualitative, and/or efficiency aspects of information; and the use of any form of rating scale or categorical grouping. This table may be useful in clinical decision making.

For example, after obtaining selected discourse measures, the clinician should review all transcripts to develop a subjective impression of the informativeness of the samples and the types of measures that may best capture the person's information output. If a set of discourse samples suggests extremely low verbal output *and* low information, simple quantitative measures of in-

Table 5–1 Classification of Speech Output of Right-Brain–Damaged Patients Based on Amount and Efficiency of Information Communication (Trupe & Hillis, 1985)

Category	Experimental Definition	Amount of Appropriate Information Communicated (CU M and SD)	Efficiency in Syllables per CU (M and SD)
Irrelevant speech	CU < 11 Syllables/ CU > 6.3	Meager (6.2 ± 2.9)	Poor (16.2 ± 13.9)
Paucity of speech	CU < 11 Syllables/ CU < 6.3	Meager (6.8 ± 2.0)	Normal (4.4 ± 1.6)
Digressive speech	CU > 11 Syllables/ CU > 6.3	Normal (15.2 ± 3.2)	Poor (9.6 ± 2.3)
Normal speech	CU > 11 Syllables/ CU < 6.3	Normal (14.5 ± 2.2)	Normal (4.2 ± 1.1)
Verbose speech	CU > 22.7	High (>1 SD above normal mean)	Normal (5.5)

Note: CU, content unit.

formation communicated may be sufficient to establish a baseline, and a priori units may be sufficient. In contrast, if a client is highly verbal but often inappropriate in information content, or if essential information is obscured by other off-target content, the clinician may wish to use a measure that allows for both qualitative and quantitative analyses and that permits some a posteriori analysis of samples. If the clinician requires a mechanism for selecting clients with similar information-based problems for group therapy purposes, procedures that allow for rating or categorization may be helpful and/or qualitative

measures will be essential. Examples throughout this chapter illustrate the different perspectives provided by various analyses and demonstrate the manner in which specific clinical populations require careful selection of information content analysis procedures.

In the Appendixes, a number of discourse samples have been provided for further practice. Some of these samples have been analyzed for information content. The reader may wish to practice on or review these samples for further experience with analyzing information content as well as other types of analyses.

Table 5-2 A Comparison of Information Discourse Analyses

Measure	Task(s)	A Priori	A Posteriori	Quantitative	Qualitative	Efficiency	Rating
Content units (Yorkston & Beukelman, 1980)	Cookie Theft picture	X		X		X	
Content units—literal and interpretive (Myers, 1979)	Cookie Theft picture	X		X	X	X	
Unscorable content (Trupe & Hillis, 1985)	Cookie Theft picture		X	X	X		X
Unscorable content (Tompkins et al, 1993)	Cookie Theft picture		X	X	X		
Essential information (Nicholas et al., 1985)	Cookie Theft picture	X		X		?	
Target lexemes and thematic units (Gleason et al., 1980)	Sequenced picture series for story retelling	X		X		?	
Propositions (Ulatowska et al., 1981)	Narrative discourse	X	?	X			
Essential steps (e.g., Ulatowska et al., 1981; Ulatowska, Doyle et al., 1983)	Procedural discourse	X	(Optional steps can be recorded)	X			
Information units (Bayles & Tomoeda, 1991)	Lady Story retelling—ABCDD	X		X	X (sequence)		
Main concepts (Nicholas & Brookshire, 1993b, 1995)	A range of discourse tasks	X		X	X		
Informational content analysis (Cherney & Canter, 1993)	A range of discourse tasks	X	X	X	X	X	
Correct information units (Nicholas and Brookshire, 1993a)	Any discourse task		X	X		X	
Content units in 1st 50 words (Arbuckle et al., 1989)	Cookie Theft picture	X		X		X	
Off-target verbosity	Interview/conversation	X		X		X	X
Five categories of speech (Trupe & Hillis, 1985)	Cookie Theft picture	X		X	?	X	X

REFERENCES

Arbuckle, T.Y., Gold, D., Frank, I., & Motard, D. (1989, November). *Speech of verbose older adults: How is it different?* Paper presented at the annual meeting of the Gerontological Society of America, Minneapolis.

Bayles, K.A., & Tomoeda, C.K. (1991). *Arizona Battery for Communication Disorders of Dementia.* Tucson, AZ: Canyonlands.

Brookshire, R.H., & Nicholas, L.E. (1993). Word choice in the connected speech of aphasic and non–brain-damaged speakers. *Clinical Aphasiology, 21,* 101–111.

Cherney, L.R. (1990). *Informational content and cohesion in the discourse of patients with probable Alzheimer's disease and patients with right brain damage.* Unpublished doctoral dissertation, Northwestern University.

Cherney, L.R., & Canter, G.J. (1993). Informational content in the discourse of patients with probable Alzheimer's disease and patients with right brain damage. *Clinical Aphasiology, 21,* 123–134.

Gleason, J.B., Goodglass, H., Obler, L., Green, E., Hyde, M.R., & Weintraub, S. (1980). Narrative strategies of aphasic and normal-speaking subjects. *Journal of Speech and Hearing Research, 23,* 370–382.

Gold, D., Andres, D., Arbuckle, T., & Schwartzman, A. (1988). Measurement and correlates of verbosity in elderly people. *Journal of Gerontology, 43,* P27–P34.

Goodglass, H. & Kaplan, E. (1972). *The Boston Diagnostic Aphasia Examination.* Boston: Lea & Febiger.

Goodglass, H., & Kaplan, E. (1983). *The Boston Diagnostic Aphasia Examination* (2nd ed.). Boston: Lea & Febiger.

Hayes, D.P. (1988). Speaking and writing: Distinct patterns of word choice. *Journal of Memory and Language, 27,* 572–585.

Hayes, D.P. (1989). *Guide to lexical analysis of texts* (Tech. Rep. Ser. 89–96). Ithaca, NY: Cornell University, Department of Sociology.

Hier, D.B., Hagenlocker, K., & Shindler, A.G. (1985). Language disintegration in dementia. *Brain and Language, 25,* 117–133.

Joanette, Y., Goulet, P., Ska, B., & Nespoulous, J. (1986). Information content of narrative discourse in right-brain-damaged right-handers. *Brain and Language, 29,* 81–105.

Kintsch, W., & van Dijk, T.A. (1978). Toward a model of text comprehension and text production. *Psychological Review, 85,* 363–394.

Kirk, S.A. (1968). Illinois Test of Psycholinguistic Abilities: Its origin and implications. In J. Hellmurth (Ed.), *Learning disorders* (Vol. 3, pp. 395–427). Seattle, WA: Special Child Publications.

Myers, P.S. (1979). Profiles of communication deficits in patients with right cerebral hemisphere damage. In R.H. Brookshire (Ed.), *Clinical aphasiology conference proceedings* (pp. 38–46). Minneapolis: BRK.

Nicholas, L.E., & Brookshire, R.H. (1993a). A system for quantifying the informativeness and efficiency of the connected speech of adults with aphasia. *Journal of Speech and Hearing Research, 36,* 338–350.

Nicholas, L.E., & Brookshire, R.H. (1993b). A system for scoring main concepts in the discourse of non-brain-damaged and aphasic speakers. *Clinical Aphasiology, 21,* 87–99.

Nicholas, L.E., & Brookshire, R.H. (1995). The presence, completeness, and accuracy of main concepts in the connected speech of non-brain-damaged and aphasic adults. *Journal of Speech and Hearing Research, 38,* 145–156.

Nicholas, M., Obler, L.K., Albert, M.L., & Helm-Estabrooks, N. (1985). Empty speech in Alzheimer's disease and fluent aphasia. *Journal of Speech and Hearing Research, 28,* 405–410.

Terrell, B.Y., & Ripich, D.N. (1989). Discourse competence as a variable in intervention. *Seminars in Speech and Language, 10,* 282–297.

Tompkins, C.A., Boada, R., McGarry, K., Jones, J., Rahn, A.E., & Ranier, S. (1993). Connected speech characteristics of right-hemisphere-damaged adults: A re-examination. *Clinical Aphasiology, 21,* 113–122.

Trupe, E.H., & Hillis, A. (1985). Paucity vs. verbosity: Another analysis of right hemisphere communication deficits. In R.H. Brookshire (Ed.), *Clinical aphasiology conference proceedings* (pp. 83–96). Minneapolis: BRK.

Ulatowska, H.K., Doyle, A.W., Freedman-Stern, R., & Macaluso-Haynes, S. (1983). Production of procedural discourse in aphasia. *Brain and Language, 18,* 315–341.

Ulatowska, H.K., Freedman-Stern, R., Doyle, A.W., Macaluso-Haynes, S., & North, A.J. (1983). Production of narrative discourse in aphasia. *Brain and Language, 19,* 306–316.

Ulatowska, H.K., North, A.J., & Macaluso-Haynes, S. (1981). Production of narrative and procedural discourse in aphasia. *Brain and Language, 13,* 345–371.

Yorkston, K.M., & Beukelman, D.R. (1980). An analysis of connected speech samples of aphasic and normal speakers. *Journal of Speech and Hearing Disorders, 45,* 27–35.

CHAPTER 6

Analysis of Story Grammar

Carl A. Coelho

Story narratives offer the possibility of an additional level of analysis beyond the microstructural (cohesion) and macrostructural (informational content) analyses previously described in Chapters 4 and 5. The superstructure or story grammar level of analysis deals with the purported regularities in the internal structure of stories. These guide an individual's comprehension and production of the logical relationships between people and events (e.g., temporal and causal). As described by Merritt and Liles (1987), story grammar consists of a set of rules that include a network of story components and relations linking the components together. The typical story involves a central figure, animate or inanimate, at a particular point in time, location, or context (*setting information*), facing an obstacle, dilemma, environmental occurrence, or personal problem (*the initiating event*). The character responds to the situation and devises a plan (*internal response*). The character then makes attempts at solving the problem (*attempt*), meeting with success or failure (*direct consequence*). Depending on the outcome, the main character may try another strategy or enlist the aid of other characters, and the story usually ends with the character's emotional response to what has occurred (*reaction*).

STORY ELICITATION TASKS

Story stimuli need to be complex enough to elicit a story that challenges the individual's story grammar abilities. Task complexity involves a number of variables, such as mode of story presentation (e.g., retelling versus generation, auditory versus auditory and visual). It is important to consider such variables when making judgments regarding story grammar abilities (i.e., whether good or poor performance is a reflection of intact or impaired abilities or a function of an excessively easy or difficult task).

In story retelling, an individual is shown a story (via pictures, filmstrip, etc.) or listens to a story and is then instructed to retell that story. In story generation, an individual is presented with a picture (e.g., a copy of a Norman Rockwell painting) or sequence of pictures and is instructed to tell a story about what he or she feels is happening in the picture(s).

Recent investigations have demonstrated differences in these elicitation tasks (Coelho, Liles, & Duffy, 1990; Liles, Coelho, Duffy, & Zalagens, 1989). The story-retelling task (as elicited by a filmstrip) provides subjects with a strategy for retelling a story presented (i.e., they recall the story frame by frame). The story generation task is more challenging, inasmuch as adequate story development requires that a speaker transpose a "static" representation (i.e., a picture) into a "dynamic" representation (i.e., a story).

ANALYSIS OF STORY NARRATIVES

There are several approaches to narrative analysis at the story grammar level. This chapter reviews two that are clinically applicable for adults with neurological damage, the analysis of episodes and Applebee's (1978) six levels of narrative structure. Both of these analysis approaches will be discussed below.

Preparation of Story Narratives for Analysis

As is the case with other types of narrative samples, stories should be recorded and then transcribed verbatim. Once transcribed, the stories should be distributed into T-units, as described in Chapter 2. Next, the entire story narrative should be read from beginning to end at least once so that the evaluator has some idea of whether the story is consistent with the target story. Do not proceed in a sentence-by-sentence fashion, because comments as well as other information interspersed between episode components may be missed. For example, the following story narrative was generated by a traumatically brain-injured adult in a story generation task. The individual was asked to tell a story about what he felt was happening in the Norman Rockwell picture *The Runaway*, which depicts a little boy sitting on a stool in a diner, with his belongings in a bandanna tied to a stick on the floor next to him. Sitting next to the boy is a large policeman who is leaning over talking to him. On the other side of the lunch counter is a cook looking at the scene with a smile on his face.

1. (Goal, Initiating Event) This little boy was thinking about running away from home.

2. And he stopped in a diner for a drink.
3. (Attempt) And a policeman in the diner talked to the little boy and tried to convince him in a friendly way that that was not the thing to do.
4. And the little boy listened to the policeman.
5. (Consequence) And the little boy turned around and went home.

Analysis of Episodes

Descriptions of story grammars differ, but the episode unit is central to virtually all models proposed by recent investigators (Frederiksen, 1975; Johnson & Mandler, 1980; Meyer, 1975; Rumelhart, 1975; Stein & Glenn, 1979; Thorndyke, 1977; Thorndyke & Yekovitch, 1980). Because the relationships among components of the episode are considered to be logical and not bound by specific content, researchers describe the organization of episodes as being within the cognitive domain. The episode components are defined as units (i.e., statements) bearing information about stated goals, attempts at solutions, and the consequences of these attempts. Stein and Glenn (1979) assign the names *initiating event, attempt*, and *direct consequence* to these components.

The episode, as previously defined, appears to be a powerful unit that guides individuals in generating and retelling stories. The three critical components of an episode—initiating events, attempts, and direct consequences—are the three most frequently used story components for both unimpaired and language-disordered children (Merritt & Liles, 1987). Additional story grammar components used within the episode structure serve to elaborate and develop the basic behavioral sequences, making the goals and outcomes more understandable or interesting (Stein & Glenn, 1979). Regardless of how they are described, the creation of episodes is evidence of story grammar knowledge, and because this unit is cognitive in nature it is reasonable to believe that it may be disrupted by brain damage.

Exhibit 6–1 Complete and Incomplete Episodes

The following narratives were taken from the stories of traumatically brain-injured adults in a story-retelling task. The individuals were each shown a filmstrip depicting a family of bears who are having dinner when a fly flies in the window. The fly irritates the father bear, so he grabs a flyswatter and begins to try and eliminate the fly. In the process, he destroys the house and knocks out the mother bear, the daughter bear, and their dog. He eventually falls off a chair that he has set up on the table and knocks himself out. The story ends as the fly flies out the window.

- Complete Episode
  1. (Initiating Event) Father bear saw the fly land on mother bear's head.
  2. (Attempt) He grabbed a flyswatter and tried to hit the fly.
  3. (Direct Consequence) He hit mother bear instead, knocking her unconscious.
- Incomplete Episode
  1. (Initiating Event) Father bear saw the fly land on mother bear's head.
  2. (Attempt) He grabbed a flyswatter and tried to hit the fly. And the whole house was a mess.

Procedures for the analysis of episodes are as follows: (a) specific episode components are identified and coded. (b) Episodes are then designated as complete (i.e., consisting of all three components: initiating event, attempt, and direct consequence) or incomplete (i.e., consisting of two of the three components). See Exhibit 6–1 for examples of complete and incomplete episodes).

Information that is logically related in terms of goal, attempt, and consequence is first identified. Keep in mind that it may be confusing at first to identify these specific episode components in a story narrative because the attempts and direct consequences may not always be action oriented. Another way to conceptualize what the components of an episode are is to think of them in terms of a statement of a goal (the initiating event), an attempt at achieving the goal (attempt), and the resolution of that attempt (direct consequence). It is also possible to have a complete episode within a single T-unit. For example:

1. Father bear's attempts with a flyswatter to kill an irritating fly disrupted the family dinner without killing the fly.

In addition to complete and incomplete episodes, other levels of story structure episodes have been described. Exhibit 6–2 provides descriptions of these levels as compiled by Hughes, McGillivray, and Schmidek (1997).

Episode-Related Measures of Story Grammar

Once episodes are identified, the number of T-units within and outside of the episode structure may be counted. Such tallies may be sensitive to a subject's ability to organize content when the number of episodes is limited, as in very short stories. Further, such measures may provide information regarding improvement or recovery of story grammar abilities for individuals who talk but only a portion of what they are saying contributes to episode structure. For example, the following is a story told by a traumatically brain-injured adult in the "Bear and the Fly" story-retelling task.

1. The story is about a family of bears.
2. They were sitting down having dinner.
3. It was supper or dinner.
4. (Initiating Event) A fly flew in.
5. (Attempt) He was going to go through anything to get rid of the fly.

Exhibit 6–2 Story Structure Levels, from Least to Most Complex

Story Structure Level	Description
Descriptive sequence	Character(s), setting(s), and actions are described without causal relationships.
Action sequence	Actions are listed chronologically but not in a causal sequence.
Reactive sequence	A series of actions are described that lead to other actions, but without a clear-cut plan; none of the activity is goal directed.
Abbreviated episode	Objectives or intentions of the character are provided, but the character's plan for achieving the objectives must be inferred.
Incomplete episode	The issue of planning is apparent; one or more of the essential components of an episode (initiating event, attempt, consequence) is missing.
Complete episode	The story contains at least the three essential components of an episode (initiating event, attempt, consequence); it may reflect planning on the part of the character to attain the objective.
Multiple episodes	There is a combination of complete and incomplete episodes.
Complex episode	There is elaboration of a complete episode by including multiple plans, attempts, or consequences within that episode.
Embedded episode	A complete episode or reactive sequence is embedded within another episode.
Interactive episode	One set of events may be described from two perspectives; a reaction or consequence for one character may serve as an initiating event for a second character.

Source: Adapted with permission from D. Hughes, L. McGillivray, and M. Schmidek, *Guide to Narrative Language: Procedures for Assessment*, p. 121, Thinking Publications.

6. He started whacking the table around.
7. (Consequence) He didn't get the fly.
8. He ended up hitting his daughter in the head, his wife in the head and his dog in the head.
9. The dog fell out.
10. And the bottom line was, the fly ended up taking off.
11. He never got him.
12. And the whole house was in chaos.

Exhibit 6–3 illustrates the analysis of a narrative, in which episode elements have been identified, coded for completeness, and scored.

Issues Related to Reliability of Episodic Analyses

Merritt and Liles (1989) have noted that narrative analysis of story samples is more reliable if a story model is available for comparison. They noted that scoring of the story generation

Exhibit 6–3 Retelling of Story, Presented via Filmstrip, by an Individual with Traumatic Brain Injury (TBI)

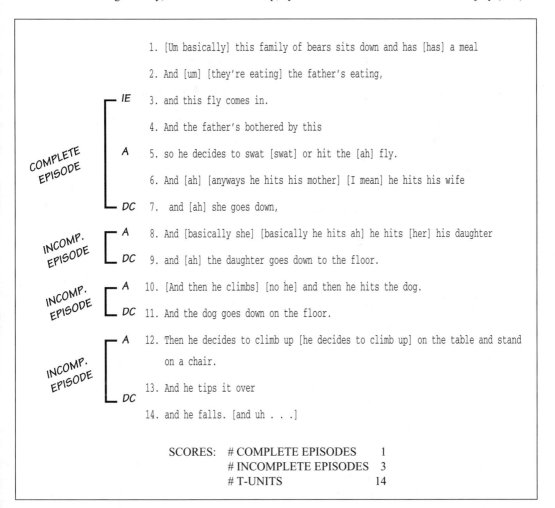

```
                              1. [Um basically] this family of bears sits down and has [has] a meal

                              2. And [um] [they're eating] the father's eating,

              ┌─ IE          3. and this fly comes in.

              │               4. And the father's bothered by this

COMPLETE      │   A           5. so he decides to swat [swat] or hit the [ah] fly.
EPISODE       │
              │               6. And [ah] [anyways he hits his mother] [I mean] he hits his wife

              └─ DC          7.  and [ah] she goes down,

INCOMP.       ┌─ A           8. And [basically she] [basically he hits ah] he hits [her] his daughter
EPISODE       └─ DC          9. and [ah] the daughter goes down to the floor.

INCOMP.       ┌─ A           10. [And then he climbs] [no he] and then he hits the dog.
EPISODE       └─ DC          11. And the dog goes down on the floor.

              ┌─ A           12. Then he decides to climb up [he decides to climb up] on the table and stand
              │                  on a chair.
INCOMP.       │
EPISODE       │              13. And he tips it over
              └─ DC          14. and he falls. [and uh . . .]
```

SCORES: # COMPLETE EPISODES   1
                # INCOMPLETE EPISODES   3
                # T-UNITS   14

samples was more difficult and less reliable because of a number of factors. For example, their subjects' generated stories often contained a greater number of descriptive details and strings of information describing the story setting. Such information may have been interesting and may have contributed to the subjective impression that spontaneously generated stories were richer, but it was irrelevant in terms of judging episode integrity or story grammar ability. In addition, many subjects became confused as they generated stories, often changing locale, introducing ambiguous characters, or dropping the story line completely.

It has also been our experience that reliability is higher for the identification of the three critical elements of an episode (initiating event, attempt, direct consequence) than for all six components (setting information, initiating event, internal response, attempt, direct consequence, reaction).

Analysis of Narrative Structure

Applebee's (1978) six levels of narrative structure reportedly parallel Vygotsky's (1962) stages of cognitive development and may be useful for analyzing types of plot structures within a given narrative. It should be noted that this analysis procedure was developed specifically for estimating cognitive development on the basis of narrative structure in children. Therefore, while the six levels may be useful for describing narrative structure following brain injury, caution should be exercised in attempting to estimate the degree of cognitive impairment on the basis of these narrative levels. Each of the six levels is described below with examples of stories produced by traumatically brain-injured adults in story-retelling or story generation tasks.

Level I—Heaps. At this level, stories are characterized by seemingly unrelated sentences with organization based on the speaker's immediate perception (Hughes et al., 1997, p. 114):

> A cop and a boy sitting on stools. They're having lunch or dinner or whichever meal is the special today, a radio playing and some meat in the refrigerator in the back and a pot. There's a pot, and a cup and a dish and something that drips out water and a duffle bag on the floor on a stick. Its color is red. And he has a gun, the cop does.

Level II—Sequences. Stories at this level tend to be concrete and factual as opposed to abstract and logical. Superficial but arbitrary sequences in time are noted in the stories, but without clear-cut causal links between events (Hughes et al., 1997, p. 114):

> This is a story about a boy and a policeman who met up in a restaurant. And the boy, I guess, had been hitchhiking or something like that. And the policeman was kind of looking at him funny. And he was kind of looking up at him, because he really couldn't arrest him there. And the waiter was covering his badge.

Level III—Primitive Narratives. At this level, narratives have a concrete core that may be expanded or clarified by a series of related statements. These statements are linked by a shared circumstance (Hughes et al., 1997, p. 114):

> It's a story about a bear family who . . . and a happy family. And one day this fly came in the window and like disrupted the whole family. And the father of the bear family started trying to hit the fly. At first they were sitting at the dinner table. And he was knocking over all these things and made a mess of the table because of the fly. And then he stood up and tried to get the fly. And he started hitting his family . . . his wife I guess. Then he hit one of his children and then the dog. And he was knocking everyone out. And then he just made a mess of the house and hurt his family. And the fly left at the end.

Level IV—Unfocused Chains. In stories at this level, events lead directly from one to another, but the components that link them shift, resulting in the listener's losing the point of the story (Hughes et al., 1997, p. 114):

> I think this cop is telling this little kid something. I don't know what. The chef probably would tell him something in a while. Neither of them had dinner. They were supposed to have spaghetti and meatballs. My father always made that. Then, I can't remember where he died. I think it was someplace in the Bradley Hospice. The last thing he told my mother was to take care of me. My brother, Sam, got there maybe two hours after my father died it was terrible for him. I think this cop is trying to tell this kid something. I don't know what. Evidently he has a gun. My brother used to have guns too. It always bothered me when he took them with him. I don't like .38 caliber revolvers, but my brother always did. There's coffee and milk. Oh and somebody's coffee cup, an old radio, three pies. I guess that's sort of it.

Level V—Focused Chains. In stories at this level, a central character is involved in a series of events, but there is nothing abstract that might indicate roles or causal relationships among characters (Hughes et al., 1997, p. 115):

> It was a story about three bears: the mother, the father and the baby . . . it looks like a daughter. And they were sitting down eating, having lunch. And a fly or a bee, either one, went through the window. Now papa bear he's gonna get rid of that fly. He don't care how. And he had a flyswatter. So in the course of swinging the flyswatter he hit mama bear in the head and knocked her out. Chased the fly. The fly landed on baby, hit the poor kid knocked her out. They had a dog. The fly was running around. It finally landed on the dog's head. He bopped the dog on the head. He was climbing on the table on chairs. He destroyed that house. He put holes in the TV set. He destroyed everything. And all mama bear was doing was laying on that table with her head on the table peeking at him with one eye open. Then the fly or the bee just flew out the window again.

Level VI—True Narratives. At this level, stories have a moral or consistent theme. The story is held together by concrete, perceptual, or abstract linkages (Hughes et al., 1997, p. 115):

> The family was having dinner. And there was a fly. And the husband tried to kill it and was disrupting the whole table, knocking over wine and stuff. And everybody left the dinner table. And he was still at it. He piled the chairs up to get it and hit the dog on the head, hit his daughter on the head. And I don't think he got it. And so he did all that for nothing. He let something like that bother him.

CONCLUSION

The multilevel analysis of story narratives (microstructural, macrostructural, and superstructural) permits an examination not only of sentence-level grammatical ability and intersentential cohesion but also of the cognitive abilities underlying the organization and production of a story text. The interactions among the levels of sentence grammar, intersentential cohesion, and story grammar knowledge required for the production of a story may place a communicative load on the brain-injured individual's performance that may reveal problems not observable in other forms of discourse. The functional validity of such multilevel analyses has been demonstrated with higher-level traumatically brain-injured individuals. Narrative stories were used to sample discourse abilities longitudinally. Two differing patterns of deficits emerged. In the first, excessive verbalization characterized by poorly organized but task-appropriate content was noted. In the second, fair to good organization but little appropriate content was noted. Prognostically, the presence of appropriate, although disorganized, content was an early indication that the individual was able to appreciate potential relationships of characters in the stimulus picture. The second pattern represented a more severe cognitive dysfunction. The individual's attempts at stories, although well organized, were merely elaborate descriptions of the picture (Coelho, Liles, & Duffy, 1991).

In the Appendixes, a variety of discourse samples have been provided for further practice. Some of these samples have been analyzed for story grammar. The reader may want to practice on or review these samples for additional experience with story grammar analysis, as well as with other types of analyses.

REFERENCES

Applebee, A. (1978). *The child's concept of story*. Chicago: University of Chicago Press.

Coelho, C.A., Liles, B.Z., & Duffy, R.J. (1990). Contextual influences on narrative discourse in normal young adults. *Journal of Psycholinguistic Research, 19*, 405–420.

Coelho, C.A., Liles, B.Z., & Duffy, R.J. (1991). Discourse analysis with closed head injured adults: Evidence for differing patterns of deficits. *Archives of Physical Medicine and Rehabilitation, 72*, 465–468.

Frederiksen, C.H. (1975). Representing logical and semantic structures of knowledge acquired from discourse. *Cognitive Psychology, 7*, 371–458.

Hughes, D., McGillivray, L, & Schmidek, M. (1997). *Guide to narrative language*. Eau Claire, WI: Thinking Publications.

Johnson, N.S., & Mandler, J.M. (1980). A tale of two structures: Underlying and surface forms in stories. *Poetics, 9*, 51–86.

Liles, B.Z., Coelho, C.A., Duffy, R.J., & Zalagens, M.R. (1989). Effects of elicitation procedures on the narratives of normal and closed head-injured adults. *Journal of Speech and Hearing Disorders, 54*, 356–366.

Merritt, D.S., & Liles, B.Z. (1987). Story grammar ability in children with and without language disorder: Story generation, story retelling, and story comprehension. *Journal of Speech and Hearing Research, 30*, 539–551.

Merritt, D.S., & Liles, B.Z. (1989). Clinical applications of story generation and story retelling. *Journal of Speech and Hearing Disorders, 54*, 438–447.

Meyer, B.J.F. (1975). Identification of the structure of prose and its implications for the study of reading and memory. *Journal of Reading Behavior, 7*, 7–47.

Rumelhart, D.E. (1975). Notes on the schema for stories. In D.G. Bobrow & A.M. Collins (Eds.), *Representation and understanding: Studies in cognitive science* (pp. 211-236). Hillsdale, NJ: Lawrence Erlbaum.

Stein, N.L., & Glenn, C.G. (1979). An analysis of story comprehension in elementary school children. In R.O. Freedle (Ed.), *New directions in discourse processing* (pp. 53–120). Norwood, NJ: Ablex.

Thorndyke, P.W. (1977). Cognitive structures in comprehension and memory of narrative discourse. *Cognitive Psychology, 9*, 77–110.

Thorndyke, P.W., & Yekovitch, F.R. (1980). A critique of schemata as a theory of human story memory. *Poetics, 9*, 23–49.

Vygotsky, L.S. (1962). *Thought and language*. Cambridge, MA: MIT Press.

CHAPTER 7

Analysis of Conversation

Carl A. Coelho

The analysis of conversational discourse is of particular interest for the investigation of brain-injured populations because it involves a functionally oriented and commonly occurring communicative activity. Conversational discourse closely approximates the social-interactional nature of communication. Each of us engages in conversational behavior on a nearly daily basis. We negotiate our needs and wants, with varying degrees of success, through conversation. Educational achievement, vocational performance, and the establishment of social relationships frequently hinge on conversational proficiency. Few communicative behaviors are as critical as conversation.

A variety of analyses for conversation have been described. These include turn taking, response adequacy and appropriateness, topic management, and conversational breakdown and repair. Each of these analyses will be discussed and illustrated through various transcripts of conversations. First, however, a few comments regarding obtaining the conversational sample as well as preparing transcriptions for analysis are offered.

CONVERSATIONAL SAMPLING AND TRANSCRIPTION PREPARATION

Several issues related to obtaining a sample of conversation need to be addressed before con-

sidering analyses. These include conversational partners, locale of conversation, topic, audio-taping versus videotaping, and length of sample. The purpose for obtaining the conversational sample will determine many of these factors. For example, if the purpose of the sample is to describe a population, the procedures used for obtaining the samples will be structured for simplicity and ease in handling multiple subjects or brain-injured individuals. The conversational partner may be the researcher or an assistant, the locale may be the investigator's office or lab, and each sample may be audiotaped only. On the other hand, if the purpose for obtaining the sample is to gather baseline data on a single individual before initiating a treatment procedure, very different procedures may be employed. For example, the examiner may choose to recruit a family member or friend to serve as the conversational partner, the locale of the sample may be the subject's home, and conversations may be videotaped. Regardless of how these factors are configured, if groups of individuals are studied or if a single individual is studied longitudinally, the partner, locale, mode of recording, and sample length should be the same for each conversational sample. If this consistency is maintained, it may be concluded that any differences or changes in performance noted are not due to differences in the sampling procedure. Furthermore, in an effort to minimize the effect of topic selection on the conversation sample across subjects, some investigators have used a predetermined set of topic questions and comments appropriate to the subject's remarks (Campbell & Dollaghan, 1990).

In general, conversational partner and locale will be dictated by the degree to which the examiner wishes to simulate a natural everyday interaction. For example, a conversation with a family member at home will be more true to life than an interaction in the clinic; however, logistical constraints may not always permit the staging of such interactions. Once again, the purpose of the sample will determine how much naturalness can be compromised in the interest of practicality.

Similarly, the decision regarding recording mode (i.e., audio versus audio and video recordings) may be decided on the basis of very practical issues such as what equipment is available to the examiner. On the other hand, the degree of analysis that is required for the information that is sought will determine the type of recording that is necessary. For example, Simmons-Mackie and Damico (1996) have described compensatory strategies employed by moderately to severely impaired aphasic speakers to overcome communication barriers in conversation. Analysis of gestures and other nonverbal behaviors was an important aspect of their investigation; therefore, video recordings were utilized.

The length of the conversational sample will also be dictated by the purpose of the sample. If, for example, the examiner is interested in the range of conversational topics introduced over the course of a lunch, the entire lunch period should be recorded. However, if the examiner is interested simply in getting a sample of conversational behavior, a 10-minute recording may be adequate. The issue of practicality also needs to be addressed, in that the time required to transcribe and analyze a 10-minute sample of conversation can be as much as three hours. In an attempt to determine how long a sample is necessary, Boles, Holland and Beeson (1993) analyzed conversational samples of aphasic subjects from 2 to 12 minutes in duration and determined that 6-minute samples yielded information that was representative of the 12-minute samples.

CONVERSATIONAL ANALYSIS

In the discussion that follows, a variety of conversational analyses are reviewed. Several of these analysis approaches are illustrated in conversational samples. Although a conversation may involve numerous participants, in the interest of simplifying the explanations, only conversations involving two participants will be illustrated. However, any of the analysis procedures discussed may be applied to conversations involving more than two participants.

Pragmatic Rating Scales

In addition to the relatively structured and specific conversational analyses to be discussed below, a number of pragmatic rating scales are available that can be applied for a less formal evaluation of conversational samples. Examples of such rating scales (Halper, Cherney, Burns, & Mogil, 1996; Damico, 1985; Ehrlich & Barry, 1989; Prutting & Kirchner, 1983), as well as general guidelines for assessing pragmatics (Roth & Spekman, 1984a, 1984b), appear in Exhibit 7–1.

Turn Taking

In a conversation, for effective communication to take place, it is critical that others listen while one person speaks (Brinton & Fujiki, 1989). A variety of models have been proposed to describe the relatively efficient process of turn taking in adult conversations. Sacks, Schegloff, and Jefferson (1974) noted that such models must account for certain characteristics of conversations:

1. There are frequent speaker changes.

Exhibit 7–1 Some Pragmatic Rating Scales

Pragmatic Communication Skills: Rating Scale (Halper, Cherney, Burns, & Mogil, 1996)

NONVERBAL COMMUNICATION

Intonation

1	2	3	4
Flat/monotone or inappropriate	Limited or inconsistently appropriate	Appropriate intonation most of the time	Appropriate

---

Facial expression

1	2	3	4
Absent or inappropriate	Limited or inconsistently appropriate	Appropriate facial expression most of the time	Appropriate

---

Eye contact

1	2	3	4
Cannot establish eye contact	Needs cue to maintain eye contact	Maintains and uses eye contact appropriately most of the time; minimal cues may be needed	Appropriate

---

Gesture and proxemics

1	2	3	4
Absent or inappropriate	Limited or inconsistently appropriate	Uses gestures and proxemics appropriately most of the time	Appropriate

---

VERBAL COMMUNICATION

Conversation initiation

1	2	3	4
Inappropriate or does not initiate	Limited or inconsistently appropriate initiation	Initiates conversation appropriately most of the time	Appropriate

continues

Exhibit 7–1 continued

VERBAL COMMUNICATION continued

Turn taking

1	2	3	4
Unaware of turn-taking signals	Inconsistently responsive to signals	Uses and responds to turn-taking signals appropriately most of the time	Appropriate

Topic maintenance

1	2	3	4
Absent or inappropriate topic maintenance (maintains topic less than 50% of the time)	Maintains topic some of the time (50–75% of the time)	Maintains topic most of the time (76–90% of the time)	Appropriate

Response length

1	2	3	4
Responses are verbose or inappropriately short (more than 50% of the time)	Responses are inconsistently verbose or inappropriately short (25–49% of the time)	Appropriate response length most of the time (inappropriate only 10–24% of the time)	Appropriate response length (more than 90% of the time)

Presupposition

1	2	3	4
Presupposes too much and/or too little (more than 50% of the time)	Presupposes too much and/or too little some of the time (25–49% of the time)	Occasionally presupposes too much and/or too little (10–24% of the time)	Appropriate (more than 90% of the time)

Referencing skills

1	2	3	4
Inappropriate referencing (more than 50% of the time)	Inappropriate referencing some of the time (25–49% of the time)	Occasional inappropriate referencing (10–24% of the time)	Appropriate referencing (more than 90% of the time)

Total score _____/40

Source: Reprinted from A.S. Halper, L.R. Cherney, M.S. Burns, and S.I. Mogil, *Clinical Management of Right Hemisphere Dysfunction,* 2nd ed., © 1996, Aspen Publishers, Inc.

continues

Exhibit 7–1 continued

Pragmatically Oriented Discourse Analysis (Modified from Damico, 1985)

Does client:

Give sufficient information when giving instructions or directions?

Use nonspecific vocabulary (*thing, stuff, whatchamacallit*)?

Perseverate or provide too much redundancy when talking?

Need a lot of repetition before even simple instructions are understood?

Give inaccurate messages; seem to talk when he or she "doesn't know what he or she is talking about"?

Make rapid and inappropriate changes in conversational topic without clues to the listener?

Seem to have an independent conversational agenda or give inappropriate and unpredictable responses?

Fail to ask relevant questions to clarify unclear messages, so that communication frequently breaks down?

Use language that is inappropriate for the social situation?

Produce speech that is frequently disrupted by repetitions, unusual pauses, and hesitations?

Use many false starts, self-repetitions, and revisions in talking?

Produce long pauses or delays before responding?

Lack forethought and planning in telling stories and giving instructions?

Fail to attend to cues for conventional turns, interrupting frequently or failing to hold up his or her end of the conversation?

Use inconsistent or inappropriate eye contact in conversation?

Use inappropriate intonation?

Source: Adapted from "The Organization of Problem Behaviors under Grice's Categories in Clinical Discourse Analysis" (p. 131), by J. Damico. In C. Simon (Ed.) Communication Skills and Classroom Success, 1991, EauClaire, WI: Thinking Publications. Adapted with Permission.

continues

Exhibit 7–1 continued

Rating of Communication Behaviors (Adapted from Ehrlich & Barry, 1989)

Intelligibility: scale 1–9
 1. Speech is severely distorted and consistently requires repetition
 3. Speech is moderately distorted; can be understood approximately 30–40% of the time
 5. Speech is mildly distorted; requires repetition approximately 10% of the time
 7. Speech is minimally impaired but is generally intelligible
 9. No discernible speech impairment; always understood

Eye gaze: scale 1–9
 1. Consistently no appropriate eye gaze with another person
 3. Severely restricted eye gaze
 5. Appropriate eye gaze 50% of the time
 7. Appropriate eye gaze 75% of the time
 9. Consistent use of appropriate eye gaze

Sentence formation: scale 1–9
 1. Consistently uses ungrammatical sentences; only short phrases and "telegraphic"
 3. Omits grammatical function words often; average sentence length is reduced most of the time
 5. Uses mainly simple sentences; infrequent embedding and clauses
 7. Uses varied sentence patterns 75% of the time
 9. Mature and varied sentence patterns consistently used

Coherence of narrative: scale 1–9
 1. Consistently random and diffuse expression; incomplete thoughts
 3. Disjointed verbal style; limited connection between ideas
 5. Thoughts are expressed with a moderate amount of irrelevant and extraneous remarks and are considered incomplete 50% of the time
 7. Ideas are expressed in some order approximately 75% of the time; notice occasional incomplete thoughts
 9. Shows a well-executed expression of ideas most of the time; well-formed narrative

Topic: scale 1–9
 1. Rapid and abrupt shifting from topic to topic within a short time
 3. Able to maintain topic for at least 30 seconds
 5. Can maintain the topic for several minutes, but demonstrates difficulty in changing to a new topic
 7. Can appropriately maintain the topic most of the time; infrequently (25% of the time) shows slowness and difficulty in change of topic
 9. Demonstrates no problem in maintenance and change of topic

Initiation of communication: scale 1–9
 1. Infrequently initiates talk; only responds to others' questions
 3. Seldom initiates talk (about 25% of the time)
 5. Limited initiation of talk (about 50% of the time)
 7. Minimal problem in initiating conversational talk
 9. Freely initiates talk; good balance of communication most of the time

Source: Adapted with permission from J. Ehrlich and P. Barry, Rating Communication Behaviors in the Head-Injured Adult, *Brain Injury*, Vol. 3, pp. 193–198, © 1989.

continues

Exhibit 7–1 continued

Prutting and Kirchner's (1983) Pragmatic Protocol

Communicative Act	Approp.	Inapprop.	NA

Utterance Act

A. Verbal or paralinguistic
1. Intelligibility
2. Vocal intensity
3. Voice quality
4. Prosody
5. Fluency

B. Nonverbal
1. Physical proximity
2. Physical contacts
3. Body posture
4. Foot or leg movements
5. Hand or arm movements
6. Gestures
7. Facial expression
8. Eye gaze

Propositional Act

A. Lexical selection and use
1. Specificity and accuracy

B. Specifying relationships between words
1. Word order
2. Given and new information

C. Stylistic variations
1. Varying the communicative style

Illocutionary and Perlocutionary Acts

A. Speech acts
1. Speech act pair analysis
2. Variety of speech acts

B. Topic
1. Selection
2. Introduction
3. Maintenance
4. Change

C. Turn taking
1. Initiation
2. Response
3. Repair and revision
4. Pause time
5. Interruption and overlap
6. Feedback to speakers
7. Adjacency
8. Contingency
9. Quantity and conciseness

Source: © American Speech-Language-Hearing Association. Reprinted by permission.

continues

Exhibit 7–1 continued

Roth and Spekman's (1984a, 1984b) Suggestions for Assessing Pragmatics

Area Assessed	Suggested Activity
Communicative intentions Expression	Engage in conversation about topics that are familiar and meaningful to client.
Comprehension	Make indirect requests.
Presupposition	Employ barrier tasks (referential communication). Assess extended discourse (looking at use of pronouns, articles, ellipsis, and conjunctions). Picture description: Show client picture and ask for a description. Next, present a second picture that is just the same except for one obvious detail. Description of second picture should take into account information presupposed in first.
Social organization of discourse	Analyze turn taking, topic maintenance, and conversational initiation, termination, and repair in referential communication task used to assess presupposition. Employ role playing, e.g., asking for directions. Feign misunderstanding to assess client's ability to make repairs. Use unclear messages to assess client's ability to request clarification.

Source: Data from F. Roth and N. Spekman, Assessing the Pragmatic Abilities of Children, Part I, Organizational Framework and Assessment Parameters, *Journal of Speech and Hearing Disorders*, Vol. 4, No. 9, pp. 2–11, © 1984 and F. Roth and N. Spekman, Assessing the Pragmatic Abilities of Children, Part II, Guidelines, Considerations, and Specific Evaluation Procedures, *Journal of Speech and Hearing Disorders*, Vol. 4, No. 9, pp. 12–17, © 1984.

2. Typically just one individual speaks at a time.
3. When two individuals talk simultaneously, such overlap is usually of short duration.
4. As speaking turns shift from one speaker to another, this typically occurs without significant gaps.
5. The order in which speakers talk, the length of turns, and the overall duration of the conversation are not preestablished and may be quite variable.
6. Turn content and distribution are not set before the conversation.
7. Turns may follow each other in succession (continuous talk), or there may be pauses in which no speaker talks (discontinuous talk).
8. Turn allocation is regulated by specific procedures.
9. Speakers and listeners employ repair mechanisms to handle turn-taking errors.

Sacks et al. (1974) have described a sequential production model of turn taking. One component of this model is the turn constructional component, which pertains to length of turn. Turns are constructed from unit types, which may vary in length from a single word to several sentences. Once a speaker has initiated a unit type, it is possible for a listener to anticipate the unit type being constructed and thus the unit's completion point. The completion point of a turn is referred to as the *transition relevance place*. It marks that point in a conversation at which a listener may initiate a speaking turn. Therefore, the listener does not simply wait for a pause in the conversation to initiate a turn but rather estimates a possible completion point and is ready to offer new information at that point.

A second component of Sacks et al.'s (1974) model is the turn allocation component. As soon as a speaker reaches the transition relevance place, three guidelines determine who takes the next turn:

1. The current speaker selects a person to be the next speaker (e.g., by glancing at a particular individual).
2. If no speaker is selected by the current speaker, then whoever speaks first takes the next turn.
3. If no one self-selects and takes the turn, the current speaker may continue talking.

Although it is unclear how speakers are consistently able to anticipate transition relevance places, Duncan and Fiske (1977) described how speakers and listeners often signal turn exchanges. These signals consist of the following:

1. use of a certain set of intonation contours (rising or falling)
2. utterance of stereotyped phrases such as "you know"
3. completion of a grammatical clause
4. prolongation of a syllable
5. completion of a hand gesture or relaxation of a tensed hand position

Analysis

Turn-Taking Errors. Inappropriate turn taking may be the most disruptive and often the most apparent difficulty in ineffective communication. This aspect of conversational behavior is commonly rated in pragmatic scales (e.g., see Ehrlich & Barry, 1989). However, while it is often easily detected, as summarized above, the underlying basis for the difficulty may be less apparent. For example, turn taking may be ineffective because an individual is inattentive to his or her listener and consequently is missing the listener's signals. On the other hand, if a speaker has not established a predictable unit type (i.e., length of turn), the listener may be erroneously anticipating transition relevance places and initiating a turn before the speaker has completed his

or her turn. Therefore, it is important, when analyzing ineffective/inefficient turn-taking behaviors, that the context of the turn-taking error be recorded or somehow coded. In other words, merely counting turn-taking errors would not allow the identification of turn-taking patterns over the course of the conversation. It is preferable to mark turn-taking errors on the transcript of the conversation and to note if these errors are consistent and predictable (e.g., Do they occur after long turns? Or do they occur when the subject is functioning as a listener? Or as a responder?).

Number and Length of Turns. An additional measure that may be used is the number of turns for each participant per conversation. Within any conversation each participant functions as an initiator and a responder. Turns, therefore, account for all utterances produced by each participant in a conversation. Number and length of turns are related. A higher number of turns is often indicative of shorter utterances and fewer turns of longer utterances. This is illustrated by recent investigations that have demonstrated that conversations between aphasic and closed–head–injured subjects and the same examiner were characterized by a higher number of turns per conversation than those between the same examiner and normal control subjects (Coelho, Liles, & Duffy, 1991; Coelho, Liles, Duffy, & Clarkson, 1993).

Response Adequacy and Appropriateness

Blank and Franklin (1980) have described a procedure for evaluating the appropriateness of an utterance in a conversation. The concept of appropriateness has received some attention in the psychiatric literature because its absence is seen to be an important element in the interpersonal difficulties of both neurotic and psychotic individuals (Blank & Franklin, 1980). This issue has also recently been addressed in the assessment of brain-injured individuals (Coelho et al., 1991, 1993). Once the conversational sample or samples are obtained, and transcribed verbatim, each utterance (turn) is assigned to one of the speakers (e.g., client and examiner; see Appendix 7–A). Each utterance is then categorized as either a speaker initiation or a speaker response. By using the distinction of speaker-initiator and speaker-responder, appropriateness in a conversational interchange can be examined.

Speaker Initiation. The utterances of a speaker-initiator are evaluated according to what Blank and Franklin termed their "summoning power." Utterances that clearly summon or demand a response are designated *obliges* (e.g., "How long have you lived in Vermont?") whereas those that do not are designated *comments* (e.g., "What a beautiful day!"). Speaker initiations are classified as obliges or comments. A differential response to these conversational initiatives describes whether the speaker is appropriately extending conversation.

Speaker Responses. Speaker responses are classified in terms of adequacy, as adequate-plus, adequate, inadequate, or ambiguous. An *adequate-plus* response is one that relevantly elaborates the theme so as to provide more information than was requested (e.g., the speaker-initiator has asked, "What time is it?" and the speaker-responder replies, "It's 3:30; I know that because I just walked past the new clock at the bank on Main Street"). An *adequate* response is one that appropriately meets the speaker-initiator's verbalization (e.g., in response to the question above, the speaker-responder replies, "It's 3:30").

An *inadequate* response is one in which the information offered is invalid, irrelevant, or insufficient to meet the constraints established by the speaker-initiator's utterance (e.g., in response to the same question, the speaker-responder replies, "It's time for me to take a nap"). An *ambiguous response* is one in which the information offered is unclear or ambiguous, so that one cannot determine whether it is adequate or not (e.g., in response to the same question, the speaker-responder replies "Why should I tell you?"). (See Appendix 7–A for examples of this coding procedure in a transcribed conversation.)

Although the determination of speaker initiations versus speaker responses is typically based upon where in the sequence of a conversation the utterance occurs (i.e., whether the utterance is produced to solicit information or to respond to another's query) or the role of the speaker at the time the utterance is produced (i.e., initiator or responder), some utterances may be classified as both responses and initiations.

Analysis

In examining the number of speaker initiations (obliges and comments) and speaker responses (adequate-plus, adequate, inadequate, and ambiguous) produced by a subject and examiner in a conversation, it is most meaningful to discuss them as a percentage of the number of turns per conversation. (See end of Appendix 7–A for summary of data from the conversational analysis.)

Speaker Initiations. In Appendix 7–A's summary, it can be seen that the clinician (designated as T in the transcript) produced a much larger percentage of obliges than comments (83% and 17% of total turns respectively) during the conversation, while the brain-injured individual (designated as S in the transcript) produced very few of either type of initiation (obliges = 2% and comments = 12% of total turns). These data confirm that the clinician had to assume a greater proportion of the communicative burden (i.e., the responsibility that each participant of a conversation must carry to ensure the successful exchange of information) in this conversation. This is illustrated by the clinician's adapting a rather structured or assistive mode of interaction, as seen in the high number of obliges produced.

Speaker Responses. Depending on the population studied, the number of inadequate or ambiguous responses may be high or low. For example, Coelho et al. (1993) noted that for groups of mildly impaired closed-head–injured and aphasic subjects, the occurrence of both types of responses was very low (i.e., less than 2% of total responses). These type of responses are more prevalent in more severely impaired individuals or those in more acute stages of recovery. For example, in Appendix 7–A's summary, it can be seen that the brain-injured individual, who was moderately impaired, produced no ambiguous or inadequate responses.

Adequate-plus and adequate responses reflect the ability of the speaker-responder to extend the conversation in an appropriate, meaningful fashion. Coelho et al. (1993) observed that in conversations between an examiner and normal controls, nearly 50% of all responses were categorized as adequate-plus. In the same study, and in conversations with the same examiner, closed-head–injured subjects produced adequate-plus responses approximately 30% of the time and aphasic subjects 22% of the time. The percentage of adequate-plus responses will most likely vary with the familiarity of the participants and the firsthand knowledge that participants have about the topic being discussed. Appendix 7–A's summary illustrates that of the responses produced by the brain-injured individual, 62% were judged as adequate and 24% as adequate-plus. The majority of the brain-injured individual's turns were devoted to responding to the clinician's obliges.

Topic Management

Topic refers to what conversations are about and how what they are about changes as an interaction proceeds (Brinton & Fujiki, 1989). *Topic management* pertains to how topics are introduced and continued over the course of a conversation. Mentis (1994) has noted that any individual who is unable to share responsibility for introducing and developing topics in a conversation, who changes topics abruptly without signaling the listener, or who adds inappropriate irrelevant information to an ongoing discussion will quickly be judged as an ineffective communicator. Topic management will be discussed in terms of topic initiation and topic maintenance.

Analyses of Topic Initiation

Topic initiation refers to how an individual initiates or introduces topics into a conversation. In the typical conversation, topics may be introduced by either participant. Initiation of a new topic is often marked by the introduction of propositional content. For example, a speaker simply begins talking about something else, or a speaker may use special devices known as opening markers, such as "By the way . . . " or questions, that signal the listener that the topic is changing (Hurtig, 1977). Topics may be changed in one of three ways: (a) by a *novel introduction*, which may be at the beginning of the conversation or which ends discussion of one topic and initiates another; (b) by a *smooth shift*, in which discussion of one topic is subtly switched to another; or (c) by a *disruptive shift*, in which discussion of one topic is abruptly or illogically switched to another topic. The total number of novel introductions produced by each participant over the course of the conversation, as well as the total number of topic shifts, both smooth and disruptive, may be tallied.

Appendix 7–A provides examples of novel introductions and topic shifts within the transcribed conversation. In this conversational sample, the clinician's supportive or assistive approach to the conversation, noted above in the discussion of speaker initiations, is also apparent when topic initiations are examined. A total of 36 topics were introduced over the course of this conversation. Of that total, the clinician introduced 35, or 97% of all topics, while the brain-injured individual introduced one. Subtle shifts were the predominant means used by the clinician to introduce new topics (74%), followed by novel topic introductions.

Garcia and Joanette (1994) have observed that conversational partners must continually adjust their information-processing skills from speaker to listener and vice versa. As speakers, they must make contributions that will be relevant to their own interpretation of the macroproposition (i.e., topic or gist) under discussion on the basis of various processing strategies and information stored in memory. As speakers, they must interpret, on line, what the speaker presents to them by forming a new macroproposition and comparing it with information already stored in memory, thereby attaching relevance to the speaker's utterance. This process is highly complex when the array of topic shifts that occur in a typical conversation is considered. Further, if an individual must hold propositions in memory to process additional incoming propositions, it is apparent that individuals with memory deficits will have difficulty participating meaningfully in conversation. These authors have elaborated the analysis of topic shifts by coding each topic shift for place, type, reason for shift, and the context in which it occurred. This system of analysis has proven to be sensitive to the conversational breakdowns that occur in individuals with dementia secondary to Alzheimer's disease (Garcia & Joanette, 1994). Descriptions of these topic shift coding categories are presented in Exhibit 7–2.

Mentis and Prutting (1991) have described a far more elaborate multidimensional topic analysis system. They reported that the procedure is able to reliably identify, quantify, and describe topic management problems. This system also addresses topic and subtopic introduction, using somewhat different but related terminology. For example, types of topics or subtopics introduced are classified as new, related, or reintroduced. A *topic* is defined as a clause or noun phrase that identifies the content of a sequence of utterances. A *subtopic* is a sequence in which the focus of discussion is part of and related to the topic sequence.

There is evidence to suggest that the number of topics introduced during a conversation decreases with age and that this developmental trend continues through adolescence (Brinton & Fujiki, 1984). Similarly, recent investigations have indicated that conversations involving aphasic and traumatically brain-injured subjects are characterized by more frequent topic changes than those of normal controls (Coelho et al., 1991, 1993).

Analyses of Topic Maintenance

A topic is said to be "maintained" when it is continued (Brinton & Fujiki, 1989). Topics may be maintained by a single speaker or by both participants in a conversational dyad. Topics may be discontinued when (a) speakers stop talking or (b) speakers change topics. Topics may be discontinued and a new topic initiated subtly, a process referred to as *topic shading*. Topic shading may be characterized by the production of smooth or disruptive topic shifts as described above.

In Mentis and Prutting's (1991) analysis, the basic unit for analyzing topic and subtopic maintenance is the *intonation unit*, as described by Chafe (1987). Chafe defined an intonation unit as "a sequence of words combined under a single, coherent intonation contour, usually preceded by a pause" (p. 22). According to Chafe, each intonation unit expresses only one new concept at a time. Therefore, the intonation unit may be used as a measure of the amount of information conveyed within a single topic, as well as the individual contributions of each participant in a conversation to topic maintenance.

Mentis and Prutting (1991) categorized intonation units as *ideational* (i.e., carrying propositional, ideational information) or *textual* or *interpersonal* (i.e., serving a primarily textual or interpersonal function in the conversation). The ideational intonation units were further classified into four categories: (a) *new information ideational units*, measuring the extent to which each participant contributed to the development of the conversation by adding novel and relevant information; (b) *no new information*, measuring the extent to which each participant maintained the topic of discussion but did not further develop the topic through the addition of novel information; (c) *side sequence units*, measuring the number of intonation units inserted by each participant within a topic sequence that did not contribute to topic maintenance but were not considered a new topic introduction; and (d) *problematic ideational units*, measuring the ex-

Exhibit 7–2 Topic Shift Categories

Place of Shift

1. Within Turn:	Topic shift that occurs in the same turn as the preceding topic.
2. Across Turn:	Topic shift that occurs across turn boundaries.

Type of Shift

1. Topic Initiation:	Attempt at initiating new topic either after a prior topic has been terminated or after a period of nontopical talk or silence.
2. Topic Shading:	New topic is introduced by first establishing its relevance to the topic currently under discussion. Relevance is established through repetition of a referent, pronominal referencing, or use of connecting phrasing like "Speaking of . . . "
3. Renewal:	A shift back to an earlier topic after one or more other topics have been introduced. These may not always be marked, as in "Getting back to . . . "
4. Insert:	An abrupt, frequently tangential, shift, most often within a turn, that does not succeed in gaining the topical floor. It may appear as if the speakers did not want to drop the last topic.
5. Unexpected:	An abrupt shift that succeeds in gaining the topical floor.
6. Undetermined:	Topic shift in which it is evident that the topic has been switched but in which it is difficult to identify what the new topic is.

Reason for Shift

1. End of Topic:	Topic shift occurs because the speakers have nothing more to say about the topic. May be signaled by a passing of turns in which no new semantic information is added or a period of silence.
2. Decreased Comprehension:	Listener does not appear to have understood the speaker and changes topic. Comprehension problems may result from the listener's not paying attention, difficulty identifying the referent or understanding the gist of what is said, or difficulties in the delivery of the message.
3. Failure To Continue:	Occurs when a member of the dyad either decides not to continue or cannot continue the current topic, leading the other member of the dyad to change the topic.
4. Outside Event:	Occurs because something happens in the immediate environment like a telephone ringing or the appearance of an object/person.
5. Repetition of an Idea:	Occurs because of a need to repeat a previously discussed idea.
6. Anecdotal:	Occurs because of a desire to share a short, usually biographical, story.
7. Undetermined:	Reason for topic shift does not fit into any of the categories above.

continues

Exhibit 7–2 continued

Relation to Context
1. Text: Related to something previously stated (knowledge that had already
                          been shared) in the conversation.
2. Environment: Related to an object or an event in the immediate environment.
3. Specific Knowledge: Related to knowledge within speaker's (or speakers') repertoire—for
                          example, personal experience.
4. General Knowledge: Related to knowledge assumed to be within the general public's
                          repertoire—for example, current events.
5. Unknown: Unable to determine what topic shift relates to.

Source: Adapted with permission from L.J. Garcia and Y. Joanette, Conversational Topic-Shifting Analysis in Dementia, in *Discourse Analysis and Application: Studies in Adult Clinical Populations*, R.L. Bloom et al., eds., pp. 161–
183, © 1994, Lawrence Erlbaum Associates, Inc.

tent to which each participant contributed information units judged to have a negative effect on
the conversation through the addition of ambiguous, unrelated, or incomplete fragmented
intonation units. Mentis and Prutting (1991) further subdivided each of these four categories
into descriptive subcategories (see Exhibit 7–3).

The utility of this multidimensional analysis
system has been demonstrated in recent studies.
In an investigation of one closed–head–injured
adult and a matched control, Mentis and Prutting
(1991) found that the head-injured individual's
topic management abilities were disrupted, as
evidenced by his production of noncoherent
topic changes and ambiguous, unrelated, and incomplete ideational units. These problems resulted in a decrease in overall coherence and
continuity of topic development. The topic management abilities of two groups of older adults,
one with the diagnosis of senile dementia of the
Alzheimer's type (SDAT) and the other of normal elderly, have also been analyzed using the
same procedures. Results indicated that the topic
management skills of the SDAT group were
characterized by a reduced ability to change topics while preserving discourse flow, difficulty in
actively contributing to the development of topics, and problems in consistently maintaining
topics in a coherent manner (Mentis, Briggs-
Whittaker, & Gramigna, 1995).

Conversational Repair

Conversational repair mechanisms allow listeners to indicate when they have not understood
and allow speakers to revise their ongoing production and to provide clarification (Brinton &
Fujiki, 1989). Four major types of repair mechanisms have been described by Schegloff,
Jefferson, and Sacks (1977) according to who
initiated the repair and who provided the clarification or repair:

1. *Other-initiated other-repair*, in which the
   listener identifies a problem and repairs
   it.
   Example:
   Listener: "You've lost me. I think you really mean. . . ."
2. *Other-initiated self-repair*, in which the
   listener requests clarification and the
   speaker provides it.
   Example:
   Listener: "What do you mean by that?"
   Speaker: "What I mean is. . . ."
3. *Self-initiated other-repair*, in which the
   speaker identifies a problem and the listener repairs it.
   Example:
   Speaker: "I can't really explain it."
   Listener: "What you really mean is. . . ."

Exhibit 7–3 Mentis and Prutting's (1991) Analysis of Topic Categories

---

Topic Introduction
  Type topic/subtopic introduction
    New
    Related
    Reintroduced
  Manner topic/subtopic introduction
    Shifts
    Changes
    Noncoherent changes

Topic Maintenance
  Intonation unit categories
    Textual
    Interpersonal
    Ideational
      New information
        Requests for novel information
        Provides requested information
        Unsolicited novel information
        Other
      No new information
        Agreement/acknowledgment
        Clarification requests
        Provides requested information
        Repeats old information
        Confirmation requests
        Passes
        Clarification statement
        Summary statement
        Other
  Side sequence units
    Environmentally triggered
    Politeness markers
    Word search
  Problematic ideational units
    Ambiguous units
    Unrelated units
    Incomplete units

Source: Data from M. Mentis and C.A. Prutting, Analysis of Topic as Illustrated in a Head-Injured and Normal Adult, *Journal of Speech and Hearing Research*, Vol. 34, pp. 583–595, © 1991.

---

4. *Self-initiated self-repair*, in which the speaker identifies a problem and also repairs it.
   Example:
   Speaker: "I haven't explained that very clearly. . . . What I am trying to say is. . . ."

It is important to note that these repair mechanisms also reflect the degree to which a conversational participant is dependent on the other participant for repairing a breakdown during conversation. The repair mechanisms are listed from most dependent (other-initiated other-repair) to least dependent (self-initiated self-repair).

In the analysis of conversational repair mechanisms, the occurrence of a breakdown is first identified on the conversational transcript, and the type of repair implemented may then be noted, as well as its success. A tally of each type of repair mechanism will reflect the style and effectiveness of the repair strategy adopted by the participants in a given conversation. (See Appendix 7–A for examples of conversational repairs within the transcribed conversation.)

A somewhat different approach to the analysis of conversational breakdowns has been described by Gerber and Gurland (1990). This system was developed as an analysis of pragmatic-linguistic abilities in acquired aphasia. Known as the Assessment Protocol of Pragmatic Linguistic Skills (APPLS), it attempts first to identify the source of the conversational breakdown, which may be linguistic problems, pragmatic problems, or both. Next, the breakdown repair sequence is described by identifying partner or client strategies. Finally, the successfulness of the breakdown resolution is noted. Descriptions of the APPLS categories appear in Exhibit 7–4.

SYSTEMIC FUNCTIONAL LINGUISTICS

Systemic functional linguistics (SFL) is a theory of language use developed by Halliday

Exhibit 7–4 Assessment Protocol of Pragmatic Linguistic Skills (APPLS)

I. Breakdown

Conversational turn in which speaker's intended message is not understood by listener due to one or more factors, such as:

A. Linguistic Problems

    1. Phonological: — Deviation in the production of a phoneme manifested in a substitution, omission, distortion, transposition, or addition of a phoneme

    2. Word Retrieval: — Difficulty in retrieving a lexical item

    3. Semantic-Syntactic: — Difficulty in coding meaning and/or grammatical relations in a conventional manner

B. Pragmatic Problems

    1. Presupposition Referencing: — Utterance that fails to provide a specific referent and/or other information necessary for partner comprehension

    2. Topic Maintenance: — Difficulty sustaining a topic (e.g., limited conversational contribution)

    3. Turn Taking: — Difficulty signaling and/or maintaining speaker-listener turns (e.g., failure to take or relinquish one's conversational turn)

II. Breakdown-Repair Sequence

A. Partner Strategies (Signal To Repair) — Indication or cue provided by the listener that the intended message was not understood

    1. Nonspecific Request: — Request for repair signaled by a general question (e.g., "what?," "huh?") without specific reference to prior utterance

    2. Request for Specific Information: — Request for repair that specifies the kind of additional information needed by the partner to clarify failed message (e.g., "Who did you go with?")

    3. Conversational Directive: — Request for repair that implicitly or explicitly directs speaker to clarify message (e.g., "I don't understand what you mean. Try again.")

B. Client Strategies (Revision Attempts) — Modification of the message to clarify listener's confusion

    1. Acknowledgment/Rejection: — Simple nonverbal or verbal affirmation or denial of speaker's prior utterance (e.g., "yes," "no," or head nods)

    2. Repetition of Partner's Utterance: — Partial or complete repetition of partner's utterance; also included are speaker's repetition of his/her prior utterance

continues

Exhibit 7–4 continued

3.	Paraphrase:	Restatement of the partner's utterance, retaining meaning but changing wording; may include lexical, syntactic, and/or syntactic-semantic changes
4.	Adding Information:	Conversational turn that adds information to speaker's prior utterance
5.	Semantic-Syntactic Revision:	Restatement of the speaker's (e.g., aphasic individual's) prior utterance, retaining meaning but changing the wording; may include lexical, syntactic, and/or syntactic-semantic changes
6.	Gesture:	Nonverbal communicative signals (e.g., gestures, pointing) that may or may not be accompanied by verbalizations

III. Communication Breakdown Resolution

Outcome of the listener's signal or request for repair, the speaker's responsiveness to that signal, and the effectiveness of the speaker's repair of the intended message. The breakdown may be resolved successfully or may persist over several conversational turns until the intended message is understood or until there is a shift in the topic.

Source: Adapted with permission from S. Gerber and G. Gurland, Interactive Analysis of Pragmatic-Linguistic Abilities in Acquired Aphasia. Presented at the annual convention of American Speech Language Hearing Association in Seattle, Washington, © 1990.

(1985) based on the practical use of language and described as a system of choices. Each time an individual speaks, a choice is made regarding what is going to be said and how it is to be said according to who is being spoken to and the constraints of the speaking situation. As well as describing the effect of context on the language produced, SFL attempts to identify on what dimensions and in what ways context influences language. Eggins (1994) noted that context may be divided into a number of levels. *Register* describes the impact of the dimensions of the immediate environment on the way language is used. Three dimensions have a significant and predictable impact on language use: field, tenor, and mode. *Field* refers to the nature of the social interaction that is taking place (e.g., interview or casual conversation); *tenor* refers to those persons taking part in the interaction and their status and roles (e.g., teacher and student, two friends, salesman and customer); and *mode* refers to the manner in which the interaction is taking place (e.g., oral, written).

This approach to studying interactions has been applied to the telephone conversations of traumatically brain-injured individuals (Togher, Hand, & Code, 1997). Each subject was required to request information over the telephone from four different communication partners: a bus schedule information service, the police, the subject's mother, and a clinician. By manipulating the parameters of social distance and role, the investigators noted that traumatically brain-injured individuals' proficiency as coparticipants in interactions varied according to the tenor of the relationships. The factors of familiarity or social distance as well as status had a powerful influence on the language choices made by both normal and brain-injured subjects during the various interactions. Examining the brain-injured subjects' interactional skills in a variety of contexts afforded the subjects the opportunity to use a wider range of strategies, such as requesting clarification and confirmation, than are typically required in the therapy interview context.

CONCLUSION

This chapter has presented an overview of sampling and analysis procedures for conversational discourse. Although numerous measures can be extracted from a sample of conversation, ultimately the specific measures and level of analysis selected will be determined by the intent of the clinician for undertaking the discourse analysis. A conversational analysis may be employed broadly—for example, as an index of social skills proficiency—or narrowly, as an indicator of generalization of a very specific language ability such as word retrieval. In any event, conversational analysis is an important procedure for estimating communicative effectiveness in natural, real-world settings. In Appendix F, at the end of the book, conversational samples have been provided for further practice or review.

REFERENCES

Blank, M., & Franklin, E. (1980). Dialogue with preschoolers: A cognitively-based system of assessment. *Applied Psycholinguistics, 1,* 127–150.

Boles, L., Holland, A., & Beeson, P. (1993, November). *Conversation analysis: How much talk is enough?* Miniseminar presented at the annual meeting of the American Speech-Language-Hearing Association, Anaheim, CA.

Brinton, B., & Fujiki, M. (1984). Development of topic manipulation skills in discourse. *Journal of Speech and Hearing Research, 27,* 350–358.

Brinton, B., & Fujiki, M. (1989). *Conversational management with language-impaired children.* Gaithersburg, MD: Aspen Publishers, Inc.

Campbell, T.F., & Dollaghan, C.A. (1990). Expressive language recovery in severely brain-injured children and adolescents. *Journal of Speech and Hearing Disorders, 55,* 567–581.

Chafe, W. (1987). Cognitive constraints on information flow. In R.S. Tomlin (Ed.), *Coherence and grounding in discourse* (pp. 21–51). Philadelphia: John Benjamins.

Coelho, C.A., Liles, B.Z., & Duffy, R.J. (1991). Analysis of conversational discourse in head-injured adults. *Journal of Head Trauma Rehabilitation, 6,* 92–99.

Coelho, C.A., Liles, B.Z., Duffy, R.J., & Clarkson, J.V. (1993). Conversational patterns of aphasic, closed-head-injured and normal speakers. *Clinical Aphasiology, 21,* 183–192.

Damico, J. (1985). Clinical discourse analysis: A functional language assessment technique. In C.S. Simon (Ed.), *Communication skills and classroom success: Assessment of language-learning-disabled students* (pp. 165–206). San Diego: College-Hill.

Duncan, S.D., & Fiske, D.W. (1977). *Face to face interaction: Research, methods, and theory.* Hillsdale, NJ: Lawrence Erlbaum.

Eggins, S. (1994). *An introduction to systemic functional linguistics.* London: Pinter.

Ehrlich, J., & Barry, P. (1989). Rating communication behaviors in the head-injured adult. *Brain Injury, 3,* 193–198.

Garcia, L.J., & Joanette, Y. (1994). Conversational topic-shifting analysis in dementia. In R.L. Bloom, L.K. Obler, S. De Santi, & J.S. Ehrlich (Eds.), *Discourse analysis and applications: Studies in adult populations* (pp. 161–183). Hillsdale, NJ: Lawrence Erlbaum.

Gerber, S., & Gurland, G. (1990, November). *Interactive analysis of pragmatic-linguistic abilities in acquired aphasia.* Paper presented at the annual convention of the American Speech Language Hearing Association, Seattle, WA.

Halliday, M.A.K. (1985). *An introduction to functional grammar.* London: Edward Arnold.

Halper, A.S., Cherney, L.R., Burns, M.S., & Mogil, S.I. (1996). *Clinical management of right hemisphere dysfunction* (2nd ed.). Gaithersburg, MD: Aspen Publishers, Inc.

Hurtig, R. (1977). Toward a functional theory of discourse. In R.O. Freedle (Ed.), *Discourse production and comprehension* (pp. 89–106). Norwood, NJ: Ablex.

Mentis, M. (1994). Topic management in discourse: Assessment and intervention. *Topics in Language Disorders, 14,* 29–54.

Mentis, M., Briggs-Whittaker, J., & Gramigna, G.D. (1995). Discourse topic management in senile dementia of the Alzheimer's type. *Journal of Speech and Hearing Research, 38,* 1054–1066.

Mentis, M., & Prutting, C.A. (1991). Analysis of topic as illustrated in a head-injured and normal adult. *Journal of Speech and Hearing Research, 34,* 583–595.

Prutting, C., & Kirchner, D. (1983). Applied pragmatics. In T.M. Gallagher & C.A. Prutting (Eds.), *Pragmatic assess-*

ment and intervention issues in language (pp. 29–64). San Diego, CA: College-Hill.

Roth, F., & Spekman, N. (1984a). Assessing the pragmatic abilities of children: Part I. Organizational framework and assessment parameters. *Journal of Speech and Hearing Disorders, 49,* 2–11.

Roth, F., & Spekman, N. (1984b). Assessing the pragmatic abilities of children: Part II. Guidelines, considerations, and specific evaluation procedures. *Journal of Speech and Hearing Disorders, 49,* 12–17.

Sacks, H., Schegloff, E.A., & Jefferson, G. (1974). A sim-

plest systematics for the organization of turn-taking for conversation. *Language, 50,* 696–735.

Schegloff, E.A., Jefferson, G., & Sacks, H. (1977). The preference for self-correction in the organization of repair in conversation. *Language, 53,* 361–382.

Simmons-Mackie, N.N., & Damico, J.S. (1996). The contribution of discourse markers to communicative competence in aphasia. *American Journal of Speech-Language Pathology, 5,* 37–43.

Togher, L., Hand, L., & Code, C. (1997). Measuring service encounters in the traumatic brain injury population. *Aphasiology, 11,* 491–504.

Sample of Conversation between a Clinician (T) and a Traumatically Brain-Injured Individual (S)

Turns: designated by T (clinician) or S (patient)

Speaker Initiations: OB = oblige, COM = comment

Speaker Responses: AD = adequate, AD+ = adequate-plus, INAD = inadequate, AMB = ambiguous

Topic Initiation: N = novel introduction, SS = subtle shift, DS = disruptive shift

Conversational Repairs: OI OR = other-initiated other-repair
OI SR = other-initiated self-repair
SI OR = self-initiated other-repair
SI SR = self-initiated self-repair

Conversation Sample

COM	T: O.K. now I'd just like to have a conversation with you for a few minutes.
COM	S: Yes, certainly.
N OB	T: Um how long have you been a priest?
AD	S: About 15 years.
COM	T: Uh-huh.
COM	S: Yes.
N OB	T: And you said you grew up in New York?
AD	S: Yes.
N OB	T: Uh-huh and where did you go to seminary?
AD+	S: I started off in Orange in Orange, Connecticut, did what is called a novitiate which is sort of a the the basic for a spiritual like we learn how to pray and we learn the first person the first time we're introduced to the community life we live with others and we're also given the expla explanation of what the life of a priest is like receive a few of our classes or else I have the opportunity for doing some work with some other people in one of the local parishes maybe teaching what we call CCD religious instruction and in finishing my novitiate I made my

temporary religious vows of poverty, chastity and obedience for a span of three years then I continued my studies going to Salaminca Spain where I studied two years of what we call Humanities Liberal Arts studies Latin, Greek, Art and Literature.

SS OB T: Now where in Spain is that?

AD S: Salaminca.

O
I   **OB** T: What part of Spain was that?
S
R **AD+** S: Sort of the center an hour outside of Madrid. Used to have a the old reputation of being a higher seed of learning.

SS OB T: Uh-huh. Now while you were in Spain did you have the opportunity to travel much?

AD+ S: Well within Spain we'd go for vacations in the northern part and that's probably about it no I didn't really.

SS OB T: Now and the other uh um individuals that you were studying with . . .

S: Yes

T: Were they all from the States or were they from all over?

AD+ S: No they're from all over pretty much Mexico, Spain a few of them Ireland and a few from the United States.

SS OB T: Now did you speak Spanish before you went over?

AD S: A little bit, yes, yes.

OB T: And your instruction was it in Spanish?

AD S: Yes.

OB T: Was it easy to pick up?

AD+ S: A little bit because we are sort of encouraged any anything we had to do to ask for in Spanish to use the language as much as we could.

COM T: Yeah.

COM S: Yes.

SS OB T: Um why did you chose to go to Spain instead of somewhere in the States?

AD S: Well that's where our order that's our religious order that I belong to we would have a sort of a centers for where we go for different formation they have everything set up for us so we go there and everything um we receive all that they have to offer.

OB T: Uh-hm uh O.K. now what order are you affiliated with?

AD+ S: Legion of Christ. It's an order that's founded in Mexico at the beginning of the century and is now in about now in about seventeen countries.

SS OB T: And how did you happen to land in Cheshire?

INAD S: Well my oldest brother he entered into the order before me about four years before me he entered in Woodmont, Connecticut, so we went when he was in Woodmont I went up there to visit him and met a lot of the youngsters he was with and the priest some times they joke around with me and say well what are you going to do why don't you come up here and I sort of tried to give me they explained that they really got along well and they had hikes and they went they really made good use of their time so I liked that.

SS OB   T: Uh-huh. And um what parish were you associated with?

AD+   S: We're not usually associated with parishes as of yet cause after we're ordained we usually we just usually our founder may receive certain requests from different bishops and then the bishops will designate us where they think there would be where there's an opening where we could be most of use.

SS OB   T: Uh-huh. And what were you doing? What have you been doing?

AD   S: Yes I was working in some of our schools in Mexico then in the youth center we have in Brazil.

SS OB   T: Where in Brazil?

AD+   S: A city called Curitiba. It's got a lot of European influence there.

OB   T: What part of the country is that in?

AD   S: The central.

COM   T: Um . . .

AD   S: Or the southern.

SS OB   T: Did you ever hear of a city Juiz de Fora?

AD   S: No.

OB   T: Did you ever get to Rio?

AD   S: Yes.

OB   T: Sao Paulo?

AD   S: Yes.

OB   T: So you did you have occasion to travel around the country?

AD   S: No not too much no in Rio no no in Brazil.

OB   T: How how long were you in Brazil?

AD   S: I think two years.

OB   T: O.K. What years were you there?

AD   S: About 84, 1984.

SS OB   T: 1984, uh-hm. Did you enjoy that experience?

AD   S: Yes very much so.

OB   T: Which did you like more, Brazil or Mexico?

AD   S: Probably Mexico.

OB   T: Uh in Brazil did you pick up Portuguese?

AD+   S: Yes. It's very sim very similar to Spanish and Italian.

SS OB   T. Uh-huh. Would you ever want to go back to Brazil?

AD   S: Yes, yes.

SS OB   T: And how do you like your situation in Cheshire?

AD   S: I like it very much.

OB   T: Good group of men?

AD+ S: Yes and a place [where well I wrote it down in the book that I this place] that's accessible to a wheelchair and it's a place that's close to a place where you could receive therapy [to receive and] to better myself I have a lot of deficiencies.

COM T: You have your work cut out for you.

AD S. Yes.

SS OB T: Now what where is your brother these days?

AD S: My oldest brother is in Dublin, Ireland.

COM T: Uh-huh.

COM S: Yes.

SS OB T: Over there teaching?

AD+ S: I think he's sort of in charge of the section there language center we have there.

OB T. Uh-huh that's nice. It's called a language center?

AD S: Yes.

OB T: And what is that?

AD+ S: Well you see a lot of Mexicans go there and spend a year to learn the English language and they sort of go out and see the city and go out see certain cultural aspects of the city.

SS OB T: Uh-huh. Does your brother like Ireland?

AD S: Yes.

OB T: How long has he been there?

AD S: I think about two years.

OB T: And where was he before? You recall?

AD S: I'm not too sure I think he was in Santiago, Chile.

SS OB T: Could did you ever have the opportunity to request a placement?

AD S: No.

OB T: So you were sent where they needed you.

AD S: Yes.

SS OB T: And what's the likelihood that you'd be sent somewhere and for a prolonged period of time beyond two years, like ten years?

O I S R [**OB** S: I'd say its . . . what's the likelihood?
OB T: Yeah I mean did you know anyone who was sent somewhere for a long period of time?

AD+ S: No we usually unless it's sort of a say a stable that person is really cut out for that type of job and there's a lot of need for him like the director of the university which can't usually go for just one year something.

SS OB T: Uh-hm. Now are any individuals from your order tied in with universities in the States?

AD S: No. Not that I know of.

OB T: It's primarily Latin America or Europe.

SS AD+	S: Yes, yes. We have a we're trying to start in the United States what are called family centers where people can come youngsters and they come and receive courses and we organize different recreational activities for them as well some of the local parks are go skiing or summer time there's summer camp.
OB	T: Aren't there kids who come up and play basketball?
AD	S: Yes.
OB	T: Up in Cheshire?
AD	S: Yes. St. Bridgets I think.
COM	T: Uh-huh.
COM	S: Parish in Cheshire.
SS OB	T: Now were you teaching any CCD there?
AD	S: No.
OB	T: Oh you've only been in Cheshire since you've been injured.
AD	S: I've been in Cheshire since I've been injured.
COM	T: Well this has worked out pretty well for you.
AD	S: Yes.
SS OB	T: Cause you're uh do you still have family in New York?
AD	S: Yes.
OB	T: So you're relatively close to family.
AD	S: Yes, yes, they come up.
SS OB	T: How big is your family other than your older brother?
AD+	S: I have five sisters and three other brothers.
COM	T: Holy cow.
COM	S: Yes.
SS OB	T: Are they all in the Northeast?
AD+	S: Yes. My oldest sister is in Pittsburgh, Pennsylvania, my youngest daughters in my youngest sister is in New Rochelle.
SS OB	T: Uh-huh now uh where do you fall in the . . .
AD	S: Fourth from the top.
OB	T: So the . . .
AD	S: Fourth oldest.
COM	T: Fourth oldest.
COM	S: Yes.
OB	T: And what's the age span what's the oldest and the youngest?
AD	S: . . . Say from just me guessing there's probably 25 years difference between the oldest and the youngest.

O
I
S
R bracket grouping: OB / AD / COM

OB   T: Now how old is the oldest? Roughly?

AD   S: Probably about 42.

OB   T: 42 to about a teenager.

AD   S: Yes about 20 in their 20s probably 25.

OB   T: Quite a family huh that was a house full huh.

AD   S: Yes. A lot of fun growing up.

COM   T: I'll bet.

COM   S: Yes.

COM   T: You've always been a ready team.

COM   S: Yes, yes.

SS OB   T: Any of your sisters uh go in to become nuns?

AD   S: No.

OB   T: So just the two of you.

AD   S: Yes, yes, yes.

SS OB   T: Anybody else in your family, uncles or aunts?

AD   S: No, not that I know of.

SS OB   T: Now did you go to Catholic schools growing up?

AD+   S: Yes I went to the Irish Christian Brothers in New Rochelle then after that I went to the public school Marinak, New York.

OB   T: For high school?

AD   S: Yes.

SS OB   T: Were you involved in sports?

AD   S: Yes, yes a lot.

OB   T: Uh-huh. What did you do?

AD+   S: Well I've always swam and I used to play golf, water ski and snow ski and that's probably about then around my house sometimes I played baseball or touch football or some of those things but those were the basic sports were swimming and skiing and then I used to sometimes also play golf in the summer and tennis.

COM   T: Good.

Summary of Conversational Analysis Performed on Conversation Sample

	TBI Individual (S)	*Clinician (T)*
Speaker Initiations		
Obliges	1 (2%)	62 (83%)
Comments	9 (12%)	13 (17%)
Response Adequacy		
Adequate-plus	18 (24%)	0
Adequate	46 (62%)	0
Inadequate	0	0
Ambiguous	0	0
Total Turns	74 (100%)	75 (100%)
Topic Initiatives		
Novel	0	9 (26%)
Subtle shift	1	26 (74%)
Disruptive shift	0	0
Total	1	35
Conversational Repairs		
Other-initiated other-repaired	0	0
Other-initiated self-repaired	2	1
Self-initiated other-repaired	0	0
Self-initiated self-repaired	2	0

Note: TBI, traumatically brain-injured. Percentage scores reflect proportion of total turns.

CHAPTER 8

Discourse Characteristics of Neurologically Impaired Adults: An Annotated Bibliography

Leora Reiff Cherney, Carl A. Coelho, and Barbara B. Shadden

In previous chapters, discourse behavior and specific discourse types have been defined, and procedures for the different discourse analyses have been outlined. Clearly, there is pronounced variability in discourse performance, with task differences contributing to widely different cognitive and linguistic demands being placed on the individual patient. Further, there is variability in the type of analyses that may be selected for a given task. As a result, research data concerning discourse performance in various clinical populations may be expected to show a fair degree of heterogeneity, depending on task attributes, the level of analysis, and the specific profile of patient deficits.

This expected variability has one critical implication. The search for the ultimate "normative" database concerning discourse performance in adult neurologically impaired populations is in its infancy at best. Further, there may never be a clean, readily referenced set of norms for aspects of discourse behavior. The heterogeneity of language and communication functioning in the normal older adult population alone may preclude the development of the kinds of assessment norms that we associate with children's language development (Shadden, Burnette, Eikenberry, & DiBrezzo, 1991).

Nevertheless, one major contention of this book is that discourse performance measures not only provide one of the best indices of communicative performance available for neurologi-

cally impaired adults, but also offer important clues as to the nature of underlying deficits central to communicative success or breakdown (whether due to linguistic or cognitive domains). Some response to concerns about variability in so-called "normative" discourse performance must be offered.

The answer to the dilemmas posed here lies in an examination of *patterns* of discourse performance. For clinicians, there is a need to know which discourse patterns suggest which diagnoses, as part of the differential diagnostic process. Conversely, clinicians may require guidance in determining which discourse analysis domains will yield the most productive information, given a particular patient diagnosis. Further, discourse analysis becomes a primary tool for quantifying those factors contributing to communication performance breakdown. In this context, an understanding of general *patterns* of discourse performance in specific clinical populations is all that is needed to guide clinical assessment and intervention activities.

The purpose of this chapter, then, is to provide the clinician with a sampling of research literature that illustrates aspects of discourse functioning in four neurologically impaired populations typically seen by the speech-language pathologist. The patterns that emerge for each population may indicate where the most predictable domains for discourse analysis and subsequent interventions may lie. The four populations are:

1. individuals with dementia, especially individuals with probable Alzheimer's disease (see Table 8–1)
2. individuals with aphasia (see Table 8–2)
3. individuals with right-hemisphere neurological impairment (see Table 8–3)
4. individuals with traumatic brain injury (see Table 8–4)

For each population, the representative literature is summarized so that, at a glance, the clinician can determine the types of subjects, the discourse task used, the level of analysis, and the results of each study. The primary emphasis is on discourse production, since the book focuses on analysis of discourse output.

No attempt has been made to interpret the literature or to provide a definitive textbook review. The reader is encouraged to seek out the original articles as well as additional information about the discourse skills of these and other clinical populations of particular interest. In view of the growing literature on discourse behavior in adults, readers are also encouraged to keep their own ongoing summaries of any new studies of interest.

Summarizing and highlighting patterns of discourse performance in these populations may assist in the process of differential diagnosis and may provide an appreciation of those discourse behaviors that are appropriate targets for intervention.

REFERENCE

Shadden, B.B., Burnette, R.B., Eikenberry, B.R., & DiBrezzo, R. (1991). All discourse tasks are not created equal. *Clinical Aphasiology*, *20*, 327–341.

Table 8–1 Discourse Deficits Secondary to Dementia of the Alzheimer's Type (DAT)

Reference	Subjects	Discourse Tasks	Level of Analysis	Results for Subjects with DAT
Chapman et al. (1995)	12 early stage DAT 12 normal old-elderly (over 80 years) 12 normal controls (mean age 65.7, range 47–78)	Narrative discourse (story generation from Norman Rockwell pictures)	Informational content (propositions)	Significant impairment associated with mild DAT on coherence measures (application of a typical frame of interpretation and generation of frame-supporting information).
			Coherence	
			Presence of narrative story structure	Production of fewer narratives (but more partial narratives or nonnarratives) than the other two groups.
			Reference (use of pronouns)	
Chenery & Murdoch (1994)	7 early DAT 7 matched controls	Narrative (computer generated animations)	Informational content	Produced fewer total propositions with fewer core pieces of information; made significantly more ambiguous and incorrect errors, and fewer errors of elaboration, but did not differ on the frequency of irrelevant errors.
			Story grammer	Consistently omitted setting information, mention of a complicating action, and reference to a resolution.
			Cohesion	Produced similar numbers of pronominal referents; produced many types of disrupted cohesion.

continues

Table 8–1 continued

Reference	Subjects	Discourse Tasks	Level of Analysis	Results for Subjects with DAT
Cherney & Canter (1993)	10 DAT 10 RHD 10 health controls	Descriptive (pictures and objects) Narrative (story retelling) Procedural	Informational content	Significantly different from normals in all categories of informational content, but similar to subjects with RHD; large number of irrelevant utterances produced with somewhat more redundant information than RHD. In early stages, DAT could be differentiated from normal status on basis of rate of speech and proportion of essential information produced.
DeSanti et al. (1994)	2 midstage DAT 2 normal controls	Conversation	Cohesion	Use of as many cohesive devices as controls but proportionally more lexical cohesion (e.g., repetition) than normals. All speakers displayed different styles of repetition use.
Ehrlich et al. (1997)	16 DAT 16 matched controls	Narrative (from single pictures and picture sequences)	Informational content Cohesion Sentential/surface level	Produced fewer propositions and lexical items. Amount of target content was influenced by the amount of information pictorially represented; DAT performed better when the stimuli contained relatively less information. Produced shorter sentence lengths, with more sentence fragments and reference errors.

Study	Subjects	Task/Genre	Discourse measure	Findings
Garcia & Joanette (1994)	4 DAT 5 normal elderly 1 conversational partner for all subjects	Conversation	Topic shifting	Lower percentages of topic shading shifts. In subjects with DAT, more shifts occurred as a result of a failure to continue the topic of conversation; in normal subjects more shifts occurred because of a desire to tell an anecdote.
Heller et al. (1992)	16 questionable mild DAT 16 healthy controls	Narrative (retold the story of a silent video cartoon while watching the events as they were occurring)	Sentential/surface level Informational content	Produced fewer clauses. Described fewer thematically important events.
Hier et al. (1985)	26 DAT 13 stroke-related dementia 20 aphasics 15 healthy controls	Cookie theft picture description	Sentential/surface level analysis Informational content	Fewer total words, fewer unique words, fewer prepositional phrases, fewer subordinate clauses, and more incomplete sentence fragments. Mild DAT showed similarities to anomic aphasia; moderate DAT to Wernicke's or transcortical aphasia; the more severe stroke-related dementia to Broca's aphasia.
Illes (1989)	10 DAT 10 Huntington's disease 10 Parkinson's disease 10 healthy controls	Answered open-ended autobiographical questions	Analysis of silent and filled hesitations Rate Syntactic complexity	Each neurodegenerative disease displayed a unique profile of spontaneous language production. Temporal interruptions of varying types occurred in DAT and Huntington's disease; long-duration silent hesitations occurred in Parkinson's disease only. Syntactic complexity was reduced in Huntington's disease. Verbal paraphasias were present in DAT and moderately advanced Huntington's disease.

continues

Reference	Subjects	Discourse Tasks	Level of Analysis	Results for Subjects with DAT
Lamar et al. (1994)	10 end-stage DAT	Conversation (with familiar and unfamiliar speakers)	Pragmatic parameters	Small set of pragmatic behaviors spared in all subjects—giving a relevant response about a topic introduced by the partner, making appropriate informative contributions to the conversation, and taking turns of appropriate length in response to familiar questions. Most subjects did not make spontaneous comments or requests, or express feelings.
Mentis et al. (1995)	12 DAT 12 elderly controls	Conversation	Topic management	More limited and disrupted topic introduction skills, difficulty maintaining topic, and limited contributions to propositional development of topic sequences.
Nicholas et al. (1985)	19 DAT 16 Wernicke's 8 anomics 30 normal controls	Cookie theft picture description	Informational content Cohesion	Like those with Wernicke's aphasia, DAT subjects produced many deictic terms, pronouns without antecedents, semantic paraphasias, and repetitions. Wernicke's aphasia and DAT could be distinguished, as subjects with Wernicke's aphasia produced more neologisms and more literal and verbal (not semantic) paraphasias.
Orange et al. (1996)	5 early stage DAT 5 middle stage DAT 6 normal controls	Conversation (with a family member over mealtime)	Conversational repair	Subjects with early DAT similar to normal controls in proportion and types of trouble sources and repair strategies produced. Subjects with middle stage DAT also engaged in speaker-generated repair and self-repair, generally with success.

Study	Subjects	Type of discourse	Discourse measures	Findings
Ripich & Terrell (1988)	6 DAT, 6 normal controls	Topic-directed interviews	Turns; Informational content (complete propositions, incomplete propositions, nonpropositions); Cohesion; Coherence	More words and more turns; no significant difference in propositional form or cohesion devices, but a pattern of disrupted cohesion associated with DAT. Interviews with DAT subjects were judged to be significantly less coherent than those with normal controls.
Ripich et al. (1991)	11 DAT, 11 normally elderly	Conversation (same examiner conversed with each DAT and control subject)	Speech acts; Conversational turns	Used more requestives and fewer assertives. Had shorter turns and more occurrences of unintelligible utterances; overall, maintained interaction patterns so the discourse genre of conversation was sustained.
Smith et al. (1989)	18 DAT, 18 normal controls	Picture description (from Western Aphasia Battery)	Surface structure analysis; Informational content	No difference in number or complexity of clauses. Conveyed as much information as controls, but were less concise (more time, fewer content units per minute, more syllables per content unit).
Tomoeda & Bayles (1993)	3 DAT, 3 matched normal controls	Picture description (Norman Rockwell's "Easter Morning"; longitudinally over 5 years. This is one of the very few longitudinal studies.)	Informational content; Verbal fragmentation (revisions and aborted phrases)	Common pattern of deterioration marked by reductions in total output and in amount and quality of information. Conciseness best distinguished the discourse of subjects with mild DAT from normals.

continues

Table 8–1 continued

Reference	Subjects	Discourse Tasks	Level of Analysis	Results for Subjects with DAT
Ulatowska & Chapman (1991)	5 DAT 5 matched controls 5 old-elderly persons (over 85 years old)	Narrative discourse (elicited by single frame pictures and picture sequences)	Informational content	Reduction of information; performance similar to that of old-elderly, but more incomplete propositions.
			Story grammar	Increased amount of setting information; action sequences poorly developed; resolutions rarely produced.
			Coherence	Reference without an antecedent or ambiguous referents were especially evident in old-elderly subjects and some DAT subjects. Other variables such as incomplete propositions, false starts, and poorly developed story lines reduced coherence in DAT.

RHD, right hemisphere damage.

REFERENCES

Chapman, S.B., Ulatowska, H.K., Franklin, L.R., King, K., Johnson, J., & McIntire, D.D. (1995). Discourse in early Alzheimer's disease versus normal advanced aging. *American Journal of Speech Language Pathology, 4*, 125–129.

Chenery, H.J., & Murdoch, B.E. (1994). The production of narrative discourse in response to animations in persons with dementia of the Alzheimer's type: Preliminary findings. *Aphasiology, 7*, 159–171.

Cherney, L.R., & Canter, G.J. (1993). Informational content in the discourse of patients with probable Alzheimer's disease and patients with right brain damage. *Clinical Aphasiology, 21*, 123–134.

DeSanti, S., Koenig, L., Obler, L.K., & Goldberger, J. (1994). Cohesive devices and conversational discourse in Alzheimer's disease. In R. Bloom, L.K. Obler, S. DeSanti, & J.S. Ehrlich (Eds.), *Discourse analysis and applications: Studies in adult clinical populations* (pp. 210–215). Hillsdale, NJ: Lawrence Erlbaum.

Ehrlich, J.S., Obler, L.K., & Clark, L. (1997). Ideational and semantic contributions to narrative production in adults with dementia of the Alzheimer's type. *Journal of Communication Disorders, 30*, 79–99.

Garcia, L.J., & Joanette, Y. (1994). Conversational topic shifting analysis in dementia. In R. Bloom, L.K. Obler, S. DeSanti, & J.S. Ehrlich (Eds.), *Discourse analysis and applications: Studies in adult clinical populations* (pp. 161–183). Hillsdale, NJ: Lawrence Erlbaum .

Heller, R.B., Dobbs, A.R., & Rule, B.G. (1992). Communicative function in patients with questionable Alzheimer's disease. *Psychology and Aging, 7*, 395–400.

Hier, D.B., Hagenlocker, K., & Shindler, A.G. (1985). Language disintegration in dementia: Effects of etiology and severity. *Brain and Language, 25*, 117–133.

Illes, J. (1989). Neurolinguistic features of spontaneous language production dissociate three forms of neurodegenerative disease: Alzheimer's, Huntington's, and Parkinson's. *Brain and Language, 37*, 628–642.

Lamar, M.A.C., Obler, L.K., Knoefel, J.E., & Albert, M.L. (1994). Communication patterns in end-stage Alzheimer's disease: Pragmatic analysis. In R. Bloom, L.K. Obler, S. DeSanti, & J.S. Ehrlich (Eds.), *Discourse analysis and applications: Studies in adult clinical populations* (pp. 217–235). Hillsdale, NJ: Lawrence Erlbaum.

Mentis, M., Briggs-Whitaker, J., & Gramigna, G.D. (1995). Discourse topic management in senile dementia of the Alzheimer's type. *Journal of Speech and Hearing Research, 38*, 1054–1066.

Nicholas, M., Obler, L.K., Albert, M.L., & Helm-Estabrooks, N. (1985). Empty speech in Alzheimer's disease and fluent aphasia. *Journal of Speech and Hearing Research, 28*, 405–410.

Orange, J.B., Lubinski, R., & Higginbotham, D.J. (1996). Conversational repair by individuals with dementia of the Alzheimer's type. *Journal of Speech and Hearing Research, 39*, 881–895.

Ripich, D.N., & Terrell, B.Y. (1988). Patterns of discourse cohesion and coherence in Alzheimer's disease. *Journal of Speech and Hearing Disorders, 53*, 8–14.

Ripich, D.N., Vertes, D., Whitehouse, P., Fulton, S., & Ekelman, B. (1991). Turn-taking and speech act patterns in the discourse of senile dementia of the Alzheimer's type patients. *Brain and Language, 40*, 330–343.

Smith, S.R., Chenery, H.J., & Murdoch, B.E. (1989). Semantic abilities in dementia of the Alzheimer's type. *Brain and Language, 36*, 533–542.

Tomoeda, C.K., & Bayles, K.A. (1993). Longitudinal effects of Alzheimer's disease on discourse production. *Alzheimer Disease and Associated Disorders, 7*, 223–236.

Ulatowska, H.K., & Chapman, S.B. (1991). Discourse studies. In R. Lubinski (Ed.), *Dementia and communication* (pp. 115–132). Philadelphia: BC Decker.

Table 8–2 Discourse Deficits Secondary to Aphasia

Reference	Subjects	Discourse Tasks	Level of Analysis	Results for Subjects with Aphasia
Berko Gleason et al. (1980)	5 Broca's aphasia 5 Wernicke's 5 matched controls	Narrative (while looking at pictures, retelling a story that was heard)	Sentential/surface level analysis (syntactic and lexical) Cohesion—reference Informational content— number of themes	Fewer themes, smaller proportion of target lexemes, and more pronouns without antecedents than controls. Those with Wernicke's used as many words as controls, but had concatenated sentences, deixis, and verbs rather than nouns. Those with Broca's used few words, more direct speech, and more nouns than verbs.
Bottenberg & Lemme (1990)	14 mild-moderate aphasics 14 normal controls	Narrative (from colored sequenced pictures under conditions of shared or unshared knowledge of the story by the listener)	Cohesion story grammar	No differences for either group under shared or unshared conditions; more errors of cohesion and less complete stories associated with aphasia.
Brenneise-Sarshad et al. (1991)	5 nonfluent 5 fluent 10 normal controls	Narrative (from picture sequences under knowledgeable and naive listener conditions)	Informational content (correct information units) Cohesion	Listener condition did not affect performance of either group. Aphasics produced significantly fewer words, shorter grammatical units, and less relevant and accurate information than controls. No difference between groups on use of cohesive ties.

Study	Subjects	Task	Measures	Findings
Brookshire & Nicholas (1994)	6 nonfluent 14 fluent 20 non–brain-damaged controls	Descriptive, narrative, and procedural discourse elicited by single pictures, picture sequences, requests for personal information, and requests for procedural information (Each task done three times, twice on the same day and then 7–10 days later.)	Informational content—percent correct information units and words per minute	Test–retest stability increased as sample size increased. Recommended that samples be elicited from 4 or 5 stimuli (an average of 300–400 words).
Brookshire & Nicholas (1995)	10 fluent 10 nonfluent 40 non–brain-damaged controls	Descriptive, narrative, and procedural discourse elicited by single pictures, picture sequences, requests for personal information, and requests for procedural information	Informational content (e.g., correct information units, main concepts). Performance deviations (e.g., false starts, repetitions, fillers, irrelevancies)	Significantly greater percentages of inaccurate words, false starts, and part-word or unintelligible productions than controls. Fluent aphasics produced greater percentages of nonexact repetitions; nonfluent aphasics produced greater percentages of the word *and* and nonword fillers.
Busch et al. (1988)	7 non-fluent 7 anomic 7 mixed (fluent speech with literal and verbal paraphasias) 7 nonaphasic controls	Picture description	Informational content	No difference in ability to produce crucial information; aphasic subjects were less accurate than controls, but like the controls, modified their descriptions in response to communication failure.

continues

Table 8–2 continued

Reference	Subjects	Discourse Tasks	Level of Analysis	Results for Subjects with Aphasia
Coehlo et al. (1994)	1 anomic, followed longitudinally over 12 months 3 normal controls	Narrative discourse (from a 19-frame film strip with no sound track)	Sentential/surface level Cohesion Story grammar	Complexity of sentence-level grammar variable, but close to that of normals. Cohesion improved over time as language improved until comparable to normals. Story grammar remained relatively impaired and did not improve with time.
Correia et al. (1988, 1990)	3 Broca's aphasia 4 anomic 5 fluent mixed 12 nonaphasic controls	Picture description	Informational content and efficiency	Male-biased pictures elicited significantly more words and more correct information units than female-biased pictures: aphasic and control speakers differentiated by two measures (words per minute and percent words that are correct information units).
Craig et al. (1993)	103 aphasics (i.e. 15 mild, 39 moderate, 49 severe)	Cookie Theft Picture description	Informational content (amount and efficiency)	Content units and content units/minute differentiated all severity levels; syllable rate did not distinguish mild and moderate groups. There was an inverse relationship between number of content units and aphasia severity; inverse relationship between syllable rate and severity was present for nonfluent, but not fluent aphasia.
Doyle et al. (1995)	9 Broca's aphasia 1 transcortical motor 8 anomics 2 conduction	Descriptive, procedural, and narrative discourse elicited under structured conditions; Conversation (topic-open and topic-constrained conditions)	Informational content (e.g., correct information units and main concepts)	Significantly greater percentages of informative words in conversation; percent correct information units produced in structured discourse tasks predicted performance under conversational conditions.

Study	Subjects	Discourse type	Variables	Findings
Doyle et al. (1994)	12 Broca's aphasia 1 conduction 12 normals	Conversation (with familiar and unfamiliar partners, and open and constrained topics)	Communicative function	Lower proportion of statements and requests, higher proportion of answers and ambiguous communicative attempts relative to normals. Familiarity of conversational partner, number of conversational participants, or physical setting had no significant effect. Sampling procedure affected performance—proportionately more statements under topic constrained, more requests and answers under topic open.
Ernst-Baron et al. (1987)	5 Broca's aphasia 5 anomics 5 mixed fluent 5 normals	Narrative	Informational content	Less information retold by aphasic subjects, but no significant difference from amount retold by nonaphasic subjects; type of aphasia did not affect information units retold; more information central to story retold than information peripheral to story; amount of information increased on repeated retellings of story.
Ferguson (1993)	7 fluent 14 normals	Conversation	Trouble-indicating behaviors, repair by listener (supplying words)	Trouble-indicating behaviors more frequent for normal–aphasic dyads than for normal–normal dyads; less familiar communicative partners more likely to guess and supply a word than familiar partners; about half of the supplied words explicitly requested by the aphasic subject.
Hinkley & Craig (1992)	6 chronic aphasics (4 nonfluent, 2 fluent) 6 matched controls	Responses to comments about picture stimuli Responses to comments in conversation	Frequency of responses Types of responses (passing moves, successive remarks)	Both picture and conversational tasks elicited similar response profiles for aphasic and control groups.

continues

Table 8–2 continued

Reference	Subjects	Discourse Tasks	Level of Analysis	Results for Subjects with Aphasia
Klippi (1991)	2 nonfluent 3 fluent	Group conversation (aphasic patients and one speech-language pathologist)	Number of moves, total speech time, active conversational moves (initiation), reactive moves (continuation), deviant conversational moves	Variety of different interactive profiles demonstrated; no differences between fluent and nonfluent aphasics in active and reactive moves; more deviant moves demonstrated by nonfluent aphasics.
Li et al (1995)	5 Broca's aphasia 7 conduction 10 anomic 10 normal controls	Narrative (story retelling) Procedural	Informational content Story grammar	Topic familiarity influenced output in both tasks. With familiar topics, more optional steps were given in procedural discourse; more action and resolution clauses were included in story retelling. Listener familiarity affected story retelling only; more settings were provided when listeners were familiar.
Nicholas & Brookshire (1993a)	6 nonfluent 14 fluent 20 normals	Descriptive, narrative, and procedural discourse elicited by single pictures, picture sequences, requests for personal information, and requests for procedural information	Informational content and efficiency	Significant difference between aphasic and nonaphasic subjects on each measure derived from correct information units (CIUs) and word counts. The three measures that more dependably separated aphasic from non–brain-damaged subjects were words per minute, percent CIUs, and CIUs per minute.

Study	Subjects	Task	Measure	Findings
Nicholas & Brookshire (1993b, 1995)	20 aphasics varying in type and severity 20 non–brain-damaged controls	Descriptive, narrative, and procedural discourse elicited by single pictures, picture sequences, requests for personal information, and requests for procedural information (Each task was done three times, twice on the same day and then 7–10 days later.)	Informational content— main concepts	Completeness and accuracy of main concepts differentiated aphasic and control groups. Acceptable interjudge and intrajudge reliability, and test–retest stability on all measures.
Roberts & Wertz (1989)	20 aphasics	Spontaneous conversation; elicited language (PICA Subtest 1)	Syntactic well-formedness Semantic accuracy	Utterance and clause length longer in conversation; syntactic well-formedness better in elicited language; semantic accuracy better in conversation.
Ulatowska et al. (1983a)	15 moderately impaired aphasics (8 anterior, 5 posterior, 2 mixed) 15 controls	Procedural	Sentential surface level Informational content (procedural steps)	Well structured procedural discourse that was reduced in complexity and amount, with selective reduction of information.
Ulatowska et al. (1983b)	15 moderately impaired aphasics (8 anterior, 5 posterior, 2 mixed) 15 controls	Narrative discourse (both self-generated and elicited from either a picture sequence or from a story that was heard)	Sentential surface level Story grammar Informational content (propositional analysis)	Well-structured narrative discourse that was reduced in complexity and amount, with selective reduction of information.

continues

Table 8–2 continued

Reference	Subjects	Discourse Tasks	Level of Analysis	Results for Subjects with Aphasia
Wambaugh et al. (1991)	6 agrammatic 60 normals	Conversation (elicited in a referential communication task and a planning activity)	Communicative function (regulation, statement, exchange, personal, conversation, miscellaneous)	Proportional representation of communicative functions influenced by sampling methods; normal range of speech acts in some aphasic subjects; communicative function usage possibly related to severity of aphasia.
Williams et al., (1994)	5 Broca's aphasia 7 conduction 10 anomic 10 normal controls	Narrative (story retelling) Procedural	Sentential/surface level	Topic familiarity influenced output. For both tasks, more t-units produced on familiar topics. For procedural discourse, greater grammatical complexity on unfamiliar topics; no change in complexity for narrative discourse. Listener familiarity did not influence verbal output.
Yorkston & Beukelman (1980)	50 aphasics 78 normals across the age span	Cookie theft picture description	Informational content (amount and efficiency)	Inverse relationship between severity of aphasia and number of content units. Mild and high-moderate aphasics produced similar number of content units as normals, but differed on measures of efficiency (speaking rate and content units per minute).

REFERENCES

Berko Gleason, J., Goodglass, H., Obler, L., Green, E., Hyde, M.R., & Weintraub, S. (1980). Narrative strategies of aphasic and normal-speaking subjects. *Journal of Speech and Hearing Research, 23,* 370–382.

Bottenberg, D., & Lemme, M. (1990). Effect of shared and unshared listener knowledge on narratives of normal and aphasic adults. *Clinical Aphasiology, 19,* 109–116.

Brenneise-Sarshad, R., Nicholas, L.E., & Brookshire, R.H. (1991). Effects of apparent listener knowledge and picture stimuli on aphasic and non–brain-damaged speaker's narrative discourse. *Journal of Speech and Hearing Research, 34,* 168–176.

Brookshire, R.H., & Nicholas, L.E. (1994). Speech sample size and test–retest stability of connected speech measures for adults with aphasia. *Journal of Speech and Hearing Research, 37,* 399–407.

Brookshire, R.H., & Nicholas, L.E. (1995). Performance deviations in the connected speech of adults with no brain damage and adults with aphasia. *American Journal of Speech Language Pathology, 4,* 118–123.

Busch, C.R., Brookshire, R.H., & Nicholas, L.E. (1988). Referential communication by aphasic and nonaphasic adults. *Journal of Speech and Hearing Disorders, 53,* 475–482.

Coelho, C.A., Liles, B.Z., Duffy, R.J., Clarkson, J.V., & Elia, D. (1994). Longitudinal assessment of narrative discourse in a mildly aphasic adult. *Clinical Aphasiology, 22,* 145–155.

Correia, L., Brookshire, R.H., & Nicholas, L.E. (1988). The effects of picture content on descriptions by aphasic and non–brain-damaged speakers. *Clinical Aphasiology, 18,* 447–472.

Correia, L., Brookshire, R.H., & Nicholas, L.E. (1990). Aphasic and non–brain-damaged adults' descriptions of aphasia test pictures and gender-biased pictures. *Journal of Speech and Hearing Disorders, 55,* 713–720.

Craig, H.K., Hinckley, J.J., Winkelseth, M., Carry, L., Walley, J., Bardach, L., Higman, B., Hilfinger, P., Schall, C., & Sheimo, D. (1993). Quantifying connected speech samples of adults with chronic aphasia. *Aphasiology, 7,* 155–163.

Doyle, P.J., Goda, A.J., & Spencer, K.A. (1995). The communicative informativeness and efficiency of connected discourse in adults with aphasia under structured and conversational sampling conditions. *American Journal of Speech Language Pathology, 4,* 130–134.

Doyle, P.J., Thompson, C.K., Oleyar, K., Wambaugh, J., & Jackson, A. (1994). The effects of setting variables on conversational discourse in normal and aphasic adults. *Clinical Aphasiology, 22,* 135–144.

Ernst-Baron, C.B., Brookshire, R.H., & Nicholas, L.E. (1987). Story structure and retelling of narratives by aphasic and non–brain-damaged adults. *Journal of Speech and Hearing Research, 30,* 44–49.

Ferguson, A. (1993). Conversational repair of word-finding difficulty. *Clinical Aphasiology, 21,* 299–310.

Hinckley, J.J. & Craig, H.K. (1992). A comparison of picture stimulus and conversational elicitation contexts: responses to comments by adults with aphasia. *Aphasiology, 6,* 257–272.

Klippi, A. (1991). Conversational dynamics between aphasics. *Aphasiology, 5,* 373–378.

Li, E.C., Williams, S.E. & Volpe, A.D. (1995). The effects of topic and listener familiarity on discourse variables in procedural and narrative discourse tasks. *Journal of Communication Disorders, 28,* 39–55.

Nicholas, L.E., & Brookshire, R.H. (1993a). A system for quantifying the informativeness and efficiency of the connected speech of adults with aphasia. *Journal of Speech and Hearing Research, 36,* 338–350.

Nicholas, L.E., & Brookshire, R.H. (1993b). A system for scoring main concepts in the discourse of non–brain-damaged and aphasic speakers. *Clinical Aphasiology, 21,* 87–99.

Nicholas, L.E., & Brookshire, R.H. (1995). Presence, completeness and accuracy of main concepts in the connected speech of non–brain-damaged and aphasic adults. *Journal of Speech and Hearing Research, 38,* 145–156.

Roberts, J.A., & Wertz, R.T. (1989). Comparison of spontaneous and elicited oral-expressive language in aphasia. *Clinical Aphasiology, 18,* 479–488.

Ulatowska, H.K., Doyel, A.W. Freedman-Stern, R., & Macaluso-Haynes, S. (1983a). Production of procedural discourse in aphasia. *Brain and Language, 18,* 315–341.

Ulatowska, H.K., Freedman-Stern, R., Doyel, A.W., & Macaluso-Haynes, S. (1983b). Production of narrative discourse in aphasia. *Brain and Language, 19,* 317–334.

Wambaugh, J.L., Thompson, C.K., Doyle, P.J., & Camarata, S. (1991). Conversational discourse of aphasic and normal adults: An analysis of communicative functions. *Clinical Aphasiology, 20,* 343–353.

Williams, S.E., Li, E.C., Volpe, A.D. and Ritterman, S.I. (1994). The influence of topic and listener familiarity on aphasic discourse. *Journal of Communication Disorders, 27,* 207–222.

Yorkston, K.M., & Beukelman, D.R. (1980). An analysis of connected speech samples of aphasic and normal speakers. *Journal of Speech and Hearing Disorders, 45,* 27–36.

Table 8–3 Discourse Deficits Secondary to Right Hemisphere Damage (RHD)

Reference	Subjects	Discourse Tasks	Level of Analysis	Results for Subjects with RHD
Bloom et al. (1992)	9 RHD 12 LHD (mild to moderate aphasia) 12 normal controls	Narrative discourse (sequential line drawings designed to elicit neutral/procedural content, visual–spatial content, and emotional content)	Informational content	RHD subjects produced significantly fewer content elements than normal controls in all conditions; fewer content units produced in emotional condition than in visual–spatial and neutral/procedural conditions. There were no within-group differences for LHD subjects and normals.
Bloom et al. (1993)	9 RHD 12 LHD (mild to moderate aphasia) 12 normal controls	Narrative discourse (sequential line drawings designed to elicit neutral/procedural content, visual–spatial content, and emotional content)	Appropriateness of topic maintenance, conciseness, specificity, lexical selection, revision strategy, relevancy, and quantity	Overall, no significant difference between RHD subjects and normals; RHD subjects more impaired on emotional condition than visual–spatial and procedural/neutral; no within-group difference for normals; LHD subjects less impaired in emotional condition than visual–spatial and procedural/neutral.
Cherney & Canter (1993)	10 RHD 10 DAT 10 normal controls	Descriptive (cookie theft picture description and object description task) Procedural discourse with no visual stimulus Narrative (story retelling from a one-paragraph auditory stimulus)	Informational content	Overall, no difference between RHD and DAT subjects in any category of informational content; RHD and DAT subjects produced less essential and elaborative information, and more irrelevant, redundant, off-topic, and incorrect information than normals.

Study	Subjects	Discourse task	Analysis	Results
Cherney et al. (1997)	5 RHD assessed longitudinally 25 normal controls	Narrative (story retelling from an auditory stimulus)	Informational content	RHD subjects with persistent unilateral neglect produced more total content units, characterized by more elaborations, irrelevancies, and redundancies than did normals; informational content of subjects with transient unilateral neglect was similar to that of normals.
Joanette et al. (1986)	36 RHD 20 normal controls	Narrative discourse (from an eight-frame series of black and white drawings)	Surface level analysis; Informational content (simple and complex propositions)	No difference in number of words or T-units. RHD subjects produced significantly fewer simple and complex propositions; the production of a smaller amount of information did not appear related to reduced verbal output or presence of a visual neglect.
Kennedy et al. (1994)	12 RHD 11 normal controls	Conversation (first encounters)	Topic skills and turn-taking skills	No differences in topic skills; RHD subjects produced significantly more turns, but fewer words per turn; more representative statements (facts, opinions), but fewer questions.
Mackenzie et al. (1997)	17 RHD 64 normal controls	Cookie theft picture description	Informational content	Informational content of normals affected by education; RHD subjects used fewer words, spoke for less time, and produced less information
		Conversation	5-point pragmatic rating scale	Conversations of RHD subjects were characterized by limited facial expression and eye contact, and monotonous intonation. Verbosity, poor turn-taking, and tangentiality were not characteristic.

continues

Table 8–3 continued

Reference	Subjects	Discourse Tasks	Level of Analysis	Results for Subjects with RHD
Moya et al. (1986)	18 RHD 10 normal controls	Narrative discourse (recall from orally presented paragraph length passages)	Informational content (i.e., details and intrusive errors, such as perseveration, substitution, confabulation, inappropriate reference)	Significantly impaired in recall of individual details and intrusion of elements of inappropriate reference; correlations between certain aspects of verbal narrative recall for details and inclusion of details in a visual–spatial task.
Myers & Brookshire (1994, 1996)	24 RHD 30 normal controls	Picture description (Norman Rockwell pictures varying in visual and inferential complexity)	Informational content	Generation of fewer main concepts in all conditions; deficits more related to the inferential than the visual complexity of the picture stimuli; moderate to strong correlation between neglect scores and number of main concepts produced.
Sheratt & Penn (1990)	1 RHD 1 normal control	Narrative discourse (single and sequenced picture description, self-generated memorable experience)	Surface level analysis: syntactic complexity	More words than control, with no difference in syntactic complexity (words and clauses per T-unit).
			Verbal disruptions	More verbal disruptions (repetition of ideas, intrusive words and phrases) and empty phrases.
		Procedural discourse with no visual stimulus	Narrative/procedural superstructure (rated on a 5-point scale)	Difficulty with the resolution component (i.e., drawing threads of the story together); more difficulty with procedural than narrative discourse; reduced topic control and reduced relevance (with unnecessary detail).
			Organizational skills, including topic control, temporal sequencing, relevance, tense use (rated on a 5-point scale)	
			Cohesion	No differences in cohesion.

Study	Subjects	Task	Analysis	Findings
Tompkins et al. (1993)	26 RHD, 26 LHD, 26 normal controls	Cookie theft picture description	Surface level analysis (rate, phrase-length ratio)	No significant differences between RHD subjects and normals; LHD subjects had slower rate and phrase-length ratios than the other two groups.
			Informational content (literal, interpretive, unscorable) and efficiency measures	No significant differences in informational content.
Trupe & Hillis (1985)	RHD, Normal controls	Cookie theft picture description	Informational content	Based on number of content units and an efficiency ratio of syllables per content unit, subjects could be categorized into five groups: irrelevant speech, paucity of speech, digressive speech, verbose speech, or normal speech.
Uryase et al. (1990)	22 RHD, 12 LHD, 20 normal controls	Narrative discourse (about a 9-minute video to a naive listener)	Surface structure	RHD subjects produced significantly fewer T-units than normals.
			Cohesion	Smaller proportion of complete and greater proportion of incomplete cohesive markers.
			Narrative story grammar	Fewer complete episodes; more missing episodes; significant differences for all components of story grammar structure.

LHD, left hemisphere damage; DAT, dementia of the Alzheimer's type.

continues

REFERENCES

Bloom, R.L., Borod, J.C., Obler, L.K., & Gerstman, L.J. (1992). Impact of emotional content on discourse production in patients with unilateral brain damage. *Brain and Language, 42*, 153–164.

Bloom, R.L., Borod, J.C., Obler, L.K., & Gerstman, L.J. (1993). Suppression and facilitation of pragmatic performance: Effects of emotional content on discourse following right and left brain damage. *Journal of Speech and Hearing Research, 36*, 1227–1235.

Cherney, L.R., & Canter, G.J. (1993). Informational content in the discourse of patients with probable Alzheimer's disease and patients with right brain damage. *Clinical Aphasiology, 21*, 123–134.

Cherney, L.R., Drimmer, D.P., & Halper, A.S. (1997). Informational content and unilateral neglect: A longitudinal investigation of five subjects with right hemisphere damage. *Aphasiology, 11*, 351–363.

Glosser, G., Deser, T., & Weinstein, C. (1992). Structural organization of discourse production following right hemisphere damage. *Journal of Clinical and Experimental Neuropsychology, 14*, 40.

Joanette, Y., Goulet, P., Ska, B., & Nespoulous, J-L. (1986). Informative content of narrative discourse in right brained damaged right handers. *Brain and Language, 29*, 81–105.

Kennedy, M., Strand, E., Burton, W., & Peterson, C. (1994). Analysis of first-encounter conversations of right-hemisphere–damaged adults. *Clinical Aphasiology, 22*, 67–80.

Mackenzie, C., Begg, T., Brady, M., & Lees, K.R. (1997). The effects on verbal communication skills of right hemisphere stroke in middle age. *Aphasiology, 11*, 929–945.

Moya, K.L., Benowitz, L.I., Levine, D.N. & Finklestein, S. (1986). Covariant defects in visuospatial abilities and recall of verbal narrative after right hemisphere stroke. *Cortex, 22*, 381–397.

Myers, P.S., & Brookshire, R.H. (1994). The effects of visual and inferential complexity on the picture descriptions of non–brain-damaged and right-hemisphere–damaged adults. *Clinical Aphasiology, 22*, 25–34.

Myers, P.S., & Brookshire, R.H. (1996). Effect of visual and inferential variables on scene descriptions by right-hemisphere–damaged and non–brain-damaged adults. *Journal of Speech and Hearing Research, 39*, 870–880.

Sheratt, S.M., & Penn, C. (1990). Discourse in a right-hemisphere brain-damaged subject. *Aphasiology, 4*, 539–560.

Tompkins, C.A., Boada, R., McGarry, K., Jones, J., Rahn, A.E., & Ranier, S. (1993). Connected speech characteristics of right hemisphere damaged adults: A reexamination. *Clinical Aphasiology, 21*, 113–122.

Trupe, E.H., & Hillis, A. (1985). Paucity vs. verbosity: Another analysis of right hemisphere communication deficits. In R.H. Brookshire (Ed.), *Clinical Aphasiology Conference Proceedings* 83–96.

Uryase, D., Duffy, R.J., & Liles, B.Z. (1990). Analysis and description of narrative discourse in right-hemisphere–damaged adults: A comparison with neurologically normal and left-hemisphere–damaged aphasic adults. *Clinical Aphasiology, 19*, 125–137.

Table 8–4 Discourse Deficits Secondary to Traumatic Brain Injury (TBI)

Reference	Subjects	Discourse Tasks	Level of Analysis	Results for Subjects with TBI
Biddle et al. (1996)	20 TBI (10 children, 10 adults) 20 matched controls	Story generation (personal narratives)	Dependency analysis	Significantly more dysfluent, and their performance revealed a striking listener burden.
Bond & Godfrey (1997)	62 TBI 25 matched controls	Conversation	Impression ratings, prompt frequency, turn duration	Conversations rated as less interesting, less appropriate, and less rewarding, as well as more effortful.
Campbell & Dollaghan (1990)	8 CHI, 1 open head injury Matched controls	Conversation	Phonologic and/or lexical production, Syntax, productivity	Accuracy of consonant production, syntactic complexity, and total utterance remained depressed for some subjects up to 13 mos. post onset.
Chapman et al. (1992)	19 CHI, 1 gunshot wound Matched controls	Story retelling	Syntax Story structure, Coherence Productivity	Syntactic complexity comparable to that of normals. Reduction in story components. Loss of core information. Severely injured group produced less language.
Coelho et al. (1991a)	5 CHI Matched controls	Conversation	Response appropriate-ness, topic mainte-nance	More turns with shorter utterances, decreased response adequacy, and difficulty initiating and sustaining conversation.
Coelho et al. (1991b)	2 CHI 23 college students	Story generation	Cohesion Story structure	One subject demonstrated poor cohesive adequacy and meaningful content; other subject had good cohesion and poor content.
Ehrlich (1988)	10 head injury Matched controls	Picture description	Informational content	Slower rate of information production, more words and time required to convey important spoken information.

continues

Table 8–4 continued

Reference	Subjects	Discourse Tasks	Level of Analysis	Results for Subjects with TBI
Ehrlich & Barry (1989)	18 CHI	Conversation	Pragmatic rating	Rating scale useful for evaluation of selected communication behaviors.
Gajar et al. (1984)	2 head trauma	Conversation	Response appropriateness following feedback	Feedback and self-monitoring had positive effects on conversation behavior.
Giles et al. (1988)	1 head injury	Conversation	Coherence, productivity	Greater coherence following treatment to improve response succinctness (decrease in number of words/min.).
Glosser & Deser (1990)	9 CHI 9 fluent aphasia 9 DAT 17 normal	Descriptive	Lexical production Syntax Cohesion Coherence	More paraphasias and grammatical errors; global coherence more impaired than local.
Hartley & Jensen (1991)	11 CHI 21 matched controls	Story generation, story retelling, procedural	Lexical production Cohesion Informational content	Fluency and naming most impaired language skills; also fewer cohesive ties, fewer meaningful words, shorter communication units, larger percent of syllables in mazes, less accurate content.
Liles et al. (1989)	4 CHI 23 college students	Story generation, story retelling	Syntax Cohesion Story structure	Decreased proportional use of referential and increased use of lexical ties, poor story structure in story generation.
McDonald (1993)	2 CHI 12 matched controls	Referential	Cohesion, coherence Informational rating	Multiple problems with coherence, irrelevant propositions, and difficulty organizing content.
Mentis & Prutting (1987)	3 CHI Matched controls	Conversation, descriptive, procedural	Cohesion	Fewer cohesive ties, more incomplete ties.

Study	Subjects	Genre	Topic	Findings
Mentis & Prutting (1991)	1 CHI Matched control	Conversation, monologue	Topic	Problems with topic management, fewer new information units, inability to maintain topics through addition of novel information.
Milton et al. (1984)	5 head injury Matched controls	Conversation	Pragmatic rating	Communication problems with illocutionary/perlocutionary and propositional acts.
Parsons et al. (1989)	11 CHI	Answers to questions, picture description, descriptive, procedural	Pragmatic rating	Problems initiating, organizing, and maintaining of conversation.
Penn & Cleary (1988)	6 CHI	Conversation	Compensatory strategies	Use of self-initiated strategies to compensate for cognitive and language deficits with varying success.
Snow et al. (1997a)	26 TBI 26 matched orthopedic patients 26 college students	Conversation	Damico's (1985) Clinical Discourse Analysis	All members of TBI group made errors of information transfer; only more severely injured subgroup made fundamental errors of conversational interaction.
Snow et al. (1997b)	26 TBI 26 matched orthopedic patients 26 college students	Procedural	Informational content Pragmatic measures	Content and productivity in TBI group not different from those in orthopedic group although different from those of college students; pragmatic errors in TBI group different from those of both groups.
Togher et al. (1997)	5 TBI Matched controls	Telephone conversation	Exchange structure	Factors of familiarity (i.e., social distance) and status or power influenced language choices made by all subjects in the varied interactions.

Note: CHI, closed head injury; DAT, dementia of the Alzheimer's type.

continues

REFERENCES

Biddle, K.R., McCabe, A., & Bliss, L.S. (1996). Narrative skills following traumatic brain injury in children and adults. *Journal of Communication Disorders, 29,* 447–469.

Bond, F., & Godfrey, H.P.D. (1997). Conversation with traumatically brain-injured individuals: A controlled study of behavioral changes and their impact. *Brain Injury, 11,* 319–329.

Campbell, T.F., & Dollaghan, C.A. (1990). Expressive language recovery in severely brain-injured children and adolescents. *Journal of Speech and Hearing Disorders, 55,* 567–581.

Chapman, S.B., Culhane, K.A., Levin, H.S., Harward, H., Mendelsohn, D., Ewing-Cobbs, L., Fletcher, J.M., & Bruce, D. (1992). Narrative discourse after closed head injury in children and adolescents. *Brain and Language, 43,* 42–65.

Coelho, C.A., Liles, B.Z., & Duffy, R.J. (1991a). Analyses of conversational discourse in head-injured adults. *Journal of Head Trauma Rehabilitation, 6,* 92–99.

Coelho, C.A., Liles, B.Z., & Duffy, R.J. (1991b). Discourse analyses with closed head injured adults: Evidence for differing patterns of deficits. *Archives of Physical Medicine and Rehabilitation, 72,* 465–468.

Damico, J.S. (1985). Clinical discourse analysis: A functional approach to language assessment. In C.S. Simon (Ed.) *Communication Skills and Classroom Success.* (pp. 165–203). London: Taylor & Francis.

Ehrlich, J.S. (1988). Selective characteristics of narrative discourse in head-injured and normal adults. *Journal of Communication Disorders, 21,* 1–9.

Ehrlich, J., & Barry, P. (1989). Rating communication behaviors in the head-injured adult. *Brain Injury, 3,* 193–198.

Gajar, A., Schloss, P.J., & Thompson, C.K. (1984). Effects of feedback and self-monitoring on head trauma youths' conversational skills. *Journal of Applied Behavior Analysis, 17,* 353–358.

Giles, G.M., Fussey, I., & Burgess, P. (1988). The behavioral treatment of verbal interaction skills following severe head injury: A single case study. *Brain Injury, 2,* 75–79.

Glosser, G., & Deser, T. (1990). Patterns of discourse production among neurological patients with fluent language disorders. *Brain and Language, 40,* 67–88.

Hartley, L.L., & Jensen, P.J. (1991). Narrative and procedural discourse after closed head injury. *Brain Injury, 5,* 267–285.

Liles, B.Z., Coelho, C.A., Duffy, R.J., & Zalagens, M.R. (1989). Effects of elicitation procedures on the narratives of normal and closed head-injured adults. *Journal of Speech and Hearing Disorders, 54,* 356–366.

McDonald, S. (1993). Pragmatic language skills after closed head injury: Ability to meet the informational needs of the listener. *Brain and Language, 44,* 28–46.

Mentis, M., & Prutting, C.A. (1987). Cohesion in the discourse of normal and head-injured adults. *Journal of Speech and Hearing Research, 30,* 88–98.

Mentis, M., & Prutting, C.A. (1991). Analysis of topic as illustrated in a head-injured and a normal adult. *Journal of Speech and Hearing Research, 34,* 583–595.

Milton, S.B., Prutting, C.A., & Binder, G.M. (1984). Appraisal of communicative competence in head-injured adults. *Clinical Aphasiology Conference Proceedings, 14,* 114–123.

Parsons, C.L., Snow, P., Couch, D., & Mooney, L. (1989). Conversational skills in closed head injury: Part 1. *Australian Journal of Human Communication Disorders, 17,* 37–46.

Penn, C., & Cleary, J. (1988). Compensatory strategies in the language of closed head injured patients. *Brain Injury, 2,* 3–17.

Snow, P., Douglas, J., & Ponsford, J. (1997a). Conversational assessment following brain injury: A comparison across two control groups. *Brain Injury, 11,* 409–429.

Snow, P., Douglas, J., & Ponsford, J. (1997b). Procedural discourse following traumatic brain injury. *Aphasiology, 11,* 947–967.

Togher, L., Hand, L., & Code, C. (1997). Measuring service encounters in the traumatic brain injury population. *Aphasiology, 11,* 491–505.

Cookie Theft Picture Description

Three unanalyzed samples are included for practice. Then, each sample is coded into *T-units* and analyzed for *informational content*. Refer to Chapter 5 for additional information about other informational content analyses.

Transcript 3 has also been coded for *cohesion*. The reader should remember that cohesion analysis is most appropriate for narrative discourse. There are some limitations with the use of cohesion analysis with picture description tasks because of the shared visual reference. Therefore, the results of cohesion should be interpreted cautiously.

CODES:

Informational Content
ESS = Essential units
ELAB = Elaborations
IRR = Irrelevancies
RED = Redundancies
OFF-TOPIC = Off-topic units
INC = Incorrect units

Cohesive Adequacy
Comp = Complete
Inc = Incomplete
Inc-T = Incomplete tie
Err = Error
Err-T = Error tie

Cohesive Marker Types
Rp = Personal reference
Rd = Demonstrative reference
Lex = Lexical
Ca = Additive conjunction
Ct = Temporal conjunction
Ccau = Causal conjunction
Cadv = Adversative conjunction

COOKIE THEFT PICTURE DESCRIPTION
SAMPLE TRANSCRIPT 1

There's a lot of accidents just about ready to happen . . . just carelessness and lack of uh education . . . well first thing I notice is that the kitchen sink the water is overflowing out of the sink onto the floor and the woman in the picture is drying a dish while standing in a puddle of water so there's a potential there that she could slip and fall . . . then over on the other side of the kitchen there's the two children . . . the boy ha- has stepped up on a on a stool a very wobbly stool and he wasn't balanced very well while trying to reach the top shelf in a cabinet to get a cookie and he looks like he's gonna fall and could really hurt himself if he hits his head on the counter . . . and his sister looks like she's saying be quiet now . . . you know mother doesn't see us so we're sneaking in here . . . although if that were my house and my children we- were allowed to have a cookie during the day I would take the cookie jar out of the top cabinet and put it on the sink counter to make it more convenient where provide less of a chance of having an accident from somebody slipping and falling . . . okay and the kitchen window above the sink is open to get a little bit of a breeze . . . I can see the the walkway going out past the looks like part of the house or a garage

(2 minutes, 57 seconds)

SAMPLE TRANSCRIPT 2

This is an old picture from 1983 . . . it's a picture of a suburban scene in probably some middle class semi-affluent community . . . mother . . . daughter . . . son . . . the place is a t- . . . she's a the woman appears to be kind of an incompetent . . . the soap the dishes the water's running out over the sink and she's looking out the window and the kids are falling off the chairs while they're getting a cookie uh then it it's just a complete scene of uh negatives . . . except that the gr- it looks nice outside the window but inside the house looks kind of like a mess . . . there's the water running over the sink the kid getting ready to fall and break his head and the mother paying no attention . . . she does appear to be wearing an apron like she knows what she's doing . . . uh and I don't think that there's much more to say about it except the drapes are pulled evenly apart so you see out the window . . . evenly . . . any more than that I don't know

(1 minutes, 25 seconds)

SAMPLE TRANSCRIPT 3

It is a black and white ink drawing on an eight and a half by ellevenish sheet of paper . . . it depicts a young boy standing on a stool getting cookies from a cookie jar and giving one to his si-sister . . . the tool stool is tipping . . . it is evident that he will fall if unless something changes quickly . . . there is an older female in the picture . . . one can assume it is the mother . . . she is washing a dish . . . there is a sink in the picture that is showing water flowing over the edge and water is still flowing into the sink so we will continue to get more water on the floor . . . there are dishes on the counter . . . the window over the sink shows outdoor area with a sidewalk grass and tree and bush . . . there are curtains on the window . . . the older female is wearing a dress and an apron . . . the young boy is wearing shorts and a t-shirt . . . the younger girl is wearing a t-shirt and a skirt . . . shoes and socks . . . the boy is wearing shoes and socks . . . the woman is wearing just shoes . . . based on the female or the facial features of the three they appear Caucasian . . . it appears to be warm outside for they have the window open . . . the woman is drawn without a ring on her left hand which indicates she may not be married . . . she may be a single mother or a single parent . . . the picture indicates a suburban setting.

(2 minutes, 11 seconds)

COOKIE THEFT PICTURE DESCRIPTION
SAMPLE TRANSCRIPT 1

There's a lot of accidents just about ready to happen . . . just carelessness and lack of uh
education . . . well first thing I notice is that the kitchen sink the water is overflowing out of the sink
onto the floor and the woman in the picture is drying a dish while standing in a puddle of water so there's a
potential there that she could slip and fall . . . then over on the other side of the kitchen there's the two
children . . . the boy ha- has stepped up on a on a stool a very wobbly stool and he wasn't balanced very
well while trying to reach the top shelf in a cabinet to get a cookie and he looks like he's gonna fall and
could really hurt himself if he hits his head on the counter . . . and his sister looks like she's saying be
quiet now . . . you know mother doesn't see us so we're sneaking in here . . . although if that were my house
and my children we- were allowed to have a cookie during the day I would take the cookie jar out of the top
cabinet and put it on the sink counter to make it more convenient where provide less of a chance of having an
accident from somebody slipping and falling . . . okay and the kitchen window above the sink is open to get a
little bit of a breeze . . . I can see the the walkway going out past the looks like part of the house or a
garage

IRR	1. there's a lot of accidents just about to happen . . . just carelessness . . . and lack of (uh) education
ESS	2. well first thing I notice is that (the kitchen sink) the water is overflowing out of the sink onto the floor
ESS/IRR	3. and the woman in the picture is drying a dish while standing in a puddle of water so there's a potential there that she could slip and fall
ELAB/ESS	4. then over on the other side of the kitchen there's the two children
ESS	5. the boy (ha-) has stepped up (on a) on a (stool a) very wobbly stool
ELAB/ESS	6. and he wasn't balanced very well while trying to reach the top shelf in a cabinet to get a cookie
ESS/IRR	7. and he looks like he's gonna fall and could really hurt himself if he hits his head on the counter
ESS/ELAB	8. and his sister looks like she's saying "be quiet now . . . you know mother doesn't see us so we're sneaking in here"
IRR	9. although if that were my house and my children (we- were allowed to have a cookie during the day) I would take the cookie jar out of the top cabinet and put it on the sink counter to make it more convenient where provide less of a chance of having an accident from somebody slipping and falling
ELAB	10. okay and the kitchen window above the sink is open to get a little bit of a breeze
ELAB	11. I can see (the) the walkway going out past (the looks like) part of the house or a garage

COOKIE THEFT PICTURE DESCRIPTION
SAMPLE TRANSCRIPT 2

This is an old picture from 1983 . . . it's a picture of a suburban scene in probably some middle class
semi-affluent community . . . mother . . . daughter . . . son . . . the place is a t- . . . she's a the woman
ESS
appears to be kind of an incompetent . . . the soap the dishes the water's running out over the sink and
ESS
she's looking out the window and the kids are falling off the chairs while they're getting a cookie uh then
ELAB   **ESS**   **ESS**
it it's just a complete scene of uh negatives . . . except that the gr- it looks nice outside the window but
inside the house looks kind of like a a mess . . . there's the water running over the sink the kid getting
ESS
ready to fall and break his head and the mother paying no attention . . . she does appear to be wearing an
apron like she knows what she's doing . . . uh and I don't think that there's much more to say about it
except the drapes are pulled evenly apart so you see out the window . . . evenly . . . any more than that I
don't know

IRR	1. this is an old picture from 1983
IRR	2. it's a picture of a suburban scene in probably some middle class semi-affluent community
ESS/IRR	3. (mother . . . daughter . . . son . . . the place is a t- . . . she's a) the woman appears to be kind of an incompetent
ESS	4. (the soap the dishes) the water's running out over the sink
ELAB	5. and she's looking out the window
ESS	6. and the kids are falling off the chairs while they're getting a cookie
IRR	7. (uh) then (it) it's just a complete scene of (uh) negatives except that (the gr-) it looks nice outside the window
IRR	8. but inside the house looks (kind of like a) a mess
RED/ESS	9. there's the water running over the sink the kid getting ready to fall and break his head and the mother paying no attention
ELAB/IRR	10. she does appear to be wearing an apron like she knows what she's doing
IRR/ELAB	11. (uh) and I don't think that there's much more to say about it except the drapes are pulled evenly apart so you see out the window . . . evenly
IRR	12. any more than that I don't know

COOKIE THEFT PICTURE DESCRIPTION
SAMPLE TRANSCRIPT 3

It is a black and white ink drawing on an eight and a half by elevenish sheet of paper . . . it depicts a
ESS   ESS   ESS
young boy standing on a stool getting cookies from a cookie jar and giving one to his si-sister . . . the
ESS
tool stool is tipping . . . it is evident that he will fall if unless something changes quickly . . . there
                                                          ESS   ESS
is an older female in the picture . . . one can assume it is the mother . . . she is washing a
                                                          ESS
dish . . . there is a sink in the picture that is showing water flowing over the edge and water is still
flowing into the sink so we will continue get more water on the floor . . . there are dishes on the
counter . . . the window over the sink shows outdoor area with a sidewalk grass and tree and bush . . . there
are curtains on the window . . . the older female is wearing a dress and a apron . . . the young boy is
wearing shorts and a t-shirt . . . the younger girl is wearing a t-shirt and a skirt . . . shoes and
socks . . . the boy is wearing shoes and socks . . . the woman is wearing just shoes . . . based on the
female or the facial features of the three they appear Caucasian . . . it appears to be warm outside for they
have the window open . . . the woman is drawn without a ring on her left hand which indicates she may not be
married . . . she may be a single mother or a single parent . . . the picture indicates a suburban setting.

In the following T-unit segmented transcript, cohesive markers are underlined; the categorization of the markers follows on subsequent pages

IRR	1. It is a black and white ink drawing on an eight and a half by elevenish sheet of paper
ESS/ESS/ESS	2. it depicts a young boy standing on a stool getting cookies from a cookie jar and giving one to his (si-) sister
ESS	3. the (tool) stool is tipping
IRR	4. it is evident that he will fall (if) unless something changes quickly
ELAB	5. there is an older female in the picture
ESS	6. one can assume it is the mother
ESS	7. she is washing a dish
ESS	8. there is a sink in the picture that is showing water flowing over the edge
ELAB	9. and water is still flowing into the sink so we will continue get more water on the floor
ELAB	10. there are dishes on the counter
ELAB	11. the window over the sink shows outdoor area with a sidewalk grass and tree and bush
ELAB	12. there are curtains on the window
ELAB	13. the older female is wearing a dress and a apron
ELAB	14. the young boy is wearing shorts and a t-shirt
ELAB	15. the younger girl is wearing a t-shirt and a skirt . . . shoes and socks

ELAB   16. <u>the</u> boy is wearing shoes and socks

ELAB   17. <u>the</u> woman is wearing just shoes

IRR   18. based on <u>the</u> female or <u>the</u> facial features of <u>the</u> three <u>they</u> appear Caucasian

IRR/ELAB   19. <u>it</u> appears to be warm outside for <u>they</u> have <u>the</u> window open

ELAB/IRR   20. <u>the</u> woman is drawn without a ring on her left hand which indicates she may not be married

IRR   21. <u>she</u> may be a single mother or a single parent

IRR   22. <u>the</u> picture indicates a suburban setting.

Cookie Theft
3

SUBJ ID _____ TASK_____ SCORED BY _____ DATE_____   Page____1 of 2____

T-U #	Item (Word)	COHESIVE MARKER TYPE							COHESIVE ADEQUACY				
		Rp	Rd	Lex	Ca	Ct	Ccau	Cadv	Comp	Inc	Inc-T	Error	Error-T
1	IT	**(Rp)**	Rd	Lex	Ca	Ct	Ccau	Cadv	**(Comp)**	Inc	Inc-T	Error	Error-T
2	IT	**(Rp)**	Rd	Lex	Ca	Ct	Ccau	Cadv	**(Comp)**	Inc	Inc-T	Error	Error-T
3	THE	Rp	**(Rd)**	Lex	Ca	Ct	Ccau	Cadv	**(Comp)**	Inc	Inc-T	Error	Error-T
4	IT	**(Rp)**	Rd	Lex	Ca	Ct	Ccau	Cadv	Comp	**(Inc)**	Inc-T	Error	Error-T
	HE	**(Rp)**	Rd	Lex	Ca	Ct	Ccau	Cadv	**(Comp)**	Inc	Inc-T	Error	Error-T
5	THERE	Rp	**(Rd)**	Lex	Ca	Ct	Ccau	Cadv	Comp	**(Inc)**	Inc-T	Error	Error-T
	THE	Rp	**(Rd)**	Lex	Ca	Ct	Ccau	Cadv	**(Comp)**	Inc	Inc-T	Error	Error-T
6	ONE	**(Rp)**	Rd	Lex	Ca	Ct	Ccau	Cadv	Comp	**(Inc)**	Inc-T	Error	Error-T
	IT	**(Rp)**	Rd	Lex	Ca	Ct	Ccau	Cadv	Comp	Inc	Inc-T	**(Error)**	Error-T
	THE	Rp	**(Rd)**	Lex	Ca	Ct	Ccau	Cadv	Comp	**(Inc)**	Inc-T	Error	Error-T
7	SHE	**(Rp)**	Rd	Lex	Ca	Ct	Ccau	Cadv	Comp	Inc	**(Inc-T)**	Error	Error-T
8	THERE	Rp	**(Rd)**	Lex	Ca	Ct	Ccau	Cadv	Comp	Inc	**(Inc-T)**	Error	Error-T
	THE	Rp	**(Rd)**	Lex	Ca	Ct	Ccau	Cadv	**(Comp)**	Inc	Inc-T	Error	Error-T
	THE	Rp	**(Rd)**	Lex	Ca	Ct	Ccau	Cadv	Comp	**(Inc)**	Inc-T	Error	Error-T
9	AND	Rp	Rd	Lex	**(Ca)**	Ct	Ccau	Cadv	**(Comp)**	Inc	Inc-T	Error	Error-T
	THE	Rp	**(Rd)**	Lex	Ca	Ct	Ccau	Cadv	**(Comp)**	Inc	Inc-T	Error	Error-T
	THE	Rp	**(Rd)**	Lex	Ca	Ct	Ccau	Cadv	Comp	**(Inc)**	Inc-T	Error	Error-T
10	THERE	Rp	**(Rd)**	Lex	Ca	Ct	Ccau	Cadv	Comp	Inc	**(Inc-T)**	Error	Error-T
	THE	Rp	**(Rd)**	Lex	Ca	Ct	Ccau	Cadv	Comp	**(Inc)**	Inc-T	Error	Error-T
11	THE	Rp	**(Rd)**	Lex	Ca	Ct	Ccau	Cadv	Comp	**(Inc)**	Inc-T	Error	Error-T
	THE	Rp	**(Rd)**	Lex	Ca	Ct	Ccau	Cadv	**(Comp)**	Inc	Inc-T	Error	Error-T
12	THERE	Rp	**(Rd)**	Lex	Ca	Ct	Ccau	Cadv	Comp	Inc	**(Inc-T)**	Error	Error-T
	THE	Rp	**(Rd)**	Lex	Ca	Ct	Ccau	Cadv	Comp	Inc	**(Inc-T)**	Error	Error-T
13	THE	Rp	**(Rd)**	Lex	Ca	Ct	Ccau	Cadv	**(Comp)**	Inc	Inc-T	Error	Error-T
14	THE	Rp	**(Rd)**	Lex	Ca	Ct	Ccau	Cadv	**(Comp)**	Inc	Inc-T	Error	Error-T

Cookie Theft

 # 3

SUBJ ID _____ TASK_____ SCORED BY _____ DATE_____   Page___*2 of 2*___

T-U #	Item (Word)	COHESIVE MARKER TYPE							COHESIVE ADEQUACY				
15	THE	Rp	(Rd)	Lex	Ca	Ct	Ccau	Cadv	Comp	(Inc)	Inc-T	Error	Error-T
16	THE	Rp	(Rd)	Lex	Ca	Ct	Ccau	Cadv	(Comp)	Inc	Inc-T	Error	Error-T
17	THE	Rp	(Rd)	Lex	Ca	Ct	Ccau	Cadv	(Comp)	Inc	Inc-T	Error	Error-T
18	THE	Rp	(Rd)	Lex	Ca	Ct	Ccau	Cadv	(Comp)	Inc	Inc-T	Error	Error-T
	THE	Rp	(Rd)	Lex	Ca	Ct	Ccau	Cadv	Comp	(Inc)	Inc-T	Error	Error-T
	THE	Rp	(Rd)	Lex	Ca	Ct	Ccau	Cadv	(Comp)	Inc	Inc-T	Error	Error-T
	THEY	(Rp)	Rd	Lex	Ca	Ct	Ccau	Cadv	(Comp)	Inc	Inc-T	Error	Error-T
19	IT	(Rp)	Rd	Lex	Ca	Ct	Ccau	Cadv	Comp	Inc	(Inc-T)	Error	Error-T
	THEY	(Rp)	Rd	Lex	Ca	Ct	Ccau	Cadv	(Comp)	Inc	Inc-T	Error	Error-T
	THE	Rp	(Rd)	Lex	Ca	Ct	Ccau	Cadv	Comp	Inc	(Inc-T)	Error	Error-T
20	THE	Rp	(Rd)	Lex	Ca	Ct	Ccau	Cadv	(Comp)	Inc	Inc-T	Error	Error-T
21	SHE	(Rp)	Rd	Lex	Ca	Ct	Ccau	Cadv	(Comp)	Inc	Inc-T	Error	Error-T
22	THE	Rp	(Rd)	Lex	Ca	Ct	Ccau	Cadv	(Comp)	Inc	Inc-T	Error	Error-T
		Rp	Rd	Lex	Ca	Ct	Ccau	Cadv	Comp	Inc	Inc-T	Error	Error-T
		Rp	Rd	Lex	Ca	Ct	Ccau	Cadv	Comp	Inc	Inc-T	Error	Error-T
		Rp	Rd	Lex	Ca	Ct	Ccau	Cadv	Comp	Inc	Inc-T	Error	Error-T
		Rp	Rd	Lex	Ca	Ct	Ccau	Cadv	Comp	Inc	Inc-T	Error	Error-T
		Rp	Rd	Lex	Ca	Ct	Ccau	Cadv	Comp	Inc	Inc-T	Error	Error-T
		Rp	Rd	Lex	Ca	Ct	Ccau	Cadv	Comp	Inc	Inc-T	Error	Error-T
		Rp	Rd	Lex	Ca	Ct	Ccau	Cadv	Comp	Inc	Inc-T	Error	Error-T
		Rp	Rd	Lex	Ca	Ct	Ccau	Cadv	Comp	Inc	Inc-T	Error	Error-T
		Rp	Rd	Lex	Ca	Ct	Ccau	Cadv	Comp	Inc	Inc-T	Error	Error-T
		Rp	Rd	Lex	Ca	Ct	Ccau	Cadv	Comp	Inc	Inc-T	Error	Error-T
		Rp	Rd	Lex	Ca	Ct	Ccau	Cadv	Comp	Inc	Inc-T	Error	Error-T
		Rp	Rd	Lex	Ca	Ct	Ccau	Cadv	Comp	Inc	Inc-T	Error	Error-T
		Rp	Rd	Lex	Ca	Ct	Ccau	Cadv	Comp	Inc	Inc-T	Error	Error-T

APPENDIX B

Story Retelling: Lost Wallet

Three unanalyzed samples are included for practice. Then, each sample is coded into *T-units* and analyzed for *informational content* and *cohesion*. Cohesive markers are underlined in the T-unit segmented transcript and categorized on subsequent pages. Refer to Chapters 4 and 5 for information about these and other relevant analyses.

CODES:

Informational Content
ESS = Essential units
ELAB = Elaborations
IRR = Irrelevancies
RED = Redundancies
OFF-TOPIC = Off-topic units
INC = Incorrect units

Cohesive Adequacy
Comp = Complete
Inc = Incomplete
Inc-T = Incomplete tie
Err = Error
Err-T = Error tie

Cohesive Marker Types
Rp = Personal reference
Rd = Demonstrative reference
Lex = Lexical
Ca = Additive conjunction
Ct = Temporal conjunction
Ccau = Causal conjunction
Cadv = Adversative conjunction

STORY RETELLING-LOST WALLET
SAMPLE TRANSCRIPT 1

The lady gave the child a reward for calling her and bringing her back her wallet . . . it doesn't say that . . . that that was the end of the line I was waiting for you to say . . . and a lady lost her wallet in the store . . . when she went to pay for her groceries she discovered her wallet was missing . . . she had to put the groceries back coz she had no money . . . but when she was going home just as she opened the door the phone rang . . . it's a small child on the phone saying that she had found her wallet . . . the woman was relieved it saved her a lot of headaches . . . she'd have to get all new license and everything else and do a lot of running around to replace the cards that were missing in her wallet . . . I think she should have said to the child "Give me your name and address I'd like to send you something" . . . that little child could have taken the money and thrown the wallet away and said no more . . . we had some real honest people left in this gray world of ours . . . uh people don't think so but I do and I think you ought to reward them as as to help them . . . it isn't the money matter it's the being grateful for what they did . . . you got better stories than that I know you do

(2 minutes 6 seconds)

SAMPLE TRANSCRIPT 2

A woman went shopping . . . bought all her groceries . . . but lost her wallet in the supermarket . . . she put all the groceries back . . . went home . . . when she got home she got a telephone call and was informed that a small child had found her wallet . . . she was very relieved . . . she could have paid for the groceries with a Visa . . . she might have not lost her wallet if she had a purse . . . and if she had a checking account she could have wrote a check

(1 minute 23 seconds)

SAMPLE TRANSCRIPT 3

While the lady was shopping she had . . . I guess as she began . . . got to where she had to pay for them she noticed that she did not have her wallet . . . she was unaware that she had it had fallen on the floor . . . so she . . . you know to follow through she put the groceries away that she could and proceeded on home . . . and from what I understand when she got home she received a call call from a young person who told her she had found her wallet . . . I know she was very relieved that that her wallet was found but I don't recall in the st- story what she did . . . whether she went to meet this young person to receive the wallet or gave them a reward or what

(1 minute 25 seconds)

STORY RETELLING-LOST WALLET
SAMPLE TRANSCRIPT 1

INC   1. The lady gave the child a reward for calling her and bringing her back her wallet

IRR   2. it doesn't say that

IRR   3. (that) that was the end of the line I was waiting for you to say

ESS   4. and a lady lost her wallet in the store

ESS   5. when she went to pay for her groceries she discovered her wallet was missing

ESS   6. she had to put the groceries back coz she had no money

ESS   7. but when she was going home just as she opened the door the phone rang

ESS   8. it's a small child on the phone saying that she had found her wallet

ESS   9. the woman was relieved

IRR   10. it saved her a lot of headaches

IRR   11. she'd have to get all new license and everything else and do a lot of running around to replace the cards that were missing in her wallet

IRR   12. I think she should have said to the child "Give me your name and address I'd like to send you something"

IRR   13. that little child could have taken the money and thrown the wallet away and said no more

OFF-TOPIC   14. we had some real honest people left in this gray world of ours

OFF-TOPIC   15. (uh) people don't think so but I do

OFF-TOPIC   16. and I think you ought to reward them (as as) to help them

OFF-TOPIC   17. it isn't the money matter

OFF-TOPIC   18. it's the being grateful for what they did

IRR   19. you got better stories than that

IRR   20. I know you do

Story Retelling (ABCDD, Bayles & Tomoeda, 1991)
Essential Information Units

Lady (woman)	+
Was shopping (at the store; went shopping; went to the grocery store)	+
Her wallet (billfold; coin purse)	___
Wallet fell (dropped; lost; lost her purse)	+
Out of her purse (handbag; pocketbook)	___
She did not see it fall (she didn't know it)	___
At the checkout counter (when she went to pay; at the cashiers)	+
No way to pay (she had no money; she didn't have her wallet)	+
Put the groceries away (put the groceries back)	+
Went home to her house (she went back to her house)	+
As she opened the door (when she got home; just as she got inside)	+
Phone rang (she got a call)	+
Little (young)	+
Girl (lass)	+
Told her (said; reported)	+
She found wallet (coin purse; billfold)	+
Lady relieved (happy; delighted; grateful)	+

Total: *14/17*

In the following cohesion analysis, only the narrative portion of the story retelling has been coded; off topic information and asides that do not contribute to the story are not analyzed.

Lost Wallet
1

SUBJ ID _____ TASK _____ SCORED BY _____ DATE _____ Page___ *1 of 2*___

T-U #	Item (Word)	COHESIVE MARKER TYPE							COHESIVE ADEQUACY				
4	AND	Rp	Rd	Lex	(Ca)	Ct	Ccau	Cadv	Comp	(Inc)	Inc-T	Error	Error-T
	HER	Rp	(Rd)	Lex	Ca	Ct	Ccau	Cadv	(Comp)	Inc	Inc-T	Error	Error-T
	THE	Rp	(Rd)	Lex	Ca	Ct	Ccau	Cadv	Comp	(Inc)	Inc-T	Error	Error-T
5	SHE	(Rp)	Rd	Lex	Ca	Ct	Ccau	Cadv	(Comp)	Inc	Inc-T	Error	Error-T
	HER	Rp	(Rd)	Lex	Ca	Ct	Ccau	Cadv	(Comp)	Inc	Inc-T	Error	Error-T
	SHE	(Rp)	Rd	Lex	Ca	Ct	Ccau	Cadv	(Comp)	Inc	Inc-T	Error	Error-T
	HER	Rp	(Rd)	Lex	Ca	Ct	Ccau	Cadv	(Comp)	Inc	Inc-T	Error	Error-T
6	SHE	(Rp)	Rd	Lex	Ca	Ct	Ccau	Cadv	(Comp)	Inc	Inc-T	Error	Error-T
	THE	Rp	(Rd)	Lex	Ca	Ct	Ccau	Cadv	Comp	Inc	(Inc-T)	Error	Error-T
	SHE	(Rp)	Rd	Lex	Ca	Ct	Ccau	Cadv	(Comp)	Inc	Inc-T	Error	Error-T
7	BUT	Rp	Rd	Lex	Ca	Ct	Ccau	(Cadv)	Comp	Inc	Inc-T	(Error)	Error-T
	SHE	(Rp)	Rd	Lex	Ca	Ct	Ccau	Cadv	(Comp)	Inc	Inc-T	Error	Error-T
	SHE	(Rp)	Rd	Lex	Ca	Ct	Ccau	Cadv	(Comp)	Inc	Inc-T	Error	Error-T
	THE	Rp	(Rd)	Lex	Ca	Ct	Ccau	Cadv	Comp	(Inc)	Inc-T	Error	Error-T
	THE	Rp	(Rd)	Lex	Ca	Ct	Ccau	Cadv	Comp	(Inc)	Inc-T	Error	Error-T
8	IT'S	(Rp)	Rd	Lex	Ca	Ct	Ccau	Cadv	Comp	Inc	Inc-T	(Error)	Error-T
	THE	Rp	(Rd)	Lex	Ca	Ct	Ccau	Cadv	Comp	Inc	(Inc-T)	Error	Error-T
	SHE	Rp	Rd	Lex	Ca	Ct	Ccau	Cadv	Comp	Inc	Inc-T	(Error)	Error-T
	HER	Rp	Rd	Lex	Ca	Ct	Ccau	Cadv	Comp	Inc	Inc-T	(Error)	Error-T
9	THE	Rp	(Rd)	Lex	Ca	Ct	Ccau	Cadv	(Comp)	Inc	Inc-T	Error	Error-T
10	IT	(Rp)	Rd	Lex	Ca	Ct	Ccau	Cadv	Comp	Inc	Inc-T	(Error)	Error-T
	HER	(Rp)	Rd	Lex	Ca	Ct	Ccau	Cadv	(Comp)	Inc	Inc-T	Error	Error-T
11	SHE'D	(Rp)	Rd	Lex	Ca	Ct	Ccau	Cadv	(Comp)	Inc	Inc-T	Error	Error-T
	AND	Rp	Rd	Lex	(Ca)	Ct	Ccau	Cadv	(Comp)	Inc	Inc-T	Error	Error-T
	HER	Rp	(Rd)	Lex	Ca	Ct	Ccau	Cadv	(Comp)	Inc	Inc-T	Error	Error-T

Lost Wallet
 # 1

SUBJ ID _____ TASK_____ SCORED BY _____ DATE_____   Page___*2 of 2*___

T-U #	Item (Word)	COHESIVE MARKER TYPE							COHESIVE ADEQUACY				
12	SHE	(Rp)	Rd	Lex	Ca	Ct	Ccau	Cadv	(Comp)	Inc	Inc-T	Error	Error-T
	THE	Rp	(Rd)	Lex	Ca	Ct	Ccau	Cadv	(Comp)	Inc	Inc-T	Error	Error-T
	ME	(Rp)	Rd	Lex	Ca	Ct	Ccau	Cadv	(Comp)	Inc	Inc-T	Error	Error-T
	YOUR	Rp	(Rd)	Lex	Ca	Ct	Ccau	Cadv	(Comp)	Inc	Inc-T	Error	Error-T
	I"D	(Rp)	Rd	Lex	Ca	Ct	Ccau	Cadv	(Comp)	Inc	Inc-T	Error	Error-T
	YOU	(Rp)	Rd	Lex	Ca	Ct	Ccau	Cadv	(Comp)	Inc	Inc-T	Error	Error-T
13	THAT	Rp	(Rd)	Lex	Ca	Ct	Ccau	Cadv	(Comp)	Inc	Inc-T	Error	Error-T
	THE	Rp	(Rd)	Lex	Ca	Ct	Ccau	Cadv	Comp	(Inc)	Inc-T	Error	Error-T
	THE	Rp	(Rd)	Lex	Ca	Ct	Ccau	Cadv	(Comp)	Inc	Inc-T	Error	Error-T

STORY RETELLING: LOST WALLET
SAMPLE TRANSCRIPT 2

ESS   1. A woman went shopping . . . bought all her groceries . . . but lost her wallet in the supermarket

ESS   2. she put all the groceries back . . . went home

ESS   3. when she got home she got a telephone call and was informed that a small child had found her wallet

ESS   4. she was very relieved

IRR   5. she could have paid for the groceries with (a) a Visa

IRR   6. she might have not lost her wallet if she had a purse

IRR   7. and if she had a checking account she could have wrote a check

---

Story Retelling (ABCDD, Bayles & Tomoeda, 1991)
Essential Information Units

Lady (woman)	+
Was shopping (at the store; went shopping; went to the grocery story)	+
Her wallet (billfold; coin purse)	+
Wallet fell (dropped; lost her purse)	+
Out of her purse (handbag; pocketbook)	+
She did not see it fall (she didn't know it)	
At the check-out counter (when she went to pay; at the cashiers)	
No way to pay (she had no money; she didn't have her wallet)	
Put the groceries away (put the groceries back)	+
Went home to her house (she went back to her house)	+
As she opened the door (when she got home; just as she got inside)	+
Phone rang (she got a call)	+
Little (young)	+
Girl (lass)	
Told her (said; reported)	+
She found wallet (coin purse; billfold)	+
Lady relieved (happy; delighted; grateful)	+

Total: 12/17

Lost Wallet
2   Page 1 of 1

SUBJ ID _____ TASK_____ SCORED BY _____ DATE_____

T-U #	Item (Word)	COHESIVE MARKER TYPE							COHESIVE ADEQUACY				
		Rp	Rd	Lex	Ca	Ct	Ccau	Cadv	Comp	Inc	Inc-T	Error	Error-T
1	NO ITEMS	Rp	Rd	Lex	Ca	Ct	Ccau	Cadv	Comp	Inc	Inc-T	Error	Error-T
2	SHE	(Rp)	Rd	Lex	Ca	Ct	Ccau	Cadv	(Comp)	Inc	Inc-T	Error	Error-T
	THE	Rp	(Rd)	Lex	Ca	Ct	Ccau	Cadv	(Comp)	Inc	Inc-T	Error	Error-T
3	SHE	(Rp)	Rd	Lex	Ca	Ct	Ccau	Cadv	(Comp)	Inc	Inc-T	Error	Error-T
	SHE	(Rp)	Rd	Lex	Ca	Ct	Ccau	Cadv	(Comp)	Inc	Inc-T	Error	Error-T
	HER	(Rp)	Rd	Lex	Ca	Ct	Ccau	Cadv	(Comp)	Inc	Inc-T	Error	Error-T
4	SHE	(Rp)	Rd	Lex	Ca	Ct	Ccau	Cadv	(Comp)	Inc	Inc-T	Error	Error-T
5	SHE	(Rp)	Rd	Lex	Ca	Ct	Ccau	Cadv	(Comp)	Inc	Inc-T	Error	Error-T
	THE	Rp	(Rd)	Lex	Ca	Ct	Ccau	Cadv	(Comp)	Inc	Inc-T	Error	Error-T
6	SHE	(Rp)	Rd	Lex	Ca	Ct	Ccau	Cadv	(Comp)	Inc	Inc-T	Error	Error-T
	HER	Rp	(Rd)	Lex	Ca	Ct	Ccau	Cadv	(Comp)	Inc	Inc-T	Error	Error-T
	SHE	(Rp)	Rd	Lex	Ca	Ct	Ccau	Cadv	(Comp)	Inc	Inc-T	Error	Error-T
7	AND IF	Rp	Rd	Lex	Ca	Ct	(Ccau)	Cadv	(Comp)	Inc	Inc-T	Error	Error-T
	SHE	(Rp)	Rd	Lex	Ca	Ct	Ccau	Cadv	(Comp)	Inc	Inc-T	Error	Error-T
	SHE	(Rp)	Rd	Lex	Ca	Ct	Ccau	Cadv	(Comp)	Inc	Inc-T	Error	Error-T
		Rp	Rd	Lex	Ca	Ct	Ccau	Cadv	Comp	Inc	Inc-T	Error	Error-T
		Rp	Rd	Lex	Ca	Ct	Ccau	Cadv	Comp	Inc	Inc-T	Error	Error-T
		Rp	Rd	Lex	Ca	Ct	Ccau	Cadv	Comp	Inc	Inc-T	Error	Error-T
		Rp	Rd	Lex	Ca	Ct	Ccau	Cadv	Comp	Inc	Inc-T	Error	Error-T
		Rp	Rd	Lex	Ca	Ct	Ccau	Cadv	Comp	Inc	Inc-T	Error	Error-T
		Rp	Rd	Lex	Ca	Ct	Ccau	Cadv	Comp	Inc	Inc-T	Error	Error-T
		Rp	Rd	Lex	Ca	Ct	Ccau	Cadv	Comp	Inc	Inc-T	Error	Error-T
		Rp	Rd	Lex	Ca	Ct	Ccau	Cadv	Comp	Inc	Inc-T	Error	Error-T
		Rp	Rd	Lex	Ca	Ct	Ccau	Cadv	Comp	Inc ·	Inc-T	Error	Error-T

STORY RETELLING: LOST WALLET
SAMPLE TRANSCRIPT 3

ESS   1. while the lady was shopping she had (I guess as she began) got to where she had to pay for them

ESS   2. she noticed that she did not have her wallet

ESS   3. she was unaware that (she had) it had fallen on the floor

ESS   4. so (she . . . you know to follow through) she put the groceries away that she could and proceeded on home

ESS   5. and from what I understand when she got home she received a call (call) from a young person who told her she had found her wallet

ESS   6. I know she was very relieved (that) that her wallet was found

IRR   7. but I don't recall in the (st-) story what she did . . . whether she went to meet this young person to receive the wallet or gave them a reward or what

Story Retelling (ABCDD, Bayles & Tomoeda, 1991)
Essential Information Units

Lady (woman)	+
Was shopping (at the store; went shopping; went to the grocery story)	+
Her wallet (billfold; coin purse)	+
Wallet fell (dropped; lost; lost her purse)	+
Out of her purse (handbag; pocketbook)	
She did not see it fall (she didn't know it)	+
At the checkout counter (when she went to pay; at the cashiers)	+
No way to pay (she had no money; she didn't have her wallet)	
Put the groceries away (put the groceries back)	+
Went home to her house (she went back to her house)	+
As she opened the door (when she got home; just as she got inside)	+
Phone rang (she got a call)	+
Little (young)	+
Girl (lass)	+
Told her (said; reported)	+
She found wallet (coin purse; billfold)	+
Lady relieved (happy; delighted; grateful)	+

Total: 15/17

Lost Wallet

 # 3

SUBJ ID _____ TASK _____ SCORED BY _____ DATE _____   Page___ *1 of 2*___

T-U #	Item (Word)	COHESIVE MARKER TYPE							COHESIVE ADEQUACY				
1	THE	(Rp)	Rd	Lex	Ca	Ct	Ccau	Cadv	Comp	(Inc)	Inc-T	Error	Error-T
	SHE	(Rp)	Rd	Lex	Ca	Ct	Ccau	Cadv	Comp	Inc	(Inc-T)	Error	Error-T
	SHE	(Rp)	Rd	Lex	Ca	Ct	Ccau	Cadv	Comp	Inc	(Inc-T)	Error	Error-T
	THEM	(Rp)	Rd	Lex	Ca	Ct	Ccau	Cadv	Comp	(Inc)	Inc-T	Error	Error-T
2	SHE	(Rp)	Rd	Lex	Ca	Ct	Ccau	Cadv	Comp	Inc	(Inc-T)	Error	Error-T
	SHE	(Rp)	Rd	Lex	Ca	Ct	Ccau	Cadv	Comp	Inc	(Inc-T)	Error	Error-T
	HER	Rp	(Rd)	Lex	Ca	Ct	Ccau	Cadv	Comp	Inc	(Inc-T)	Error	Error-T
3	SHE	(Rp)	Rd	Lex	Ca	Ct	Ccau	Cadv	Comp	Inc	(Inc-T)	Error	Error-T
	IT	(Rp)	Rd	Lex	Ca	Ct	Ccau	Cadv	(Comp)	Inc	Inc-T	Error	Error-T
	THE FLOOR	Rp	Rd	(Lex)	Ca	Ct	Ccau	Cadv	(Comp)	Inc	Inc-T	Error	Error-T
4	SO	Rp	Rd	Lex	Ca	Ct	(Ccau)	Cadv	(Comp)	Inc	Inc-T	Error	Error-T
	SHE	(Rp)	Rd	Lex	Ca	Ct	Ccau	Cadv	Comp	Inc	(Inc-T)	Error	Error-T
	THE	Rp	(Rd)	Lex	Ca	Ct	Ccau	Cadv	Comp	Inc	(Inc-T)	Error	Error-T
	SHE	(Rp)	Rd	Lex	Ca	Ct	Ccau	Cadv	Comp	Inc	(Inc-T)	Error	Error-T
5	AND	Rp	Rd	Lex	(Ca)	Ct	Ccau	Cadv	(Comp)	Inc	Inc-T	Error	Error-T
	SHE	(Rp)	Rd	Lex	Ca	Ct	Ccau	Cadv	Comp	Inc	(Inc-T)	Error	Error-T
	SHE	(Rp)	Rd	Lex	Ca	Ct	Ccau	Cadv	Comp	Inc	(Inc-T)	Error	Error-T
	HER	(Rp)	Rd	Lex	Ca	Ct	Ccau	Cadv	Comp	Inc	(Inc-T)	Error	Error-T
	SHE	(Rp)	Rd	Lex	Ca	Ct	Ccau	Cadv	Comp	Inc	Inc-T	(Error)	Error-T
	HER	Rp	(Rd)	Lex	Ca	Ct	Ccau	Cadv	Comp	Inc	(Inc-T)	Error	Error-T
6	SHE	(Rp)	Rd	Lex	Ca	Ct	Ccau	Cadv	Comp	Inc	(Inc-T)	Error	Error-T
	HER	Rp	(Rd)	Lex	Ca	Ct	Ccau	Cadv	Comp	Inc	(Inc-T)	Error	Error-T
7	BUT	Rp	Rd	Lex	Ca	Ct	Ccau	(Cadv)	(Comp)	Inc	Inc-T	Error	Error-T
	SHE	(Rp)	Rd	Lex	Ca	Ct	Ccau	Cadv	Comp	Inc	(Inc-T)	Error	Error-T
	SHE	(Rp)	Rd	Lex	Ca	Ct	Ccau	Cadv	Comp	Inc	(Inc-T)	Error	Error-T

Lost Wallet
 # 3

SUBJ ID _____ TASK_____ SCORED BY _____ DATE_____ Page___*2 of 2*___

T-U #	Item (Word)	COHESIVE MARKER TYPE							COHESIVE ADEQUACY				
	THIS	Rp	(Rd)	Lex	Ca	Ct	Ccau	Cadv	(Comp)	Inc	Inc-T	Error	Error-T
	THE	Rp	(Rd)	Lex	Ca	Ct	Ccau	Cadv	Comp	Inc	(Inc-T)	Error	Error-T
	THEM	(Rp)	Rd	Lex	Ca	Ct	Ccau	Cadv	Comp	Inc	Inc-T	(Error)	Error-T
		Rp	Rd	Lex	Ca	Ct	Ccau	Cadv	Comp	Inc	Inc-T	Error	Error-T
		Rp	Rd	Lex	Ca	Ct	Ccau	Cadv	Comp	Inc	Inc-T	Error	Error-T
		Rp	Rd	Lex	Ca	Ct	Ccau	Cadv	Comp	Inc	Inc-T	Error	Error-T
		Rp	Rd	Lex	Ca	Ct	Ccau	Cadv	Comp	Inc	Inc-T	Error	Error-T
		Rp	Rd	Lex	Ca	Ct	Ccau	Cadv	Comp	Inc	Inc-T	Error	Error-T
		Rp	Rd	Lex	Ca	Ct	Ccau	Cadv	Comp	Inc	Inc-T	Error	Error-T
		Rp	Rd	Lex	Ca	Ct	Ccau	Cadv	Comp	Inc	Inc-T	Error	Error-T
		Rp	Rd	Lex	Ca	Ct	Ccau	Cadv	Comp	Inc	Inc-T	Error	Error-T
		Rp	Rd	Lex	Ca	Ct	Ccau	Cadv	Comp	Inc	Inc-T	Error	Error-T
		Rp	Rd	Lex	Ca	Ct	Ccau	Cadv	Comp	Inc	Inc-T	Error	Error-T
		Rp	Rd	Lex	Ca	Ct	Ccau	Cadv	Comp	Inc	Inc-T	Error	Error-T
		Rp	Rd	Lex	Ca	Ct	Ccau	Cadv	Comp	Inc	Inc-T	Error	Error-T
		Rp	Rd	Lex	Ca	Ct	Ccau	Cadv	Comp	Inc	Inc-T	Error	Error-T
		Rp	Rd	Lex	Ca	Ct	Ccau	Cadv	Comp	Inc	Inc-T	Error	Error-T
		Rp	Rd	Lex	Ca	Ct	Ccau	Cadv	Comp	Inc	Inc-T	Error	Error-T
		Rp	Rd	Lex	Ca	Ct	Ccau	Cadv	Comp	Inc	Inc-T	Error	Error-T
		Rp	Rd	Lex	Ca	Ct	Ccau	Cadv	Comp	Inc	Inc-T	Error	Error-T
		Rp	Rd	Lex	Ca	Ct	Ccau	Cadv	Comp	Inc	Inc-T	Error	Error-T
		Rp	Rd	Lex	Ca	Ct	Ccau	Cadv	Comp	Inc	Inc-T	Error	Error-T
		Rp	Rd	Lex	Ca	Ct	Ccau	Cadv	Comp	Inc	Inc-T	Error	Error-T
		Rp	Rd	Lex	Ca	Ct	Ccau	Cadv	Comp	Inc	Inc-T	Error	Error-T
		Rp	Rd	Lex	Ca	Ct	Ccau	Cadv	Comp	Inc	Inc-T	Error	Error-T

APPENDIX C

Procedural Discourse: How To Make a Sandwich

Three unanalyzed samples are included for practice. Then, each sample is coded into *T-units* and analyzed for *informational content*. Refer to Chapter 5 for information about other informational content analyses.

Transcript 3 has also been coded for *cohesion*.

The reader should remember that cohesion analysis is most appropriate for narrative discourse. However, cohesion analysis of procedural discourse may provide clinically useful information, particularly about the use of temporal conjunctions.

CODES:

Informational Content
ESS = Essential units
ELAB = Elaborations
IRR = Irrelevancies
RED = Redundancies
OFF-TOPIC = Off-topic units
INC = Incorrect units

Cohesive Adequacy
Comp = Complete
Inc = Incomplete
Inc-T = Incomplete tie
Err = Error
Err-T = Error tie

Cohesive Marker Types
Rp = Personal reference
Rd = Demonstrative reference
Lex = Lexical
Ca = Additive conjunction
Ct = Temporal conjunction
Ccau = Causal conjunction
Cadv = Adversative conjunction

PROCEDURAL DISCOURSE: HOW TO MAKE A SANDWICH
SAMPLE TRANSCRIPT 1

That's another job my wife does very well . . . but how to make one I don't make them often I guess I'm just too lazy . . . need two pieces of bread with a little . . . butter or mayonnaise whatever you prefer . . . then if you're going to make cold meat then just take a a couple pieces of cold meat . . . and put it on and maybe a piece of lettuce or a slice of tomato . . . and some people like their bread toasted on sandwiches . . . some don't . . . I like rye bread better for a sandwich myself than white bread . . . and uh . . . certain rye is much better than other rye but uh . . . I would prefer rye bread sandwich and oh . . . and than white bread sandwich . . . I also enjoy rye bread toasted . . . so all in all that's how you make a sandwich . . . not much to that either

(1 minute, 2 seconds)

SAMPLE TRANSCRIPT 2

Okay, you take two pieces of bread, put whatever you're going to put on like mustard, mayonnaise or whatever on and then you get your lunch meat on there and stuff your lettuce, tomato and fold it over and then you cut it. But make sure you use a different cutting board and a different knife for every sandwich you make so that the salmonella and all that junk don't set in. That's very important. 'Cause I had to go be for the other job I had I had to go for my food certificate license and all that was in the studies. Don't use the same board for for cutting chicken today, right now, cut your chicken, clean your board off immediately and then cut another piece of meat or vegetables . . . because of all the germs that are in that cutting board . . . salmonella poisoning can set in. And never use the same knife to cut vegetables and meat that you cut the meat with because you transform germs from one thing to another, especially on your chicken. Do you know how to tell if a chicken is spoiled outside of smell? When you get it home, open it up, touch under the armpits. If it's real slimy then it's going bad already.

(1 minute, 33 seconds)

SAMPLE TRANSCRIPT 3

To make a sandwich I would first . . . determine . . . the . . . type of sandwich I'd want to eat . . . so I . . . can . . . organize . . . the items . . . that go in the sandwich . . . and then I would get the items out of the refrigerator and the cabinets . . . items such as bread . . . milk . . . a plate . . . silverware . . . and I would place those items on a cabinet in the kitchen or a worktable. . . then I would take the bread . . . out of the wrapper . . . the number of slices I would need for the sandwich . . . place them on the table . . . then I would butter the number of slices I felt needed buttered . . . then if I were gonna put some condiments on the sandwich I would take them from the refrigerator if hadn't already . . . and I would spread . . . the condiments would be mayonnaise . . . ketchup . . . mustard . . . or whatever . . . on the number of bread slices . . . where it's appropriate then I would take . . . other products . . . such as meat . . . and . . . decide how many what quantity I wanted . . . and I would take those that quantity . . . and place it on . . . one of the slices of bread . . . and then I would probably take . . . two slices of bread and . . . join them . . . one on top of the other to form the sandwich. . . . I would then begin . . . returning . . . the . . . the items that I had . . . prepared for the sandwich I would return them to their original location . . . refrigerator cabinets or whatever . . . and I would clean the area . . . and prepare to wash . . . silver and china

PROCEDURAL DISCOURSE: HOW TO MAKE A SANDWICH
SAMPLE TRANSCRIPT 1

That's another job my wife does very well . . . but how to make one I don't make them often I guess I'm too lazy . . . need two <u>pieces of bread</u> *(1)* with a little . . . <u>butter or mayonnaise</u> *(2)* whatever you prefer . . . then if you're going to make cold meat then just take a a couple pieces <u>of cold meat</u> *(2)* . . . and put it on and maybe a piece of lettuce or a slice of tomato . . . and some people like their bread toasted on sandwiches . . . some don't . . . I like rye bread better for a sandwich myself than white bread . . . and uh . . . certain rye is much better than other rye but uh . . . I would prefer rye bread sandwich and oh . . . and than white bread sandwich . . . I also enjoy rye bread toasted . . . so all in all that's how you make a sandwich . . . not much to that either

Number of Essential Steps = 2/4

IRR	1. that's another job my wife does very well
IRR	2. but (how to make one) I don't make them often
IRR	3. I guess I'm too lazy
ESS	4. need two pieces of bread with a little butter or mayonnaise whatever you prefer
ESS	5. then if you're going to make cold meat then just take (a) a couple pieces of cold meat
ESS	6. and put it on and maybe a piece of lettuce or a slice of tomato
IRR	7. and some people like their bread toasted on sandwiches
IRR	8. some don't
IRR	9. I like rye bread better for a sandwich myself than white bread
IRR	10. and (uh) certain rye is much better than other rye
IRR	11. but (uh) I would prefer rye bread sandwich (and oh and) than white bread sandwich
IRR	12. I also enjoy rye bread toasted
IRR	13. so all in all that's how you make a sandwich not much to that either

PROCEDURAL DISCOURSE: HOW TO MAKE A SANDWICH
SAMPLE TRANSCRIPT 2

(1)   *(2 + 3)*   *(2)*
Okay, you take two pieces of bread, put whatever you're going to put on like mustard, mayonnaise or
                                   (2 + 3)   *(2)*   *(2)*   *(4)*
whatever on and then you get your lunch meat on there and stuff your lettuce, tomato and fold it over and

then you cut it. But make sure you use a different cutting board and a different knife for every sandwich you

make so that the salmonella and all that junk don't set in. That's very important. 'Cause I had to go be for

the other job I had I had to go for my food certificate license and all that was in the studies. Don't use

the same board for for cutting chicken today, right now, cut your chicken, clean your board off immediately

and then cut another piece of meat or vegetables . . . because of all the germs that are in that cutting

board . . . salmonella poisoning can set in. And never use the same knife to cut vegetables and meat that you

cut the meat with because you transform germs from one thing to another, especially on your chicken. Do you

know how to tell if a chicken is spoiled outside of smell? When you get it home, open it up, touch under the

armpits. If it's real slimy then it's going bad already

Number of Essential Steps = 4/4

ESS	1. (Okay) you take two pieces of bread
ESS	2. put whatever you're going to put on like mustard, mayonnaise or whatever on
ESS	3. and then you get your lunch meat on there
ESS	4. and stuff your lettuce, tomato
ESS	5. and fold it over
ELAB	6. and then you cut it
IRR	7. but make sure you use a different cutting board and a different knife for every sandwich you make so that the salmonella and all that junk don't set in
IRR	8. that's very important
OFF-TOPIC	9. 'cause (I had to go be) for the other job I had I had to go for my food certificate license
OFF-TOPIC	10. and all this was in the studies
OFF-TOPIC	11. don't use the same board (for) for cutting chicken today (right now)
OFF-TOPIC	12. cut your chicken
OFF-TOPIC	13. clean your board off immediately
OFF-TOPIC	14. and then cut another piece of meat or vegetables . . .
OFF-TOPIC	15. because of all the germs that are in that cutting board . . . salmonella poisoning can set in.
OFF-TOPIC	16. and never use the same knife to cut vegetables and meat that you cut the meat with because you transform germs from one thing or another, especially on your chicken.
OFF-TOPIC	17. do you know how to tell if a chicken is spoiled outside of smell?
OFF-TOPIC	18. when you get it home, open it up
OFF-TOPIC	19. touch under the armpits
OFF-TOPIC	20. if it's real slimy then it's going bad already.

PROCEDURAL DISCOURSE: HOW TO MAKE A SANDWICH
SAMPLE TRANSCRIPT 3

To make a sandwich I would first / determine / the / type of sandwich I'd want to eat / so I / can /
organize / the items / that go in the sandwich / and then I would get the items *(2)* out of the refrigerator and
the cabinets / items such as bread *(1)* / milk / a plate / silverware / and I would place those items on a cabinet
in the kitchen or a worktable / / then I would take the bread / out of the wrapper / the number of slices I
would need for the sandwich / place them on the table / then I would butter *(3)* the number of slices I felt
needed buttered / then if I were gonna put some condiments *(3)* on the sandwich I would take them from the
refrigerator if hadn't already / and I would spread / the condiments would be mayonnaise *(3)* / ketchup / mustard
/ or whatever / on the number of bread slices / where it's appropriate then I would take / other products / *(2)*
such as meat / and / decide how many what quantity I wanted / and I would take those that quantity / and
place it on *(3)* / one of the slices of bread / and then I would probably take / two slices of bread and / join *(4)*
them / one on top of the other to form the sandwich. . . . I would then begin / returning / the / the items
that I had / prepared for the sandwich I would return them to their original location / refrigerator cabinets
or whatever / and I would clean the area / and prepare to wash / silver and china

Number of Essential Steps = 4/4

In the following T-unit segmented transcript, cohesive markers are underlined; the categorization of the markers follows on subsequent pages.

ELAB	1. to make a sandwich I would first determine the type of sandwich I'd want to eat so I can organize the items that go in the sandwich
ESS/ELAB	2. and then I would get the items out of the refrigerator and the cabinets . . . items such as bread . . . milk . . . a plate . . . silverware
ELAB	3. and I would place those items on a cabinet in the kitchen or a work table
ESS/ELAB	4. then I would take (the bread) out of the wrapper the number of slices I would need for the sandwich
ELAB	5. place them on the table
ESS	6. then I would butter the number of slices I felt needed buttered
ESS/ELAB	7. then if I were gonna put some condiments on the sandwich I would take them from the refrigerator if hadn't already
ESS	8. and I would spread the condiments (would be) mayonnaise ketchup mustard or whatever on the number of bread slices where it's appropriate
ESS	9. then I would take other products such as meat and decide (how many) what quantity I wanted
ESS	10. and I would take (those) that quantity and place it on one of the slices of bread
ESS	11. and then I would probably take two slices of bread and join them one on top of the other to form the sandwich
ELAB	12. I would then begin returning (the) the items that I had prepared for the sandwich
ELAB	13. I would return them to their original location . . . refrigerator cabinets or whatever
ELAB	14. and I would clean the area and prepare to wash silver and china

How To Make a
Sandwich # 3

SUBJ ID _____TASK_____ SCORED BY _____ DATE_____ Page____**1 of 2**____

T-U #	Item (Word)	COHESIVE MARKER TYPE							COHESIVE ADEQUACY				
		Rp	Rd	Lex	Ca	Ct	Ccau	Cadv	Comp	Inc	Inc-T	Error	Error-T
1	NO ITEMS	Rp	Rd	Lex	Ca	Ct	Ccau	Cadv	Comp	Inc	Inc-T	Error	Error-T
2	AND THEN	Rp	Rd	Lex	Ca	(Ct)	Ccau	Cadv	(Comp)	Inc	Inc-T	Error	Error-T
3	AND	Rp	Rd	Lex	(Ca)	Ct	Ccau	Cadv	(Comp)	Inc	Inc-T	Error	Error-T
	THOSE	Rp	(Rd)	Lex	Ca	Ct	Ccau	Cadv	(Comp)	Inc	Inc-T	Error	Error-T
4	THEN	Rp	Rd	Lex	Ca	(Ct)	Ccau	Cadv	(Comp)	Inc	Inc-T	Error	Error-T
	THE	Rp	(Rd)	Lex	Ca	Ct	Ccau	Cadv	(Comp)	Inc	Inc-T	Error	Error-T
5	THEM	(Rp)	Rd	Lex	Ca	Ct	Ccau	Cadv	Comp	Inc	Inc-T	(Error)	Error-T
	THE	Rp	(Rd)	Lex	Ca	Ct	Ccau	Cadv	(Comp)	Inc	Inc-T	Error	Error-T
6	THEN	Rp	Rd	Lex	Ca	(Ct)	Ccau	Cadv	(Comp)	Inc	Inc-T	Error	Error-T
7	THEN	Rp	Rd	Lex	Ca	(Ct)	Ccau	Cadv	(Comp)	Inc	Inc-T	Error	Error-T
8	AND	Rp	Rd	Lex	(Ca)	Ct	Ccau	Cadv	(Comp)	Inc	Inc-T	Error	Error-T
	IT'S	(Rp)	Rd	Lex	Ca	Ct	Ccau	Cadv	Comp	Inc	Inc-T	(Error)	Error-T
9	THEN	Rp	Rd	Lex	Ca	(Ct)	Ccau	Cadv	(Comp)	Inc	Inc-T	Error	Error-T
10	AND	Rp	Rd	Lex	(Ca)	Ct	Ccau	Cadv	(Comp)	Inc	Inc-T	Error	Error-T
	THAT	Rp	(Rd)	Lex	Ca	Ct	Ccau	Cadv	(Comp)	Inc	Inc-T	Error	Error-T
	IT	(Rp)	Rd	Lex	Ca	Ct	Ccau	Cadv	(Comp)	Inc	Inc-T	Error	Error-T
	THE	Rp	(Rd)	Lex	Ca	Ct	Ccau	Cadv	(Comp)	Inc	Inc-T	Error	Error-T
11	AND THEN	Rp	Rd	Lex	Ca	(Ct)	Ccau	Cadv	(Comp)	Inc	Inc-T	Error	Error-T
	AND	Rp	Rd	Lex	(Ca)	Ct	Ccau	Cadv	(Comp)	Inc	Inc-T	Error	Error-T
	THEM	(Rp)	Rd	Lex	Ca	Ct	Ccau	Cadv	(Comp)	Inc	Inc-T	Error	Error-T
	THE	Rp	(Rd)	Lex	Ca	Ct	Ccau	Cadv	(Comp)	Inc	Inc-T	Error	Error-T
12	THEN	Rp	Rd	Lex	Ca	(Ct)	Ccau	Cadv	(Comp)	Inc	Inc-T	Error	Error-T
	THE	Rp	(Rd)	Lex	Ca	Ct	Ccau	Cadv	(Comp)	Inc	Inc-T	Error	Error-T
	THE	Rp	(Rd)	Lex	Ca	Ct	Ccau	Cadv	(Comp)	Inc	Inc-T	Error	Error-T
13	THEM	(Rp)	Rd	Lex	Ca	Ct	Ccau	Cadv	(Comp)	Inc	Inc-T	Error	Error-T

SUBJ ID _____ TASK _____ SCORED BY _____ DATE _____ *How To Make a Sandwich # 3* Page __2 of 2__

T-U #	Item (Word)	COHESIVE MARKER TYPE							COHESIVE ADEQUACY				
	THEIR	Rp	(Rd)	Lex	Ca	Ct	Ccau	Cadv	(Comp)	Inc	Inc-T	Error	Error-T
14	*AND*	Rp	Rd	Lex	(Ca)	Ct	Ccau	Cadv	(Comp)	Inc	Inc-T	Error	Error-T
	THE	Rp	(Rd)	Lex	Ca	Ct	Ccau	Cadv	Comp	Inc	Inc-T	(Error)	Error-T
	AND	Rp	Rd	Lex	(Ca)	Ct	Ccau	Cadv	(Comp)	Inc	Inc-T	Error	Error-T
		Rp	Rd	Lex	Ca	Ct	Ccau	Cadv	Comp	Inc	Inc-T	Error	Error-T
		Rp	Rd	Lex	Ca	Ct	Ccau	Cadv	Comp	Inc	Inc-T	Error	Error-T
		Rp	Rd	Lex	Ca	Ct	Ccau	Cadv	Comp	Inc	Inc-T	Error	Error-T
		Rp	Rd	Lex	Ca	Ct	Ccau	Cadv	Comp	Inc	Inc-T	Error	Error-T
		Rp	Rd	Lex	Ca	Ct	Ccau	Cadv	Comp	Inc	Inc-T	Error	Error-T
		Rp	Rd	Lex	Ca	Ct	Ccau	Cadv	Comp	Inc	Inc-T	Error	Error-T
		Rp	Rd	Lex	Ca	Ct	Ccau	Cadv	Comp	Inc	Inc-T	Error	Error-T
		Rp	Rd	Lex	Ca	Ct	Ccau	Cadv	Comp	Inc	Inc-T	Error	Error-T
		Rp	Rd	Lex	Ca	Ct	Ccau	Cadv	Comp	Inc	Inc-T	Error	Error-T
		Rp	Rd	Lex	Ca	Ct	Ccau	Cadv	Comp	Inc	Inc-T	Error	Error-T
		Rp	Rd	Lex	Ca	Ct	Ccau	Cadv	Comp	Inc	Inc-T	Error	Error-T
		Rp	Rd	Lex	Ca	Ct	Ccau	Cadv	Comp	Inc	Inc-T	Error	Error-T
		Rp	Rd	Lex	Ca	Ct	Ccau	Cadv	Comp	Inc	Inc-T	Error	Error-T
		Rp	Rd	Lex	Ca	Ct	Ccau	Cadv	Comp	Inc	Inc-T	Error	Error-T
		Rp	Rd	Lex	Ca	Ct	Ccau	Cadv	Comp	Inc	Inc-T	Error	Error-T
		Rp	Rd	Lex	Ca	Ct	Ccau	Cadv	Comp	Inc	Inc-T	Error	Error-T
		Rp	Rd	Lex	Ca	Ct	Ccau	Cadv	Comp	Inc	Inc-T	Error	Error-T
		Rp	Rd	Lex	Ca	Ct	Ccau	Cadv	Comp	Inc	Inc-T	Error	Error-T
		Rp	Rd	Lex	Ca	Ct	Ccau	Cadv	Comp	Inc	Inc-T	Error	Error-T
		Rp	Rd	Lex	Ca	Ct	Ccau	Cadv	Comp	Inc	Inc-T	Error	Error-T
		Rp	Rd	Lex	Ca	Ct	Ccau	Cadv	Comp	Inc	Inc-T	Error	Error-T
		Rp	Rd	Lex	Ca	Ct	Ccau	Cadv	Comp	Inc	Inc-T	Error	Error-T

Story Retelling from a Film Strip

Three samples that have been coded into T-units are included for practice. Then each sample is analyzed for *story grammar* and *cohesion*. Note that cohesive markers are underlined and categorized on subsequent pages. Refer to chapters 4 and 6 for additional information about these analyses.

CODES:

Story Grammar Episode Componants
IE = Initiating events
A = Attempts
DC = Direct consequence

Cohesive Marker Types
Rp = Personal reference
Rd = Demonstrative reference
Lex = Lexical
Ca = Additive conjunction
Ct = Temporal conjunction
Ccau = Causal conjunction
Cadv = Adversative conjunction

Cohesive Adequacy
Comp = Complete
Inc = Incomplete
Inc-T = Incomplete tie
Err = Error
Err-T = Error tie

COMPLETE EPISODE = Contains all three episode components
INCOMPLETE EPISODE = Contains two of the three episode components

RETELLING FROM A FILMSTRIP
SAMPLE 1

1. The story consists of a mother bear, a papa bear and a baby bear.

2. The baby bear is the daughter.

3. And they're at home

4. and they are [are] preparing to eat dinner.

5. They're sitting down

6. and they're getting ready to eat dinner.

7. and all of a sudden a fly comes in and flies all around.

8. The father bear grabs a fly swatter and tries to swat it and misses

9. and [then it] [he misses his part] [you know] so he hits [his tray] his plate

10. it flies up

11. and it goes all over the place

12. and then [the fly itself] [of course] he misses the fly.

13. And fly itself flies around the wife

14. and he's getting ready [to flat] to swat the fly, swats the wife.

15. Then he misses the fly because the fly escapes.

16. Then the fly flies around the daughter

17. and [the] he knocks the daughter out with the fly swatter because he [swats the fly] misses the fly and hits the daughter.

18. Then it flies around his dog.

19. And the father's real mad now because he missed all them other times

20. and now he's thinking "let me get [this bear] this fly."

21. He swats at it

22. and he hits his dog

23. so [he knocks out his wife] [I mean] he knocks out his dog and his daughter

24. and the fly's still buzzing around

25. and he puts a chair on the table

26. and he tries to swat it

27. and that's when he falls and knocks over everything on the table.

28. Plus his daughter and his dog are knocked out

29. and the fly escapes and goes out the window [and thats the end of the story]

SAMPLE 2

1. [Um basically] this family of bears sits down and has [has] a meal

2. And [um] [they're eating,

3. and this fly comes in.

4. And the father's bothered by this

5. so he decides to swat [swat] or hit the [ah] fly.

6. And [ah] [anyways he hits his mother] [I mean] he hits his wife

7. and [ah] she goes down,

8. And [basically she [basically he hits ah] he hits [her] his daughter

9. and [ah] the daughter goes down to the floor.

10. [And then he climbs] [no he] and then he hits the dog.

11. And the dog goes down on the floor.

12. Then he decides to climb up [he decides to climb up] on the table and stand on a chair.

13. And he tips it over

14. and he falls. [and uh . . .]

SAMPLE 3

1. [OK] It's about a family of three bears.

2. And they're all cooking dinner and getting along amiably.

3. And along comes a little pesty fly.

4. And the papa bear pulls out a fly swatter attempts to [hit the bear] hit the fly.

5. And he misses and knocks out his wife.

6. And the fly still [is] [is] aggravates him.

7. so [he keeps] [he doesn't] he doesn't give up

8. he keeps on flying

9. And a couple more swats and passes and he knocks out his child.

10. [then] and then [then] he leaves the kid's table

11. and he keeps on hitting at the fly.

12. And [ah] he [he] has a dog nipping at his heels

13. and it really looks like a nice [a nice] little dog.

14. And then [and then] the fly lands on the ceiling

15. and so papa bear gets [a chair]

16. and he goes to put it down on the kid's table

17. and unknown [unknown] to him his wife is now awake and watching him.

18. and [she says] she knows he's gonna fall off the table

19. but she doesn't say a word,

20. so he does so.

21. And then he lands on the floor and knocks his self out.

22. And the fly goes out the window.

23. All this for a measly, pesky fly.

RETELLING FROM A FILMSTRIP
SAMPLE TRANSCRIPT 1

1. The story consists of a mother bear, a papa bear and a baby bear.

2. The baby bear is the daughter.

3. And they're at home.

4. and they are [are] preparing to eat dinner.

5. They're sitting down

6. and they're getting ready to eat dinner.

COMPLETE EPISODE

- IE 7. and all of a sudden a fly comes in and flies all around.

- A 8. The father bear grabs a fly swatter and tries to swat it and misses

  9. and [then it] [he misses his part] [you know] so he hits [his tray] his plate

  10. it flies up

- DC 11. and it goes all over the place

  12. and then [the fly itself] [of course] he misses the fly.

COMPLETE EPISODE

- IE 13. And fly itself flies around the wife

- A 14. and he's getting ready [to flat] to swat the fly, swats the wife.

- DC 15. Then he misses the fly because the fly escapes.

COMPLETE EPISODE

- IE 16. Then the fly flies around the daughter

- A & DC 17. and [the] he knocks the daughter out with the fly swatter because he [swats the fly] misses the fly and hits the daughter.

COMPLETE EPISODE

- IE 18. Then it flies around his dog.

  19. And the father's real mad now because he missed all them other times

  20. and now he's thinking "let me get [this bear] this fly."

- A 21. He swats at it

  22. and he hits his dog

- DC 23. so [he knocks out his wife] [I mean] he knocks out his dog and his daughter

COMPLETE EPISODE

- IE 24. and the fly's still buzzing around

- A 25. and he puts a chair on the table

  26. and he tries to swat it

- DC 27. and that's when he falls and knocks over everything on the table.

28. Plus his daughter and his dog are knocked out

29. and the fly escapes and goes out the window [and that's the end of the story]

FILMSTRIP # 1

SUBJ ID _____ TASK_____ SCORED BY _____ DATE_____   Page___1 of 4___

T-U #	Item (Word)	COHESIVE MARKER TYPE							COHESIVE ADEQUACY				
		Rp	Rd	Lex	Ca	Ct	Ccau	Cadv	Comp	Inc	Inc-T	Error	Error-T
1	NO ITEMS	Rp	Rd	Lex	Ca	Ct	Ccau	Cadv	Comp	Inc	Inc-T	Error	Error-T
2	THE	Rp	(Rd)	Lex	Ca	Ct	Ccau	Cadv	(Comp)	Inc	Inc-T	Error	Error-T
	THE	Rp	(Rd)	Lex	Ca	Ct	Ccau	Cadv	(Comp)	Inc	Inc-T	Error	Error-T
3	AND	Rp	Rd	Lex	(Ca)	Ct	Ccau	Cadv	(Comp)	Inc	Inc-T	Error	Error-T
	THEY	(Rp)	Rd	Lex	Ca	Ct	Ccau	Cadv	(Comp)	Inc	Inc-T	Error	Error-T
4	AND	Rp	Rd	Lex	(Ca)	Ct	Ccau	Cadv	(Comp)	Inc	Inc-T	Error	Error-T
	THEY	(Rp)	Rd	Lex	Ca	Ct	Ccau	Cadv	(Comp)	Inc	Inc-T	Error	Error-T
5	THEY	(Rp)	Rd	Lex	Ca	Ct	Ccau	Cadv	(Comp)	Inc	Inc-T	Error	Error-T
	DOWN	Rp	Rd	(Lex)	Ca	Ct	Ccau	Cadv	(Comp)	Inc	Inc-T	Error	Error-T
6	AND	Rp	Rd	Lex	(Ca)	Ct	Ccau	Cadv	(Comp)	Inc	Inc-T	Error	Error-T
	THEY	(Rp)	Rd	Lex	Ca	Ct	Ccau	Cadv	(Comp)	Inc	Inc-T	Error	Error-T
7	AND	Rp	Rd	Lex	(Ca)	Ct	Ccau	Cadv	(Comp)	Inc	Inc-T	Error	Error-T
	IN	Rp	Rd	(Lex)	Ca	Ct	Ccau	Cadv	(Comp)	Inc	Inc-T	Error	Error-T
8	THE	Rp	(Rd)	Lex	Ca	Ct	Ccau	Cadv	(Comp)	Inc	Inc-T	Error	Error-T
	IT	(Rp)	Rd	Lex	Ca	Ct	Ccau	Cadv	(Comp)	Inc	Inc-T	Error	Error-T
9	AND	Rp	Rd	Lex	(Ca)	Ct	Ccau	Cadv	(Comp)	Inc	Inc-T	Error	Error-T
	HE	(Rp)	Rd	Lex	Ca	Ct	Ccau	Cadv	(Comp)	Inc	Inc-T	Error	Error-T
	HIS	(Rp)	Rd	Lex	Ca	Ct	Ccau	Cadv	(Comp)	Inc	Inc-T	Error	Error-T
10	IT	(Rp)	Rd	Lex	Ca	Ct	Ccau	Cadv	(Comp)	Inc	Inc-T	Error	Error-T
	FLIES	Rp	Rd	(Lex)	Ca	Ct	Ccau	Cadv	(Comp)	Inc	Inc-T	Error	Error-T
11	AND	Rp	Rd	Lex	(Ca)	Ct	Ccau	Cadv	(Comp)	Inc	Inc-T	Error	Error-T
	IT	(Rp)	Rd	Lex	Ca	Ct	Ccau	Cadv	(Comp)	Inc	Inc-T	Error	Error-T
	GOES	Rp	Rd	(Lex)	Ca	Ct	Ccau	Cadv	(Comp)	Inc	Inc-T	Error	Error-T
12	AND THEN	Rp	Rd	Lex	Ca	(Ct)	Ccau	Cadv	Comp	Inc	Inc-T	(Error)	Error-T
	HE	(Rp)	Rd	Lex	Ca	Ct	Ccau	Cadv	(Comp)	Inc	Inc-T	Error	Error-T

FILMSTRIP # 1

SUBJ ID _____TASK_____ SCORED BY _____ DATE_____   Page___*2 of 4*___

T-U #	Item (Word)	COHESIVE MARKER TYPE	COHESIVE ADEQUACY
	THE	Rp **(Rd)** Lex Ca Ct Ccau Cadv	**(Comp)** Inc Inc-T Error Error-T
13	AND	Rp Rd Lex **(Ca)** Ct Ccau Cadv	**(Comp)** Inc Inc-T Error Error-T
	THE	Rp **(Rd)** Lex Ca Ct Ccau Cadv	**(Comp)** Inc Inc-T Error Error-T
14	AND	Rp Rd Lex **(Ca)** Ct Ccau Cadv	**(Comp)** Inc Inc-T Error Error-T
	HE	**(Rp)** Rd Lex Ca Ct Ccau Cadv	**(Comp)** Inc Inc-T Error Error-T
	THE	Rp **(Rd)** Lex Ca Ct Ccau Cadv	**(Comp)** Inc Inc-T Error Error-T
	THE	Rp **(Rd)** Lex Ca Ct Ccau Cadv	**(Comp)** Inc Inc-T Error Error-T
15	THEN	Rp Rd Lex Ca **(Ct)** Ccau Cadv	**(Comp)** Inc Inc-T Error Error-T
	HE	**(Rp)** Rd Lex Ca Ct Ccau Cadv	**(Comp)** Inc Inc-T Error Error-T
	THE	Rp **(Rd)** Lex Ca Ct Ccau Cadv	**(Comp)** Inc Inc-T Error Error-T
	THE	Rp **(Rd)** Lex Ca Ct Ccau Cadv	**(Comp)** Inc Inc-T Error Error-T
16	THEN	Rp Rd Lex Ca **(Ct)** Ccau Cadv	**(Comp)** Inc Inc-T Error Error-T
	THE	Rp **(Rd)** Lex Ca Ct Ccau Cadv	**(Comp)** Inc Inc-T Error Error-T
	THE	Rp **(Rd)** Lex Ca Ct Ccau Cadv	**(Comp)** Inc Inc-T Error Error-T
17	AND	Rp Rd Lex **(Ca)** Ct Ccau Cadv	**(Comp)** Inc Inc-T Error Error-T
	HE	**(Rp)** Rd Lex Ca Ct Ccau Cadv	**(Comp)** Inc Inc-T Error Error-T
	THE	Rp **(Rd)** Lex Ca Ct Ccau Cadv	**(Comp)** Inc Inc-T Error Error-T
	THE	Rp **(Rd)** Lex Ca Ct Ccau Cadv	**(Comp)** Inc Inc-T Error Error-T
	HE	**(Rp)** Rd Lex Ca Ct Ccau Cadv	**(Comp)** Inc Inc-T Error Error-T
	THE	Rp **(Rd)** Lex Ca Ct Ccau Cadv	**(Comp)** Inc Inc-T Error Error-T
	THE	Rp **(Rd)** Lex Ca Ct Ccau Cadv	**(Comp)** Inc Inc-T Error Error-T
18	THEN	Rp Rd Lex Ca **(Ct)** Ccau Cadv	**(Comp)** Inc Inc-T Error Error-T
	IT	**(Rp)** Rd Lex Ca Ct Ccau Cadv	**(Comp)** Inc Inc-T Error Error-T
	HIS	**(Rp)** Rd Lex Ca Ct Ccau Cadv	Comp Inc Inc-T Error Error-T
19	AND	Rp Rd Lex **(Ca)** Ct Ccau Cadv	**(Comp)** Inc Inc-T Error Error-T

FILMSTRIP # 1

SUBJ ID _____TASK_____ SCORED BY _____ DATE_____   Page_ 3 of 4 _____

T-U #	Item (Word)	COHESIVE MARKER TYPE							COHESIVE ADEQUACY				
	THE	Rp	(Rd)	Lex	Ca	Ct	Ccau	Cadv	(Comp)	Inc	Inc-T	Error	Error-T
	NOW	Rp	Rd	(Lex)	Ca	Ct	Ccau	Cadv	(Comp)	Inc	Inc-T	Error	Error-T
	MISSED	Rp	Rd	(Lex)	Ca	Ct	Ccau	Cadv	(Comp)	Inc	Inc-T	Error	Error-T
	OTHER	Rp *R comp.*	Rd	Lex	Ca	Ct	Ccau	Cadv	(Comp)	Inc	Inc-T	Error	Error-T
	TIMES	Rp	Rd	(Lex)	Ca	Ct	Ccau	Cadv	(Comp)	Inc	Inc-T	Error	Error-T
20	AND	Rp	Rd	Lex	(Ca)	Ct	Ccau	Cadv	(Comp)	Inc	Inc-T	Error	Error-T
	NOW	Rp	Rd	(Lex)	Ca	Ct	Ccau	Cadv	(Comp)	Inc	Inc-T	Error	Error-T
	HE	(Rp)	Rd	Lex	Ca	Ct	Ccau	Cadv	(Comp)	Inc	Inc-T	Error	Error-T
	ME	(Rp)	Rd	Lex	Ca	Ct	Ccau	Cadv	(Comp)	Inc	Inc-T	Error	Error-T
	THIS	Rp	(Rd)	Lex	Ca	Ct	Ccau	Cadv	(Comp)	Inc	Inc-T	Error	Error-T
21	HE	(Rp)	Rd	Lex	Ca	Ct	Ccau	Cadv	(Comp)	Inc	Inc-T	Error	Error-T
	IT	(Rp)	Rd	Lex	Ca	Ct	Ccau	Cadv	(Comp)	Inc	Inc-T	Error	Error-T
22	AND	Rp	Rd	Lex	(Ca)	Ct	Ccau	Cadv	(Comp)	Inc	Inc-T	Error	Error-T
	HE	(Rp)	Rd	Lex	Ca	Ct	Ccau	Cadv	(Comp)	Inc	Inc-T	Error	Error-T
	HIS	(Rp)	Rd	Lex	Ca	Ct	Ccau	Cadv	(Comp)	Inc	Inc-T	Error	Error-T
23	SO	Rp	Rd	Lex	Ca	Ct	(Ccau)	Cadv	(Comp)	Inc	Inc-T	Error	Error-T
	HE	(Rp)	Rd	Lex	Ca	Ct	Ccau	Cadv	(Comp)	Inc	Inc-T	Error	Error-T
	HIS	(Rp)	Rd	Lex	Ca	Ct	Ccau	Cadv	(Comp)	Inc	Inc-T	Error	Error-T
	HIS	(Rp)	Rd	Lex	Ca	Ct	Ccau	Cadv	(Comp)	Inc	Inc-T	Error	Error-T
24	AND	Rp	Rd	Lex	(Ca)	Ct	Ccau	Cadv	(Comp)	Inc	Inc-T	Error	Error-T
	THE	Rp	(Rd)	Lex	Ca	Ct	Ccau	Cadv	(Comp)	Inc	Inc-T	Error	Error-T
	STILL	Rp	Rd	(Lex)	Ca	Ct	Ccau	Cadv	(Comp)	Inc	Inc-T	Error	Error-T
25	AND	Rp	Rd	Lex	(Ca)	Ct	Ccau	Cadv	Comp	Inc	Inc-T	(Error)	Error-T
	HE	(Rp)	Rd	Lex	Ca	Ct	Ccau	Cadv	(Comp)	Inc	Inc-T	Error	Error-T
	THE	Rp	(Rd)	Lex	Ca	Ct	Ccau	Cadv	(Comp)	Inc	Inc-T	Error	Error-T

FILMSTRIP # 1

SUBJ ID _____ TASK _____ SCORED BY _____ DATE _____

T-U #	Item (Word)	COHESIVE MARKER TYPE							COHESIVE ADEQUACY				
26	AND	Rp	Rd	Lex	(Ca)	Ct	Ccau	Cadv	(Comp)	Inc	Inc-T	Error	Error-T
	HE	(Rp)	Rd	Lex	Ca	Ct	Ccau	Cadv	(Comp)	Inc	Inc-T	Error	Error-T
	IT	(Rp)	Rd	Lex	Ca	Ct	Ccau	Cadv	(Comp)	Inc	Inc-T	Error	Error-T
27	AND	Rp	Rd	Lex	(Ca)	Ct	Ccau	Cadv	(Comp)	Inc	Inc-T	Error	Error-T
	THAT'S	Rp	(Rd)	Lex	Ca	Ct	Ccau	Cadv	(Comp)	Inc	Inc-T	Error	Error-T
	HE	(Rp)	Rd	Lex	Ca	Ct	Ccau	Cadv	(Comp)	Inc	Inc-T	Error	Error-T
	THE	Rp	(Rd)	Lex	Ca	Ct	Ccau	Cadv	(Comp)	Inc	Inc-T	Error	Error-T
28	PLUS	Rp	Rd	Lex	(Ca)	Ct	Ccau	Cadv	(Comp)	Inc	Inc-T	Error	Error-T
	HIS	(Rp)	Rd	Lex	Ca	Ct	Ccau	Cadv	(Comp)	Inc	Inc-T	Error	Error-T
	HIS	(Rp)	Rd	Lex	Ca	Ct	Ccau	Cadv	(Comp)	Inc	Inc-T	Error	Error-T
29	AND	Rp	Rd	Lex	(Ca)	Ct	Ccau	Cadv	(Comp)	Inc	Inc-T	Error	Error-T
	THE	Rp	(Rd)	Lex	Ca	Ct	Ccau	Cadv	(Comp)	Inc	Inc-T	Error	Error-T
		Rp	Rd	Lex	Ca	Ct	Ccau	Cadv	Comp	Inc	Inc-T	Error	Error-T
		Rp	Rd	Lex	Ca	Ct	Ccau	Cadv	Comp	Inc	Inc-T	Error	Error-T
		Rp	Rd	Lex	Ca	Ct	Ccau	Cadv	Comp	Inc	Inc-T	Error	Error-T
		Rp	Rd	Lex	Ca	Ct	Ccau	Cadv	Comp	Inc	Inc-T	Error	Error-T
		Rp	Rd	Lex	Ca	Ct	Ccau	Cadv	Comp	Inc	Inc-T	Error	Error-T
		Rp	Rd	Lex	Ca	Ct	Ccau	Cadv	Comp	Inc	Inc-T	Error	Error-T
		Rp	Rd	Lex	Ca	Ct	Ccau	Cadv	Comp	Inc	Inc-T	Error	Error-T
		Rp	Rd	Lex	Ca	Ct	Ccau	Cadv	Comp	Inc	Inc-T	Error	Error-T
		Rp	Rd	Lex	Ca	Ct	Ccau	Cadv	Comp	Inc	Inc-T	Error	Error-T
		Rp	Rd	Lex	Ca	Ct	Ccau	Cadv	Comp	Inc	Inc-T	Error	Error-T
		Rp	Rd	Lex	Ca	Ct	Ccau	Cadv	Comp	Inc	Inc-T	Error	Error-T
		Rp	Rd	Lex	Ca	Ct	Ccau	Cadv	Comp	Inc	Inc-T	Error	Error-T
		Rp	Rd	Lex	Ca	Ct	Ccau	Cadv	Comp	Inc	Inc-T	Error	Error-T
		Rp	Rd	Lex	Ca	Ct	Ccau	Cadv	Comp	Inc	Inc-T	Error	Error-T

RETELLING FROM A FILMSTRIP
SAMPLE TRANSCRIPT 2

1. [Um basically] this family of bears sits down and has [has] a meal

2. And [um] [they're eating] the fasther's eating

3. and this fly comes in

4. And the father's bothered by this

5. so he decides to swat [swat] or hit the [ah] fly

6. And [ah] [anyways he hits his mother] [I mean] he hits his wife

7. and [ah] she goes down

8. And [basically she] [basically he hits ah] he hits [her] his daughter

9. and [ah] the daughter goes down to the floor

10. [And then he climbs] [no he] and then he hits the dog

11. And the dog goes down on the floor

12. Then he decides to climb up [he decides to climb up] on the table and stand on a chair

13. And he tips it over

14. and he falls. [and uh . . .]

COMPLETE EPISODE:
- IE (lines 3)
- A (lines 5)
- DC (lines 7)

INCOMP. EPISODE:
- A (line 8)
- DC (line 9)

INCOMP. EPISODE:
- A (line 10)
- DC (line 11)

INCOMP. EPISODE:
- A (line 12)
- DC

FILMSTRIP # 2

SUBJ ID _____ TASK _____ SCORED BY _____ DATE _____   Page __1 of 2__

T-U #	Item (Word)	COHESIVE MARKER TYPE							COHESIVE ADEQUACY				
1	THIS	Rp	(Rd)	Lex	Ca	Ct	Ccau	Cadv	Comp	(Inc)	Inc-T	Error	Error-T
2	AND	Rp	Rd	Lex	(Ca)	Ct	Ccau	Cadv	(Comp)	Inc	Inc-T	Error	Error-T
	THE	Rp	(Rd)	Lex	Ca	Ct	Ccau	Cadv	(Comp)	Inc	Inc-T	Error	Error-T
	EATING	Rp	Rd	(Lex)	Ca	Ct	Ccau	Cadv	(Comp)	Inc	Inc-T	Error	Error-T
3	AND	Rp	Rd	Lex	(Ca)	Ct	Ccau	Cadv	(Comp)	Inc	Inc-T	Error	Error-T
	THIS	Rp	(Rd)	Lex	Ca	Ct	Ccau	Cadv	(Comp)	Inc	Inc-T	Error	Error-T
	IN	Rp	Rd	(Lex)	Ca	Ct	Ccau	Cadv	(Comp)	Inc	Inc-T	Error	Error-T
4	AND	Rp	Rd	Lex	(Ca)	Ct	Ccau	Cadv	(Comp)	Inc	Inc-T	Error	Error-T
	THE	Rp	(Rd)	Lex	Ca	Ct	Ccau	Cadv	(Comp)	Inc	Inc-T	Error	Error-T
	THIS	Rp	(Rd)	Lex	Ca	Ct	Ccau	Cadv	(Comp)	Inc	Inc-T	Error	Error-T
5	SO	Rp	Rd	Lex	Ca	Ct	(Ccau)	Cadv	(Comp)	Inc	Inc-T	Error	Error-T
	HE	(Rp)	Rd	Lex	Ca	Ct	Ccau	Cadv	(Comp)	Inc	Inc-T	Error	Error-T
	THE	Rp	(Rd)	Lex	Ca	Ct	Ccau	Cadv	(Comp)	Inc	Inc-T	Error	Error-T
6	AND	Rp	Rd	Lex	(Ca)	Ct	Ccau	Cadv	(Comp)	Inc	Inc-T	Error	Error-T
	HE	(Rp)	Rd	Lex	Ca	Ct	Ccau	Cadv	(Comp)	Inc	Inc-T	Error	Error-T
	HIS	(Rp)	Rd	Lex	Ca	Ct	Ccau	Cadv	(Comp)	Inc	Inc-T	Error	Error-T
7	AND	Rp	Rd	Lex	(Ca)	Ct	Ccau	Cadv	(Comp)	Inc	Inc-T	Error	Error-T
	SHE	(Rp)	Rd	Lex	Ca	Ct	Ccau	Cadv	(Comp)	Inc	Inc-T	Error	Error-T
	DOWN	Rp	Rd	(Lex)	Ca	Ct	Ccau	Cadv	(Comp)	Inc	Inc-T	Error	Error-T
8	HE	(Rp)	Rd	Lex	Ca	Ct	Ccau	Cadv	(Comp)	Inc	Inc-T	Error	Error-T
	HITS	Rp	Rd	(Lex)	Ca	Ct	Ccau	Cadv	(Comp)	Inc	Inc-T	Error	Error-T
	HIS	(Rp)	Rd	Lex	Ca	Ct	Ccau	Cadv	(Comp)	Inc	Inc-T	Error	Error-T
9	AND	Rp	Rd	(Lex)	Ca	Ct	Ccau	Cadv	(Comp)	Inc	Inc-T	Error	Error-T
	THE	Rp	(Rd)	Lex	Ca	Ct	Ccau	Cadv	(Comp)	Inc	Inc-T	Error	Error-T
	DOWN	Rp	Rd	(Lex)	Ca	Ct	Ccau	Cadv	(Comp)	Inc	Inc-T	Error	Error-T

FILMSTRIP # 2

SUBJ ID _____TASK_____ SCORED BY _____ DATE_____   Page___2 of 2___

T-U #	Item (Word)	COHESIVE MARKER TYPE							COHESIVE ADEQUACY				
10	AND THEN	Rp	Rd	Lex	Ca	(Ct)	Ccau	Cadv	(Comp)	Inc	Inc-T	Error	Error-T
	HE	(Rp)	Rd	Lex	Ca	Ct	Ccau	Cadv	(Comp)	Inc	Inc-T	Error	Error-T
	HITS	Rp	Rd	(Lex)	Ca	Ct	Ccau	Cadv	(Comp)	Inc	Inc-T	Error	Error-T
	THE	Rp	(Rd)	Lex	Ca	Ct	Ccau	Cadv	(Comp)	Inc	Inc-T	Error	Error-T
11	AND	Rp	Rd	Lex	(Ca)	Ct	Ccau	Cadv	(Comp)	Inc	Inc-T	Error	Error-T
	THE	Rp	(Rd)	Lex	Ca	Ct	Ccau	Cadv	(Comp)	Inc	Inc-T	Error	Error-T
	DOWN	Rp	Rd	(Lex)	Ca	Ct	Ccau	Cadv	(Comp)	Inc	Inc-T	Error	Error-T
12	THEN	Rp	Rd	Lex	Ca	(Ct)	Ccau	Cadv	(Comp)	Inc	Inc-T	Error	Error-T
	HE	(Rp)	Rd	Lex	Ca	Ct	Ccau	Cadv	(Comp)	Inc	Inc-T	Error	Error-T
	THE	Rp	(Rd)	Lex	Ca	Ct	Ccau	Cadv	(Comp)	Inc	Inc-T	Error	Error-T
13	AND	Rp	Rd	Lex	(Ca)	Ct	Ccau	Cadv	(Comp)	Inc	Inc-T	Error	Error-T
	HE	(Rp)	Rd	Lex	Ca	Ct	Ccau	Cadv	(Comp)	Inc	Inc-T	Error	Error-T
	IT	(Rp)	Rd	Lex	Ca	Ct	Ccau	Cadv	(Comp)	Inc	Inc-T	Error	Error-T
14	AND	Rp	Rd	Lex	(Ca)	Ct	Ccau	Cadv	(Comp)	Inc	Inc-T	Error	Error-T
	HE	(Rp)	Rd	Lex	Ca	Ct	Ccau	Cadv	(Comp)	Inc	Inc-T	Error	Error-T
		Rp	Rd	Lex	Ca	Ct	Ccau	Cadv	Comp	Inc	Inc-T	Error	Error-T
		Rp	Rd	Lex	Ca	Ct	Ccau	Cadv	Comp	Inc	Inc-T	Error	Error-T
		Rp	Rd	Lex	Ca	Ct	Ccau	Cadv	Comp	Inc	Inc-T	Error	Error-T
		Rp	Rd	Lex	Ca	Ct	Ccau	Cadv	Comp	Inc	Inc-T	Error	Error-T
		Rp	Rd	Lex	Ca	Ct	Ccau	Cadv	Comp	Inc	Inc-T	Error	Error-T
		Rp	Rd	Lex	Ca	Ct	Ccau	Cadv	Comp	Inc	Inc-T	Error	Error-T
		Rp	Rd	Lex	Ca	Ct	Ccau	Cadv	Comp	Inc	Inc-T	Error	Error-T
		Rp	Rd	Lex	Ca	Ct	Ccau	Cadv	Comp	Inc	Inc-T	Error	Error-T
		Rp	Rd	Lex	Ca	Ct	Ccau	Cadv	Comp	Inc	Inc-T	Error	Error-T
		Rp	Rd	Lex	Ca	Ct	Ccau	Cadv	Comp	Inc	Inc-T	Error	Error-T
		Rp	Rd	Lex	Ca	Ct	Ccau	Cadv	Comp	Inc	Inc-T	Error	Error-T

RETELLING FROM A FILMSTRIP
SAMPLE TRANSCRIPT 3

1. [OK] It's about a family of three bears
2. <u>And</u> <u>they</u>'re <u>all</u> cooking dinner and getting along amiably

IE 3. <u>And</u> along comes a little pesty fly

A 4. <u>And</u> <u>the</u> papa bear pulls out a fly swatter attempts to [hit the bear] hit <u>the</u> fly

DC 5. <u>And</u> <u>he</u> <u>misses</u> and knocks out <u>his</u> wife

IE 6. <u>And</u> <u>the</u> fly <u>still</u> [is] [is] aggravates <u>him</u>

A 7. <u>so</u> [he keeps] [he doesn't] <u>he</u> doesn't <u>give</u> <u>up</u>

8. <u>he</u> <u>keeps</u> on flying

DC 9. <u>And</u> a couple <u>more</u> swats and <u>passes</u> and <u>he</u> knocks out <u>his</u> child

IE 10. [then] <u>and then</u> [then] <u>he</u> leaves <u>the</u> kid's table

A 11. <u>and</u> <u>he</u> <u>keeps</u> <u>on</u> hitting at <u>the</u> fly

12. <u>And</u> [ah] <u>he</u> [he] has a dog nipping at <u>his</u> heels

13. <u>and</u> <u>it</u> really <u>looks like</u> a nice [a nice] little dog

IE 14. <u>And then</u> [and then] <u>the</u> fly lands on the ceiling

A 15. <u>and</u> <u>so</u> <u>papa</u> <u>bear</u> gets [a table] a chair

16. <u>and</u> <u>he</u> goes to put <u>it</u> down on <u>the</u> kid's table

17. <u>and</u> unknown [unknown] to <u>him</u> <u>his</u> wife is <u>now</u> awake and watching <u>him</u>

18. <u>and</u> [she says] <u>she</u> knows <u>he's</u> gonna fall off <u>the</u> table

19. <u>but</u> <u>she</u> doesn't say a word

20. <u>so</u> <u>he</u> <u>does</u> <u>so</u>

21. <u>And then</u> <u>he</u> lands on the floor and knocks <u>his</u> self out

22. <u>And</u> <u>the</u> fly goes out the window

23. All <u>this</u> for a measly, pesky fly

COMPLETE EPISODE (lines 3–5)

COMPLETE EPISODE (lines 6–9)

INCOMP. EPISODE (lines 10–13)

INCOMP. EPISODE (lines 14–16)

FILMSTRIP # 3

SUBJ ID _____TASK_____ SCORED BY _____ DATE_____   Page___1 of 3___

T-U #	Item (Word)	COHESIVE MARKER TYPE							COHESIVE ADEQUACY				
1	NO ITEMS	Rp	Rd	Lex	Ca	Ct	Ccau	Cadv	Comp	Inc	Inc-T	Error	Error-T
2	AND	Rp	Rd	Lex	(Ca)	Ct	Ccau	Cadv	(Comp)	Inc	Inc-T	Error	Error-T
	THEY	(Rp)	Rd	Lex	Ca	Ct	Ccau	Cadv	(Comp)	Inc	Inc-T	Error	Error-T
	ALL	Rp	Rd	(Lex)	Ca	Ct	Ccau	Cadv	(Comp)	Inc	Inc-T	Error	Error-T
3	AND	Rp	Rd	Lex	(Ca)	Ct	Ccau	Cadv	(Comp)	Inc	Inc-T	Error	Error-T
4	AND	Rp	Rd	Lex	(Ca)	Ct	Ccau	Cadv	(Comp)	Inc	Inc-T	Error	Error-T
	THE	Rp	(Rd)	Lex	Ca	Ct	Ccau	Cadv	(Comp)	Inc	Inc-T	Error	Error-T
	THE	Rp	(Rd)	Lex	Ca	Ct	Ccau	Cadv	(Comp)	Inc	Inc-T	Error	Error-T
5	AND	Rp	Rd	Lex	(Ca)	Ct	Ccau	Cadv	(Comp)	Inc	Inc-T	Error	Error-T
	HE	(Rp)	Rd	Lex	Ca	Ct	Ccau	Cadv	(Comp)	Inc	Inc-T	Error	Error-T
	MISSES	Rp	Rd	(Lex)	Ca	Ct	Ccau	Cadv	(Comp)	Inc	Inc-T	Error	Error-T
	HIS	(Rp)	Rd	Lex	Ca	Ct	Ccau	Cadv	(Comp)	Inc	Inc-T	Error	Error-T
6	AND	Rp	Rd	Lex	(Ca)	Ct	Ccau	Cadv	(Comp)	Inc	Inc-T	Error	Error-T
	THE	Rp	(Rd)	Lex	Ca	Ct	Ccau	Cadv	(Comp)	Inc	Inc-T	Error	Error-T
	STILL	Rp	Rd	(Lex)	Ca	Ct	Ccau	Cadv	(Comp)	Inc	Inc-T	Error	Error-T
	HIM	(Rp)	Rd	Lex	Ca	Ct	Ccau	Cadv	(Comp)	Inc	Inc-T	Error	Error-T
7	SO	Rp	Rd	Lex	Ca	Ct	(Ccau)	Cadv	(Comp)	Inc	Inc-T	Error	Error-T
	HE	(Rp)	Rd	Lex	Ca	Ct	Ccau	Cadv	(Comp)	Inc	Inc-T	Error	Error-T
	GIVE UP	Rp	Rd	(Lex)	Ca	Ct	Ccau	Cadv	(Comp)	Inc	Inc-T	Error	Error-T
8	HE	(Rp)	Rd	Lex	Ca	Ct	Ccau	Cadv	Comp	Inc	Inc-T	(Error)	Error-T
	KEEPS ON	Rp	Rd	(Lex)	Ca	Ct	Ccau	Cadv	(Comp)	Inc	Inc-T	Error	Error-T
9	AND	Rp	Rd	Lex	(Ca)	Ct	Ccau	Cadv	(Comp)	Inc	Inc-T	Error	Error-T
	MORE	Rp	Rd	(Lex)	Ca	Ct	Ccau	Cadv	(Comp)	Inc	Inc-T	Error	Error-T
	PASSES	Rp	Rd	(Lex)	Ca	Ct	Ccau	Cadv	Comp	(Inc)	Inc-T	Error	Error-T
	HE	(Rp)	Rd	Lex	Ca	Ct	Ccau	Cadv	(Comp)	Inc	Inc-T	Error	Error-T

SUBJ ID _____TASK_____ SCORED BY _____ DATE_____   Page___*2 of 3*___

T-U #	Item (Word)	COHESIVE MARKER TYPE							COHESIVE ADEQUACY				
	HIS	**(Rp)**	Rd	Lex	Ca	Ct	Ccau	Cadv	**(Comp)**	Inc	Inc-T	Error	Error-T
10	AND THEN	Rp	Rd	Lex	Ca	**(Ct)**	Ccau	Cadv	**(Comp)**	Inc	Inc-T	Error	Error-T
	HE	**(Rp)**	Rd	Lex	Ca	Ct	Ccau	Cadv	**(Comp)**	Inc	Inc-T	Error	Error-T
	THE	Rp	**(Rd)**	Lex	Ca	Ct	Ccau	Cadv	**(Comp)**	Inc	Inc-T	Error	Error-T
11	AND	Rp	Rd	Lex	**(Ca)**	Ct	Ccau	Cadv	**(Comp)**	Inc	Inc-T	Error	Error-T
	HE	**(Rp)**	Rd	Lex	Ca	Ct	Ccau	Cadv	**(Comp)**	Inc	Inc-T	Error	Error-T
	KEEPS ON	Rp	Rd	**(Lex)**	Ca	Ct	Ccau	Cadv	**(Comp)**	Inc	Inc-T	Error	Error-T
	THE	Rp	**(Rd)**	Lex	Ca	Ct	Ccau	Cadv	**(Comp)**	Inc	Inc-T	Error	Error-T
12	AND	Rp	Rd	Lex	**(Ca)**	Ct	Ccau	Cadv	Comp	Inc	Inc-T	**(Error)**	Error-T
	HE	**(Rp)**	Rd	Lex	Ca	Ct	Ccau	Cadv	**(Comp)**	Inc	Inc-T	Error	Error-T
	HIS	**(Rp)**	Rd	Lex	Ca	Ct	Ccau	Cadv	**(Comp)**	Inc	Inc-T	Error	Error-T
13	AND	Rp	Rd	Lex	**(Ca)**	Ct	Ccau	Cadv	**(Comp)**	Inc	Inc-T	Error	Error-T
	IT	**(Rp)**	Rd	Lex	Ca	Ct	Ccau	Cadv	Comp	**(Inc)**	Inc-T	Error	Error-T
	LOOKS LIKE	Rp	Rd	**(Lex)**	Ca	Ct	Ccau	Cadv	**(Comp)**	Inc	Inc-T	Error	Error-T
14	AND THEN	Rp	Rd	Lex	Ca	**(Ct)**	Ccau	Cadv	**(Comp)**	Inc	Inc-T	Error	Error-T
	THE	Rp	**(Rd)**	Lex	Ca	Ct	Ccau	Cadv	**(Comp)**	Inc	Inc-T	Error	Error-T
15	AND SO	Rp	Rd	Lex	Ca	Ct	**(Ccau)**	Cadv	**(Comp)**	Inc	Inc-T	Error	Error-T
	PAPA BEAR	Rp	Rd	**(Lex)**	Ca	Ct	Ccau	Cadv	**(Comp)**	Inc	Inc-T	Error	Error-T
16	AND	Rp	Rd	Lex	**(Ca)**	Ct	Ccau	Cadv	**(Comp)**	Inc	Inc-T	Error	Error-T
	HE	**(Rp)**	Rd	Lex	Ca	Ct	Ccau	Cadv	**(Comp)**	Inc	Inc-T	Error	Error-T
	IT	**(Rp)**	Rd	Lex	Ca	Ct	Ccau	Cadv	**(Comp)**	Inc	Inc-T	Error	Error-T
	THE	Rp	**(Rd)**	Lex	Ca	Ct	Ccau	Cadv	**(Comp)**	Inc	Inc-T	Error	Error-T
17	AND	Rp	Rd	Lex	**(Ca)**	Ct	Ccau	Cadv	**(Comp)**	Inc	Inc-T	Error	Error-T
	HIM	**(Rp)**	Rd	Lex	Ca	Ct	Ccau	Cadv	**(Comp)**	Inc	Inc-T	Error	Error-T
	HIS	**(Rp)**	Rd	Lex	Ca	Ct	Ccau	Cadv	**(Comp)**	Inc	Inc-T	Error	Error-T

FILMSTRIP # 3

SUBJ ID _____ TASK_____ SCORED BY _____ DATE_____   Page___3 of 3___

T-U #	Item (Word)	COHESIVE MARKER TYPE							COHESIVE ADEQUACY				
	NOW	Rp	Rd	(Lex)	Ca	Ct	Ccau	Cadv	Comp	(Inc)	Inc-T	Error	Error-T
	HIM	(Rp)	Rd	Lex	Ca	Ct	Ccau	Cadv	(Comp)	Inc	Inc-T	Error	Error-T
18	AND	Rp	Rd	Lex	(Ca)	Ct	Ccau	Cadv	(Comp)	Inc	Inc-T	Error	Error-T
	SHE	(Rp)	Rd	Lex	Ca	Ct	Ccau	Cadv	(Comp)	Inc	Inc-T	Error	Error-T
	HE	(Rp)	Rd	Lex	Ca	Ct	Ccau	Cadv	(Comp)	Inc	Inc-T	Error	Error-T
	THE	Rp	(Rd)	Lex	Ca	Ct	Ccau	Cadv	(Comp)	Inc	Inc-T	Error	Error-T
19	BUT	Rp	Rd	Lex	Ca	Ct	Ccau	(Cadv)	(Comp)	Inc	Inc-T	Error	Error-T
	SHE	(Rp)	Rd	Lex	Ca	Ct	Ccau	Cadv	(Comp)	Inc	Inc-T	Error	Error-T
20	SO	Rp	Rd	Lex	Ca	Ct	(Ccau)	Cadv	(Comp)	Inc	Inc-T	Error	Error-T
	HE	(Rp)	Rd	Lex	Ca	Ct	Ccau	Cadv	(Comp)	Inc	Inc-T	Error	Error-T
	DOES SO	Rp	Rd	(Lex)	Ca	Ct	Ccau	Cadv	(Comp)	Inc	Inc-T	Error	Error-T
21	AND THEN	Rp	Rd	Lex	Ca	(Ct)	Ccau	Cadv	(Comp)	Inc	Inc-T	Error	Error-T
	HE	(Rp)	Rd	Lex	Ca	Ct	Ccau	Cadv	(Comp)	Inc	Inc-T	Error	Error-T
	HIS	(Rp)	Rd	Lex	Ca	Ct	Ccau	Cadv	(Comp)	Inc	Inc-T	Error	Error-T
22	AND	Rp	Rd	Lex	(Ca)	Ct	Ccau	Cadv	(Comp)	Inc	Inc-T	Error	Error-T
	THE	Rp	(Rd)	Lex	Ca	Ct	Ccau	Cadv	(Comp)	Inc	Inc-T	Error	Error-T
23	THIS	Rp	(Rd)	Lex	Ca	Ct	Ccau	Cadv	(Comp)	Inc	Inc-T	Error	Error-T
		Rp	Rd	Lex	Ca	Ct	Ccau	Cadv	Comp	Inc	Inc-T	Error	Error-T
		Rp	Rd	Lex	Ca	Ct	Ccau	Cadv	Comp	Inc	Inc-T	Error	Error-T
		Rp	Rd	Lex	Ca	Ct	Ccau	Cadv	Comp	Inc	Inc-T	Error	Error-T
		Rp	Rd	Lex	Ca	Ct	Ccau	Cadv	Comp	Inc	Inc-T	Error	Error-T
		Rp	Rd	Lex	Ca	Ct	Ccau	Cadv	Comp	Inc	Inc-T	Error	Error-T
		Rp	Rd	Lex	Ca	Ct	Ccau	Cadv	Comp	Inc	Inc-T	Error	Error-T
		Rp	Rd	Lex	Ca	Ct	Ccau	Cadv	Comp	Inc	Inc-T	Error	Error-T
		Rp	Rd	Lex	Ca	Ct	Ccau	Cadv	Comp	Inc	Inc-T	Error	Error-T

Narrative Discourse: Story Generation from a Rockwell Picture

Three samples that have been coded into T-units are included for practice. Then each sample is analyzed for *story grammar* and *cohesion*. Note that cohesive markers are underlined and categorized on subsequent pages. Refer to chapters 4 and 6 for additional information about these analyses.

CODES:

Story Grammar Episode Componants
IE = Initiating events
A = Attempts
DC = Direct consequence

Cohesive Marker Types
Rp = Personal reference
Rd = Demonstrative reference
Lex = Lexical
Ca = Additive conjunction
Ct = Temporal conjunction
Ccau = Causal conjunction
Cadv = Adversative conjunction

Cohesive Adequacy
Comp = Complete
Inc = Incomplete
Inc-T = Incomplete tie
Err = Error
Err-T = Error tie

COMPLETE EPISODE = Contains all three episode components
INCOMPLETE EPISODE = Contains two of the three episode components

STORY GENERATION FROM A ROCKWELL PICTURE
SAMPLE TRANSCRIPT 1

1. [It looks like] There's a little kid running away from home

2. and [I guess] he went into some kind of coffee shop to get something to eat

3. well maybe [maybe] [uh it could be that] a police officer seen him walking down the street and thought that the kid was gonna run away

4. so he got out and started talking to the kid and took him to the coffee shop to find out what was going on, why he was running away because [when I look at it and I see that] he's got [a like] that hankerchief all packed up on a stick

5. [that's what] that's why [I get the impression] he's running away or something from the old pictures you see on TV

6. kids used to do that

7. and I see a cop sitting there

8. and they're both sitting down in a restaurant

9. and he's talking to em

10. so [I guess] there's gotta be a reason he's talking to em.

SAMPLE 2

1. [Well] one [one] day this [um] little boy was mad,

2. he was having a fight with his parents

3. and he decided to pack his bags and run away from home.

4. So he got his little knapsack

5. and he threw a bunch of clothes in it.

6. And then on the way [he says] [well] he decides well "I'm hungry."

7. "I'm going to get something to eat at the local deli."

8. So he climbs on the seat

9. and [um the um] the man he sees [um] the kid [you know] with the [um backpack I mean] knapsack.

10. and he's concerned.

11. And he thinks [oh gee] maybe I should call a police officer and maybe have him talk him [into it] [I mean] out of this idea of running away from home

12. because he realized it wasn't very safe out there alone for a little kid of his age to be.

13. And so he called up his friend who was an officer.

14. And he was on duty right by the store

15. so he [um] stopped in and sat down and started talking to the kid, just telling him [how you know] how dangerous it is out in the wild, wild world.

16. And it worked out OK.

17. The kid decided to hang in.

SAMPLE 3

1. [Oh] that's that movie

2. [oh] did you know what?

3. This is in a movie this picture as a matter of fact.

4. This [this] is [the um] the cop sittin on the stool with his son [at a] [at a] [at a] [what the heck is the word]

5. it's like a restaurant.

6. The cop is sittin in a restaurant with his son on a stool.

7. and they're probably havin [like I din't know] cake and ice cream or something like that.

8. [I think] that's his son too.

9. It's pretty cool though.

STORY GENERATION FROM A ROCKWELL PICTURE
SAMPLE TRANSCRIPT 1

INCOMP. EPISODE

IE 1. [It looks like] There's a little kid running away from home

A 2. <u>and</u> [I guess] <u>he</u> went into some kind of coffee shop to get something to eat

INCOMP. EPISODE

IE 3. <u>well</u> maybe [maybe] [uh it could be that] a police officer seen <u>him</u> walking down the street and thought that <u>the</u> kid was gonna run away

A 4. <u>so he</u> got <u>out</u> and started talking to <u>the</u> kid and took him to <u>the</u> coffee shop to find out what was going on, why he was running away because [when I look at it and I see that] he's got [a like] that hankerchief all packed up on a stick

5. [that's what] that's why [I get the impression] <u>he's</u> running away or something from the old pictures you see on TV

6. kids <u>used</u> to do <u>that</u>

7. <u>and</u> I <u>see</u> a cop sitting <u>there</u>

8. <u>and</u> <u>they</u>'re both sitting down in a restaurant

9. <u>and</u> <u>he's</u> talking to <u>em</u>

10. <u>so</u> [I guess] there's gotta be a reason <u>he's</u> talking to <u>em</u>.

ROCKWELL # 1

SUBJ ID _____ TASK _____ SCORED BY _____ DATE _____   Page___ *1 of 1*___

T-U #	Item (Word)	COHESIVE MARKER TYPE							COHESIVE ADEQUACY				
1	NO ITEMS	Rp	Rd	Lex	Ca	Ct	Ccau	Cadv	Comp	Inc	Inc-T	Error	Error-T
2	AND	Rp	Rd	Lex	(Ca)	Ct	Ccau	Cadv	(Comp)	Inc	Inc-T	Error	Error-T
	HE	(Rp)	Rd	Lex	Ca	Ct	Ccau	Cadv	(Comp)	Inc	Inc-T	Error	Error-T
3	WELL	Rp	Rd	Lex	(Ca)	Ct	Ccau	Cadv	(Comp)	Inc	Inc-T	Error	Error-T
	HIM	(Rp)	Rd	Lex	Ca	Ct	Ccau	Cadv	(Comp)	Inc	Inc-T	Error	Error-T
	THE	Rp	(Rd)	Lex	Ca	Ct	Ccau	Cadv	(Comp)	Inc	Inc-T	Error	Error-T
4	SO	Rp	Rd	Lex	(Ca)	Ct	Ccau	Cadv	(Comp)	Inc	Inc-T	Error	Error-T
	HE	(Rp)	Rd	Lex	Ca	Ct	Ccau	Cadv	(Comp)	Inc	Inc-T	Error	Error-T
	OUT	Rp	Rd	(Lex)	Ca	Ct	Ccau	Cadv	(Comp)	Inc	Inc-T	Error	Error-T
	THE	Rp	(Rd)	Lex	Ca	Ct	Ccau	Cadv	(Comp)	Inc	Inc-T	Error	Error-T
	THE	Rp	(Rd)	Lex	Ca	Ct	Ccau	Cadv	(Comp)	Inc	Inc-T	Error	Error-T
5	HE	(Rp)	Rd	Lex	Ca	Ct	Ccau	Cadv	(Comp)	Inc	Inc-T	Error	Error-T
6	USED	Rp	Rd	(Lex)	Ca	Ct	Ccau	Cadv	(Comp)	Inc	Inc-T	Error	Error-T
	THAT	Rp	(Rd)	Lex	Ca	Ct	Ccau	Cadv	(Comp)	Inc	Inc-T	Error	Error-T
7	AND	Rp	Rd	Lex	(Ca)	Ct	Ccau	Cadv	Comp	Inc	Inc-T	(Error)	Error-T
	SEE	Rp	Rd	(Lex)	Ca	Ct	Ccau	Cadv	Comp	(Inc)	Inc-T	Error	Error-T
	THERE	Rp	(Rd)	Lex	Ca	Ct	Ccau	Cadv	Comp	(Inc)	Inc-T	Error	Error-T
8	AND	Rp	Rd	Lex	(Ca)	Ct	Ccau	Cadv	(Comp)	Inc	Inc-T	Error	Error-T
	THEY	(Rp)	Rd	Lex	Ca	Ct	Ccau	Cadv	(Comp)	Inc	Inc-T	Error	Error-T
9	AND	Rp	Rd	Lex	(Ca)	Ct	Ccau	Cadv	(Comp)	Inc	Inc-T	Error	Error-T
	HE	(Rp)	Rd	Lex	Ca	Ct	Ccau	Cadv	Comp	Inc	Inc-T	(Error)	Error-T
	EM (HIM)	(Rp)	Rd	Lex	Ca	Ct	Ccau	Cadv	Comp	Inc	Inc-T	(Error)	Error-T
10	SO	Rp	Rd	Lex	Ca	Ct	(Ccau)	Cadv	(Comp)	Inc	Inc-T	Error	Error-T
	HE	(Rp)	Rd	Lex	Ca	Ct	Ccau	Cadv	Comp	Inc	Inc-T	Error	(Error-T)
	EM (HIM)	(Rp)	Rd	Lex	Ca	Ct	Ccau	Cadv	Comp	Inc	Inc-T	Error	(Error-T)

STORY GENERATION FROM A ROCKWELL PICTURE
SAMPLE TRANSCRIPT 2

1. [Well] one [one] day this [um] little boy was mad,

IE 2. he was having a fight with his parents.

3. and he decided to pack his bags and run away from home.

A 4. So he got his little knapsack

5. and he threw a bunch of clothes in it.

DC 6. And then on the way [he says] [well] he decides well "I'm hungry."

7. "I'm going to get something to eat at the local deli."

8. So he climbs up on the seat

IE 9. and [um the um] the man he sees [um] the kid [you know] with the [um backpack I mean] knapsack.

10. and he's concerned.

11. And he thinks [oh gee] maybe I should call a police officer and maybe have him talk him [into it] [I mean] out of this idea of running away from home

12. because he realized it wasn't very safe out there alone for a little kid of his age to be.

A 13. And so he called up his friend who was an officer.

14. And he was on duty right by the store

15. so he [um] stopped in and sat down and started talking to the kid, just telling him [how you know] how dangerous it is out in the wild, wild world.

DC 16. And it worked out OK.

17. The kid decided to hang in.

COMPLETE EPISODE

COMPLETE EPISODE

ROCKWELL # 2

SUBJ ID _____ TASK _____ SCORED BY _____ DATE _____   Page ___1 of 2___

Circled selections are marked with ✓.

T-U #	Item (Word)	Rp	Rd	Lex	Ca	Ct	Ccau	Cadv	Comp	Inc	Inc-T	Error	Error-T
1	NO ITEMS								✓				
2	HE	✓							✓				
	HIS	✓							✓				
3	AND				✓				✓				
	HE	✓							✓				
	HIS	✓							✓				
4	SO						✓		✓				
	HE	✓							✓				
	HIS	✓							✓				
5	AND				✓				✓				
	HE	✓							✓				
	IT	✓							✓				
6	AND THEN					✓			✓				
	WAY			✓					✓				
	HE	✓							✓				
	I'M	✓							✓				
7	I'M	✓							✓				
8	SO						✓		✓				
	HE	✓							✓				
	THE		✓						✓				
9	AND				✓				✓				
	THE		✓							✓			
	THE		✓						✓				
	THE		✓						✓				
10	AND				✓				✓				

ROCKWELL # 2

SUBJ ID _____ TASK _____ SCORED BY _____ DATE _____   Page___2 of 2___

T-U #	Item (Word)	COHESIVE MARKER TYPE							COHESIVE ADEQUACY				
	HE	**Rp**	Rd	Lex	Ca	Ct	Ccau	Cadv	Comp	Inc	**Inc-T**	Error	Error-T
11	AND	Rp	Rd	Lex	**Ca**	Ct	Ccau	Cadv	**Comp**	Inc	Inc-T	Error	Error-T
	HE	**Rp**	Rd	Lex	Ca	Ct	Ccau	Cadv	Comp	Inc	**Inc-T**	Error	Error-T
	I	**Rp**	Rd	Lex	Ca	Ct	Ccau	Cadv	Comp	Inc	**Inc-T**	Error	Error-T
	HIM	**Rp**	Rd	Lex	Ca	Ct	Ccau	Cadv	**Comp**	Inc	Inc-T	Error	Error-T
12	BECAUSE	Rp	Rd	Lex	Ca	Ct	**Ccau**	Cadv	**Comp**	Inc	Inc-T	Error	Error-T
	HE	**Rp**	Rd	Lex	Ca	Ct	Ccau	Cadv	Comp	Inc	**Inc-T**	Error	Error-T
	HIS	**Rp**	Rd	Lex	Ca	Ct	Ccau	Cadv	**Comp**	Inc	Inc-T	Error	Error-T
13	AND SO	Rp	Rd	Lex	Ca	Ct	**Ccau**	Cadv	**Comp**	Inc	Inc-T	Error	Error-T
	HE	**Rp**	Rd	Lex	Ca	Ct	Ccau	Cadv	Comp	Inc	**Inc-T**	Error	Error-T
	HIS	**Rp**	Rd	Lex	Ca	Ct	Ccau	Cadv	Comp	Inc	**Inc-T**	Error	Error-T
14	AND	Rp	Rd	Lex	**Ca**	Ct	Ccau	Cadv	**Comp**	Inc	Inc-T	Error	Error-T
	HE	**Rp**	Rd	Lex	Ca	Ct	Ccau	Cadv	**Comp**	Inc	Inc-T	Error	Error-T
	THE	Rp	**Rd**	Lex	Ca	Ct	Ccau	Cadv	Comp	**Inc**	Inc-T	Error	Error-T
15	SO	Rp	Rd	Lex	Ca	Ct	**Ccau**	Cadv	**Comp**	Inc	Inc-T	Error	Error-T
	HE	**Rp**	Rd	Lex	Ca	Ct	Ccau	Cadv	**Comp**	Inc	Inc-T	Error	Error-T
	IN	Rp	Rd	**Lex**	Ca	Ct	Ccau	Cadv	**Comp**	Inc	Inc-T	Error	Error-T
	THE	Rp	**Rd**	Lex	Ca	Ct	Ccau	Cadv	**Comp**	Inc	Inc-T	Error	Error-T
16	AND	Rp	Rd	Lex	**Ca**	Ct	Ccau	Cadv	**Comp**	Inc	Inc-T	Error	Error-T
	IT	**Rp**	Rd	Lex	Ca	Ct	Ccau	Cadv	**Comp**	Inc	Inc-T	Error	Error-T
17	THE	Rp	**Rd**	Lex	Ca	Ct	Ccau	Cadv	**Comp**	Inc	Inc-T	Error	Error-T
	IN	Rp	Rd	**Lex**	Ca	Ct	Ccau	Cadv	**Comp**	Inc	Inc-T	Error	Error-T
		Rp	Rd	Lex	Ca	Ct	Ccau	Cadv	Comp	Inc	Inc-T	Error	Error-T
		Rp	Rd	Lex	Ca	Ct	Ccau	Cadv	Comp	Inc	Inc-T	Error	Error-T
		Rp	Rd	Lex	Ca	Ct	Ccau	Cadv	Comp	Inc	Inc-T	Error	Error-T

STORY GENERATION FROM A ROCKWELL PICTURE
SAMPLE TRANSCRIPT 3

1. [Oh] that's that movie

2. [oh] did you know what?

3. This is in a movie this picture as a matter of fact.

4. This [this] is [the um] the cop sittin on the stool with his son [at a] [at a] [at a] [what the heck is the word]

5. it's like a restaurant.

6. The cop is sittin in a restaurant with his son on a stool.

7. and they're probably havin [like I din't know] cake and ice cream or something like that.

8. [I think] that's his son too.

9. It's pretty cool though.

NO COMPLETE OR INCOMPLETE EPISODES

ROCKWELL # 2

SUBJ ID _____ TASK_____ SCORED BY _____ DATE_____   Page___1 of 1___

T-U #	Item (Word)	COHESIVE MARKER TYPE	COHESIVE ADEQUACY
1	NO ITEMS	Rp Rd Lex Ca Ct Ccau Cadv	Comp Inc Inc-T Error Error-T
2	NO ITEMS	Rp Rd Lex Ca Ct Ccau Cadv	Comp Inc Inc-T Error Error-T
3	NO ITEMS	Rp Rd Lex Ca Ct Ccau Cadv	Comp Inc Inc-T Error Error-T
4	THE	Rp (Rd) Lex Ca Ct Ccau Cadv	Comp (Inc) Inc-T Error Error-T
	THE	Rp (Rd) Lex Ca Ct Ccau Cadv	Comp (Inc) Inc-T Error Error-T
5	IT'S	(Rp) Rd Lex Ca Ct Ccau Cadv	(Comp) Inc Inc-T Error Error-T
6	THE	Rp (Rd) Lex Ca Ct Ccau Cadv	Comp Inc (Inc-T) Error Error-T
7	AND	Rp Rd Lex (Ca) Ct Ccau Cadv	(Comp) Inc Inc-T Error Error-T
	THEY'RE	(Rp) Rd Lex Ca Ct Ccau Cadv	(Comp) Inc Inc-T Error Error-T
8	THAT'S	Rp (Rd) Lex Ca Ct Ccau Cadv	Comp (Inc) Inc-T Error Error-T
	HIS	(Rp) Rd Lex Ca Ct Ccau Cadv	(Comp) Inc Inc-T Error Error-T
	TOO	Rp Rd (Lex) Ca Ct Ccau Cadv	Comp (Inc) Inc-T Error Error-T
9	IT	(Rp) Rd Lex Ca Ct Ccau Cadv	Comp (Inc) Inc-T Error Error-T
		Rp Rd Lex Ca Ct Ccau Cadv	Comp Inc Inc-T Error Error-T
		Rp Rd Lex Ca Ct Ccau Cadv	Comp Inc Inc-T Error Error-T
		Rp Rd Lex Ca Ct Ccau Cadv	Comp Inc Inc-T Error Error-T
		Rp Rd Lex Ca Ct Ccau Cadv	Comp Inc Inc-T Error Error-T
		Rp Rd Lex Ca Ct Ccau Cadv	Comp Inc Inc-T Error Error-T
		Rp Rd Lex Ca Ct Ccau Cadv	Comp Inc Inc-T Error Error-T
		Rp Rd Lex Ca Ct Ccau Cadv	Comp Inc Inc-T Error Error-T
		Rp Rd Lex Ca Ct Ccau Cadv	Comp Inc Inc-T Error Error-T
		Rp Rd Lex Ca Ct Ccau Cadv	Comp Inc Inc-T Error Error-T
		Rp Rd Lex Ca Ct Ccau Cadv	Comp Inc Inc-T Error Error-T
		Rp Rd Lex Ca Ct Ccau Cadv	Comp Inc Inc-T Error Error-T
		Rp Rd Lex Ca Ct Ccau Cadv	Comp Inc Inc-T Error Error-T
		Rp Rd Lex Ca Ct Ccau Cadv	Comp Inc Inc-T Error Error-T

Conversation Samples

Two unanalyzed samples are included for practice. Then each sample is analyzed for Speaker Initiation, Response Adequacy, Topic Initiation, and Conversational Repair. Refer to Chapter 7 for additional information about conversational analyses.

CODES:

Speaker Initiation
   OB = Obliges
   COM = Comments

Response Adequacy
   AD+ = Adequate plus response
   AD = Adequate response
   INAD = Inadequate response
   AMB = Ambiguous response

Topic Initiations
   N = Novel topic introduction
   SS = Subtle shift of topic
   DS = Disruptive shift of topic

Conversational Repairs
   OIOR = Other-Initiated Other-Repaired
   OISR = Other-Initiated Self-Repaired
   SIOR = Self-Initiated Other-Repaired
   SISR = Self-Initiated Self-Repaired

CONVERSATION SAMPLE 1

T: So you're you've grown up in Stamford?

S: Yeah I've lived here all my life.

T: Uh-huh

S: Yeah

T: and do you have any brothers and sisters?

S: I have two sisters and one is married and one is going to be gettin married in April this this year.

T: OK, Now what are the age differences?

S: Um my oldest sister is 25 and my other one is 23 so I'm the youngest one, sixteen years old.

T: The baby, huh?

S: Yep that's me.

T: Now what do your sisters do?

S: Um

T: Do they work at all or . . .

S: Yeah my sister Joanne works at Royal Engineering and my sister Louise works at Central Electronics. I don't know what they do exactly they never went to college so . . .

T: And they all have gone to Stamford High?

S: Yeah

T: Un-huh. Now what do you want to do when you finish?

S: Well I either I want to go to college I want to go I want to open up my own business I don't know in what yet but that's what I'm gonna open up a business with one of my friends.

T: Good

S: Yeah

T: You guys haven't talked about what you want to do though?

S: No, not what we want to do but we know we want to open up our own business.

T: Un-huh

S: Cuz we know that we don't want to work for anybody else. If it works out we'll try.

T: Well what kinds of things, do you have any idea, clothing, jewelry or . . .

S: Um, we were kinda hoping to go into hairdressing as the owners not the workers.

T: Not doing the hair . . .

S: We'll assist, we'll, you know, we'll manage things we'll tell people what to do. That's what we want.

T: And you'll be the boss, huh?

S: Yeah, that's what we want to be.

T: Good

S: Yeah

T: And do you like Stamford? Think you'd want to stay there?

S: Um yeah, yeah it's pretty good I mean not too quiet and and it's not too loud like New York.

T: Do you get into New York much?

S: We go there for visits, like we went there for a play "Cats."

T: Uh-huh

S: You ever hear of that?

T: Sure

S: It was fun.

T: Uh-huh

S: Yeah I went with my uncle and my sister Joanne and my mom it was nice, but it's too crazy for me to live there.

T: Too busy huh?

S: Too busy and too much crime.

T: Yeah Yeah

S: Yeah

T: Now how big is Stamford High?

S: It has has they built a new building on there's like six floors

T: Wow

S: There's one, well, there's three on one building and three on the other.

T: OK

S: Yeah so um . . .

T: And one of the buildings is new?

S: Yeah

T: Yeah

S: It's a new building it was confusing at first when I first got there because the fourth floor is below the sixth floor.

T: Un-huh

S: Which is normal, but the sixth floor is on the same level as the first floor and then there's two and three because uh the first floor and the sixth floor are on the same level you have to cross a ramp I was so confused at first I was like where's the first floor? Downstairs- I was on the first floor.

T: Right

S: So I thought that the fourth floor would be upstairs.

T: Right, right

S: Yeah

T: Now is that is Stamford 9th through 12th?

S: Yep

T: So by your by your senior year you had it down, right? After three years?

S: Yeah actually I pretty much got it down by uh the end of my freshman year.

T: Yeah

S: Yeah this is my senior year so I hope I can graduate with my class I mean

T: Well we'll see what happens. Now you're working with Ralph and Mary?

S: On Thursdays and Fridays

T: Uh-huh, good

S: Yeah

T: So have they gotten any school books or are you doing any of that stuff yet?

S: School books no not yet. She's . . . they're mainly . . .

T: Doing some testing?

S: Yeah. To see like what level I'm on.

T: Un-huh. Now have they talked at all about when you're going to be leaving?

S: Ralph and Mary?

T: Well no, I mean the folks in the hospital

S: We went we went to a meeting so I'm supposed to my um leave date is October October 20th.

CONVERSATION SAMPLE 2

T: Um so you're you're home is in New London you said?

S: Oh, I that's where I did live before my accident.

T: Now did you grow up there?

S: No I grew up in upstate New York. I'm originally from thirty miles south of Albany.

T: OK

S: Chatham, New York

T: OK how'd you end up in Connecticut?

S: I always wanted to work on a boat, I always wanted to do that and my uncle was down in New London and he got me the job on the ferry.

T: Huh. What were you doing on that?

S: Engineer

T: So what did that entail?

S: Basically just keeping an eye on the engines during, while you're on your way, and basic, and just general maintenance and if anything serious went wrong or broke, then I had to repair that, but most of the time it was just monitoring the systems.

T: How long is the ride each way?

S: Hour and a half.

T: How many times a day would you do it?

S: Do four round trips a day. Start at six in the morning and get through at ten thirty at night.

T: That's a long haul. How much, how much of a lay over at each?

S: Only about half an hour

T: So all told then it's two hours each way right, with the stop over?

S: A. right. Yeah round, yeah two hours round trip.

T: So ah, did you mind the hours?

S: At times they got a little bit ah ah a little bit hard to take but I got used to it, yes.

T: Did it pay you decent wages?

S: Yes

T: They didn't have anything like split shifts or anything like that?

S: No

T: You worked the whole day?

S: I went by days. Four days on three days off I worked.

T: Well that's not bad.

S: Yeah

T: And ah did you have four runs on the weekends too?

S: Yeah, every day I had four runs

T: Not bad at all. Four on four off.

S: Four on three off.

T: Yeah, Yeah, that's what I meant. Four on three off. Um so, let me think here, what was the worst part of the job? The hours?

S: Yeah. Yeah the hours was the worst part.

T: What did you like about it?

S: Ah, I liked the people that I worked with and the people I saw everyday traveling.

T: You got to know them?

S: I got to the people, yeah. Got to see people I knew everyday, a lot of people.

T: So most of the people were coming to Connecticut to work or going out to . . .

S: Going out to Long Island for one reason or the other.

T: What's the busiest time of the year? summertime?

S: Right, this time of year it's just starting to get busy, yeah. The summertime's busiest, yeah.

T: Is this a car ferry?

S: Yes and trucks.

T: OK

S: Cars and big tractor trailers.

T: Um, how was it in heavy weather?

S: Ah it, it was interesting. I like the rough weather myself.

T: Yeah?

S: The other people, a lot of people got sick, But I I like the rou, I like when it's rough.

T: More to do? More to your job?

S: A little bit more to the job but it's more of an interesting ride rather that just a calm, calm ride across and back, you know?

T: How many ferrys were operated from that company?

S: Four

T: And each of 'em would take four a day?

S: In the summertime they, that's the schedule they have. In the winter, in the wintertime they they stop running so many boats, they run two, two boats during the week and three on the weekends. Fewer trips.

T: So it was a pretty decent job to have then, huh?

S: I liked it very much

T: Now was there any kind of test you had to take to be certified or . . . ?

S: Well it depends on what kind of license that you had, you have to have to have a Coast Guard license.

T: What did you have?

S: I have an AB, AB document. It's called a Merchant Marine document, so I was an AB.

T: Now did you know about engines before?

S: No, actually the whole job, I worked there over ten years, actually I was, I self taught myself working there over the years, ten years. I got to know, I didn't know engines that well at all, diesels I didn't know. I learned as I went along.

T: Now did you start, did you work your way up?

S: Yeah, I started working on deck, then I worked, worked my way into the engine room.

CONVERSATION SAMPLE 1

Segment of conversation between clinician (T) and individual with TBI (S)

N OB T: So you're you've grown up in Stamford?

AD S: Yeah I've lived here all my life.

COM T: Uh-huh

COM S: Yeah

N OB T. and do you have any brothers and sisters?

AD+ S: I have two sisters and one is married and one is going to be gettin married in April this this year.

OB T: OK, Now what are the age differences?

AD S: Um my oldest sister is 25 and my other one is 23 so I'm the youngest one, sixteen years old.

OB T: The baby, huh?

AD S: Yep that's me.

SS OB T: Now what do your sisters do?

INAD S: Um

OB T: Do they work at all or . . .

AD+ S: Yeah my sister Joanne works at Royal Engineering and my sister Louise works at Central Electronics. I don't know what they do exactly they never went to college so . . .

OB T: And they all have gone to Stamford High?

AD S: Yeah

SS OB T: Uh-huh. Now what do you want to do when you finish?

AMB S: Well I either I want to go to college I want to go I want to open up my own business I don't know in what yet but that's what I'm gonna open up a business with one of my friends.

COM T: Good

COM S: Yeah

OB T: You guys haven't talked about what you want to do though?

AD S: No, not what we want to do but we know we want to open up our own business.

COM T: Uh-huh

COM S: Cuz we know that we don't want to work for anybody else. If it works out we'll try.

OB T: Well what kinds of things, do you have any idea, clothing, jewelry or . . .

AD+ S: Um, we were kinda hoping to go into hairdressing as the owners not the workers.

O ⌐**OB** T: Not doing the hair . . .

I │ **AD+** S: We'll assist, we'll, you know, we'll manage things we'll tell people what to do. That's what we want.

S

R └ **OB** T: And you'll be the boss, huh?

    <u>|</u> *AD*   S: Yeah, that's what we want to be.

    COM T: Good

    COM S: Yeah

  N OB T: And do you like Stamford? Think you'd want to stay there?

    AD+ S: Um yeah, yeah it's pretty good I mean not too quiet and and it's not too loud like New York.

 SS OB T: Do you get into New York much?

SS AD+ S: We go there for visits, like we went there for a play "Cats."

    COM T: Uh-huh

     OB S: You ever hear of that?

     AD T: Sure

    COM S: It was fun.

    COM T: Uh-huh

  SS COM S: Yeah I went with my uncle and my sister Joanne and my mom it was nice, but it's too crazy for
O   me to live there.
I
S   *OB* T: Too busy huh?
R *AD+* S: Too busy and too much crime.

    COM T: Yeah Yeah

    COM S: Yeah

  N OB T: Now how big is Stamford High?

    AMB S: It has has they built a new building on there's like six floors

    COM T: Wow

    AMB S: There's one, well, there's three on one building and three on the other.

    COM T: OK

    COM S: Yeah so um . . .

O   *OB* T: And one of the buildings is new?
I
S   *AD* S: Yeah
R *COM* T: Yeah

    COM S: It's a new building it was confusing at first when I first got there because the fourth floor
                                             is below the sixth floor.

    COM T: Uh-huh

    AMB S: Which is normal, but the sixth floor is on the same level as the first floor and then there's
                                           two and three because uh the first floor and the sixth floor are on the same level you have
                                           to cross a ramp I was so confused at first I was like where's the first floor? Downstairs-
                                           I was on the first floor.

    COM T: Right

    COM S: So I thought that the fourth floor would be upstairs.

COM T: Right, right

COM S: Yeah

SS OB T: Now is that is Stamford 9th through 12th?

AD S: Yep

SS OB T: So by your by your senior year you had it down, right? After three years?

AD S: Yeah actually I pretty much got it down by uh the end of my freshman year.

COM T: Yeah

SS COM S: Yeah this is my senior year so I hope I can graduate with my class I mean

SS COM/OB T: Well we'll see what happens. Now you're working with Ralph and Mary?

AD S: On Thursdays and Fridays

COM T: Uh-huh, good

COM S: Yeah

OB T: So have they gotten any school books or are you doing any of that stuff yet?

AD S: School books no not yet. She's . . . they're mainly . . .

OB T: Doing some testing?

AD+ S: Yeah. To see like what level I'm on.

SS OB T: Uh-huh. Now have they talked at all about when you're going to be leaving?

OB S: Ralph and Mary?

AD T: Well no, I mean the folks in the hospital

AD+ S: We went we went to a meeting so I'm supposed to my um leave date is October October 20th.

O
I
S
R

CLINICIAN

CONVERSATION SAMPLE 2

Segment of conversation between clinician (T) and individual with TBI (S)

N OB   T: Um so you're you're home is in New London you said?

    AD+   S: Oh, I that's where I did live before my accident.

SS OB   T: Now did you grow up there?

    AD+   S: No I grew up in upstate New York. I'm originally from thirty miles south of Albany.

    COM   T: OK

     AD   S: Chatham, New York

SS OB   T: OK how'd you end up in Connecticut?

    AD+   S: I always wanted to work on a boat, I always wanted to do that and my uncle was down in New London and he got me the job on the ferry.

SS OB   T: Huh. What were you doing on that?

     AD   S: Engineer

     OB   T: So what did that entail?

    AD+   S: Basically just keeping an eye on the engines during, while you're on your way, and basic, and just general maintenance and if anything serious went wrong or broke, then I had to repair that, but most of the time it was just monitoring the systems.

SS OB   T: How long is the ride each way?

     AD   S: Hour and a half.

     OB   T: How many times a day would you do it?

    AD+   S: Do four round trips a day. Start at six in the morning and get through at ten thirty at night.

COM/OB   T: That's a long haul. How much, how much of a lay over at each?

     AD   S: Only about half an hour

     OB   T: So all told then it's two hours each way right, with the stop over?

     AD   S: A. right. Yeah round, yeah two hours round trip.

SS OB   T: So ah, did you mind the hours?

     AD   S: At times they got a little bit ah ah a little bit hard to take but I got used to it, yes.

SS OB   T: Did it pay you decent wages?

     AD   S: Yes

     OB   T: They didn't have anything like split shifts or anything like that?

     AD   S: No

     OB   T: You worked the whole day?

   AMB   S: I went by days. Four days on three days off I worked.

   COM   T: Well that's not bad.

   COM   S: Yeah

OB   T: And ah did you have four runs on the weekends too?

AD   S: Yeah, every day I had four runs

S ⌐   *COM*   T: Not bad at all. Four on four off.

I   *COM*   S: Four on three off.

O

R ⌐   *COM*   T: Yeah, Yeah, that's what I meant. Four on three off. Um so, let me think here, what was the

   SS OB   worst part of the job? The hours?

AD   S: Yeah. Yeah the hours was the worst part.

SS OB   T: What did you like about it?

AD+   S: Ah, I liked the people that I worked with and the people I saw everyday traveling.

OB   T: You got to know them?

AMB   S: I got to the people, yeah. Got to see people I knew everyday, a lot of people.

SS OB   T: So most of the people were coming to Connecticut to work or going out to . . .

AD   S: Going out to Long Island for one reason or the other.

SS OB   T: What's the busiest time of the year? summertime?

AD   S: Right, this time of year it's just starting to get busy, yeah. The summertime's busiest, yeah.

SS OB   T: Is this a car ferry?

AD+   S: Yes and trucks.

COM   T: OK

COM   S: Cars and big tractor trailers.

SS OB   T: Um, how was it in heavy weather?

AD+   S: Ah it, it was interesting. I like the rough weather myself.

COM   T: Yeah?

COM   S: The other people, a lot of people got sick, But I I like the rou, I like when it's rough.

OB   T: More to do? More to your job?

AD+   S: A little bit more to the job but it's more of an interesting ride rather that just a calm, calm ride across and back, you know?

SS OB   T: How many ferrys were operated from that company?

AD   S: Four

OB   T: And each of 'em would take four a day?

AD+   S: In the summertime they, that's the schedule they have. In the winter, in the wintertime they they stop running so many boats, they run two, two boats during the week and three on the weekends. Fewer trips.

SS OB   T: So it was a pretty decent job to have then, huh?

AD   S: I liked it very much

SS OB   T: Now was there any kind of test you had to take to be certified or . . . ?

AD   S: Well it depends on what kind of license that you had, you have to have to have a Coast Guard license.

OB   T: What did you have?

AD   S: I have an AB, AB document. It's called a Merchant Marine document, so I was an AB.

SS OB T: Now did you know about engines before?

AD+ S: No, actually the whole job, I worked there over ten years, actually I was, I self taught myself working there over the years, ten years. I got to know, I didn't know engines that well at all, diesels I didn't know. I learned as I went along.

SS OB T: Now did you start, did you work your way up?

AD+ S: Yeah, I started working on deck, then I worked, worked my way into the engine room.

Index